# Disorders of Human Learning, Behavior, and Communication

Ronald L. Taylor and Les Sternberg
Series Editors

James K. Luiselli   Johnny L. Matson
Nirbhay N. Singh
Editors

# Self-injurious Behavior

## Analysis, Assessment, and Treatment

With 17 Illustrations

Springer-Verlag
New York Berlin Heidelberg London Paris
Tokyo Hong Kong Barcelona Budapest

James K. Luiselli, Psychological and Educational Resource Associates, 40 Bronson Way, Concord, MA 01742, USA

Johnny L. Matson, Department of Psychology, Louisiana State University, Baton Rouge, LA 70803, USA

Nirbhay N. Singh, Department of Psychiatry, Medical College of Virginia, Richmond, VA 23298, USA

*Series Editors*: Ronald L. Taylor and Les Sternberg, Exceptional Student Education, Florida Atlantic University, Boca Raton, FL 33431-0991, USA

Library of Congress Cataloging-in-Publication Data
Self-injurious behavior: analysis, assessment, and treatment/James K. Luiselli, Johnny L. Matson, Nirbhay Nand Singh, editors.
p. cm.—(Disorders of human learning, behavior, and communication)
Includes bibliographical references and index.
ISBN-13: 978-1-4613-9132-6 e-ISBN-13: 978-1-4613-9130-2
DOI: 10.1007/978-1-4613-9130-2
1. Self-injurious behavior. 2. Self-injurious behavior—Treatment. 3. Developmentally disabled—Rehabilitation.
I. Luiselli, James K. II. Matson, Johnny L. III. Singh, Nirbhay N.
IV. Series.
[DNLM: 1. Mental Retardation. 2. Self Mutilation—diagnosis.
3. Self Mutilation—therapy. WM 307.M5 S465]
RC569.5.S48S45 1992
616.8—dc20
DNLM/DLC
for Library of Congress 91-4812

Printed on acid-free paper.



Typeset by Best-set Typesetter, Ltd., Hong Kong.

9 8 7 6 5 4 3 2 1

ISBN-13: 978-1-4613-9132-6

# Preface

This volume addresses the topic of self-injurious behavior (SIB) in persons with developmental disabilities. Among professionals and the lay public alike, there is little debate over the seriousness of self-injury, its detrimental effects, and the need for therapeutic intervention. At the same time, there are divergent views concerning its etiology and treatment. Understanding the causes of self-injury, for example, requires an analysis of biological factors, socioenvironmental variables, communication competencies, and in complex clinical cases, the interrelationships among these influences. There is also uncertainty with regard to the function of self-injury. Put simply, why would people willingly inflict injury upon themselves? Finally, although there is little disagreement about the necessity to intervene for self-injury, clinicians do not make uniform therapeutic recommendations, and, in fact, considerable differences in treatment selection are common. This fact is most apparent when one considers the ongoing controversy with regard to aversive and nonaversive programming.

Our premise for this volume is that a greater understanding of self-injurious behavior is dependent upon an empirical research base. Theories of causality must be conceptually valid and capable of being evaluated objectively. Treatment must be functionally determined, operationalized, and replicable across personnel and settings. For these reasons, we have assembled chapters by individuals who are experienced clinicians and researchers in the fields of psychology, medicine, psychiatry, education, psychopharmacology, and developmental disabilities. They provide what we think is a comprehensive and critical evaluation of the many topics that must be considered when addressing the complex phenomenon of self-injurious behavior.

The volume comprises three sections: Part 1, "General Issues," includes chapters on definition and classification of SIB and a review of prevalence data. Part 2, "Etiology and Assessment," covers the areas of neurobiological influences, psychophysiology, socioenvironmental variables, and functional analysis. In Part 3, "Treatment," several learning-based therapy approaches are examined in individual chapters, in addition to reviews of psychopharmacology, behavioral diagnostic interventions, the management of self-restraint, and formation of program review and human rights committees. This organizational format notwithstanding, we would add that most chapters provide an integrated discussion of diagnostic, assessment, and treatment concerns.

We wish to thank each of the authors for their willingness to prepare and revise chapters. We are also grateful to the staff of Springer-Verlag, Inc. for their commitment to this work. Most of all, this book is dedicated to our wives, Tracy Evans Luiselli, Deann Matson, and Judy Singh, for the constant support, care, and patience that enables us to write and edit books.

*James K. Luiselli*
*Johnny L. Matson*
*Nirbhay N. Singh*

# Contents

# Contributors

*Jon S. Bailey*, Ph.D., Department of Psychology, Florida State University, Tallahassee, FL 32310 USA

*Walter P. Christian*, Ph.D., The May Institute, Inc., 100 Sea View Street, Chatham, MA 02633 USA

*Robert M. Day*, Ph.D., Bureau of Child Research, University of Kansas, Lawrence, KS 66045 USA

*Cynthia R. Ellis*, M.D., Department of Psychiatry, Medical College ot Virginia, P.O. Box 489, Richmond, VA 23298-0489 USA

*Virginia E. Fee*, M.A., Department of Psychology, Louisiana State University, Baton Rouge, LA 70803 USA

*James C. Harris*, M.D., Division of Child Psychiatry, Kennedy Institute, Johns Hopkins University School of Medicine, Baltimore, MD 21205 USA

*Mike Houlihan*, M.A., Department of Psychology, Mt. Saint Vincent University, Halifax, Nova Scotia, Canada B2X 2V5

*Willard L. Johnson*, Ph.D., Behavior Management Services, South Mississippi Retardation Center, Long Beach, MS 39560 USA

*Joseph S. Lalli*, M.A., Department of Pediatrics, University of Pennsylvania, Philadelphia, PA 19104 USA

*Eric V. Larsson*, Ph.D., The May Institute, Inc., 100 Sea View Street, Chatham, MA 02633 USA

*Thomas R. Linscheid*, Ph.D., Department of Pediatrics, Ohio State University and Children's Hospital, 700 Children's Drive, Columbus, OH 43205 USA

*Stephanie Lockshin*, M.A., Department of Psychology, State University of New York at Binghamton, Binghamton, N.Y. 13901 USA

*Stephen C. Luce*, Ph.D., New Medico Associates, 100 Federal Street, Boston, MA 02110 USA

*James K. Luiselli*, Ed.D., Psychological and Educational Resource Associates, 40 Bronson Way, Concord, MA 01742 USA

*F. Charles Mace*, Ph.D., Graduate School of Applied and Professional Psychology, Rutgers University, P.O. Box 819, Piscataway, N.J. 08855 USA

*Elaine C. Marshburn*, M.A., Department of Psychology, Ohio State University, Columbus, OH 43210 USA

*Johnny L. Matson*, Ph.D., Department of Psychology, Louisiana State University, Baton Rouge, LA 70803 USA

*Julia O'Connor*, M.A., Department of Psychology, State University of New York at Binghamton, Binghamton, N.Y. 13901 USA

*David A. M. Pyles*, M.S., Department of Psychology, Florida State University, Tallahassee, FL 32310 USA

*Johannes Rojahn*, Ph.D., Department of Psychology, Nisonger Center for Mental Retardation and Developmental Disabilities, Ohio State University, 1581 Dodd Drive, Columbus, OH 43210-1296 USA

*Ahmos E. Rolider*, Ph.D., McMaster University, Hamilton, Ontario, Canada L8N 3Z5

*Raymond G. Romanczyk*, Ph.D., Department of Psychology, State University of New York at Binghamton, Binghamton, N.Y. 13901 USA

*Stephen R. Schroeder*, Ph.D., Director of Bureau of Child Research, 1052 Dole Human Development Center, University of Kansas, Lawrence, KS 66045 USA

*Michael C. Shea*, M.A., Graduate School of Applied and Professional Psychology, Rutgers University, P.O. Box 819, Piscataway, N.J. 08855 USA

*Nirbhay N. Singh*, Ph.D., Department of Psychiatry, Medical College of Virginia, P.O. Box 489, Richmond, VA 23298-0489 USA

*Yadhu N. Singh*, Ph.D., College of Pharmacy, South Dakota State University, Box 2202-C, Brookings, SD 57007 USA

*Ron Van Houten*, Ph.D., Department of Psychology, Mt. Saint Vincent University, Halifax, Nova Scotia, Canada B2X 2V5

# Part 1
# General Issues

# 1
# Definition, Classification, and Taxonomy

VIRGINIA E. FEE and JOHNNY L. MATSON

Self-injury is a topic currently receiving a great deal of attention from psychologists, educators, and others who work with developmentally disabled persons. Through all of this activity, some tentative conclusions have emerged. For example, self-injurious behavior (SIB) is a modifiable condition, and epidemiological data are available concerning the incidence and characteristics of those who self-injure (see Gorman-Smith & Matson, 1985; Schroeder, Schroeder, Rojahn, & Mulick, 1981). Although results have been encouraging, an evaluation of the literature suggests a multitude of avenues for investigators to follow. One such avenue, the definition and classification of SIB, is the focus of this chapter.

A chapter on definition and taxonomy in SIB research is important and is placed first in this particular volume for several reasons. Researchers have used a variety of definitions to describe the problem, and thus a somewhat heterogeneous group of behaviors has been studied. Careful description and definition of SIB is especially important in treatment research for generalization because behavior-change strategies are potentially specific to behaviors or to parametric aspects of the behaviors treated. A clear definition of the problem is an essential precursor to useful classification models leading to accurate predictions for treatment outcome (Matson, 1988).

In addition to defining the problem, a framework for viewing SIB is necessary for communicating the various multifaceted aspects of the condition, for developing exclusionary and inclusionary criteria, for making treatment decisions, and for ensuring comparability of data across studies. Although a meaningful classification system would be helpful for tying results together, only a few researchers have attempted to provide such a framework for SIB (Jones, 1987; Rojahn, 1986; Schroeder, Mulick, & Rojahn, 1980). Thus, while this research is considered important, difficulties and limitations are also apparent.

In addition to describing definitions of SIB and current taxonomies for its classification, this chapter highlights several relevant and current controversies. These include the relationship between SIB and stereotypy and the occurrence of SIB among normal infants. Also, a critique of current SIB classification systems is provided.

## Definitions

In an early attempt to define SIB, Tate and Barroff (1966) described the condition as "behavior which produces physical injury to the individual's own body." These authors stressed the outcome of behavior rather than the etiology. Because the effects of SIB are most easily studied, and because little is known about the cause, this is an appropriate emphasis. A similar definition was provided in the 1973 *Manual on Terminology and Classification in Mental Retardation* (Grossman): "to damage or disfigure a body part by one's own action." More recent definitions have continued the tradition of excluding etiological hypotheses. For example, Matson (1989) described self-injury as a class of behaviors, often highly repetitive and rhythmic, that result in physical harm to the individual displaying the behavior.

The aforementioned definitions describe responses occurring without the apparent intent of willful self-harm (Baroff, 1974). Suicidal gestures, self-neglect, and behaviors seen in Munchausen syndrome (Turner, Jacob, & Morrison, 1984) are similar to SIB because damage is self-inflicted. However, these behaviors are more likely to be willful and have therefore been excluded from most of the SIB literature (Schroeder, Schroeder, Rojahn, & Mulick, 1981). Moreover, other terms such as *self-mutilation*, *self-destructive behavior*, or *masochistic behavior* have been used to describe responses traditionally associated with the term *self-injury*. These categories are likely to include behaviors where self-harm is intentional.

Research efforts have been primarily concerned with severe SIB cases commonly found among mentally retarded, autistic, and, sometimes, schizophrenic persons. However, a subset of normal children also display forms of SIB (Baumeister & Rollings, 1976). Institutionalization results when the problem is severe (Matson, 1989).

Murphy and Wilson (1985) pointed out how similar classes of behavior displayed by mentally retarded and autistic individuals may be difficult to distinguish from SIB. For instance, stereotypies are often displayed by autistic and mentally retarded persons. Similarly, Baumeister (1978) defined stereotyped behavior as "highly consistent and repetitious motor or posturing responses which are excessive in rate, frequency, and/or amplitude and which do not appear to possess any adaptive significance."

Jones (1987) noted that the definitions of SIB and stereotyped behavior diverge primarily at the point where injury occurs. This author suggested that stereotypy and SIB are members of the same response class and are, in fact, on a continuum.

Another controversy in the definition of SIB concerns behaviors that are less directly damaging but may nevertheless be considered cases. For example, potentially injurious behaviors may not result in harm if the person is prevented from completing the response. Murphy and Wilson (1985) described two examples from the literature that could fall within the domain of SIB, depending on the particular definition used. First, a case of ruminative vomiting (Lang & Melamed, 1969) was presented. In this instance, the child's condition had become life-threatening and was of serious concern to those providing treatment. Second, a child who evinced uncontrollable climbing (Risley, 1968) was described. The severity of this child's problem was again serious because numerous and potentially life-threatening falls were likely. Some would question these examples as forms of SIB because tissue damage did not occur directly but was highly likely in a more indirect fashion (e.g., Baumeister & Rollings, 1976; Gunter, 1984). According to Murphy and Wilson (1985), these behaviors should be considered forms of SIB because the same treatment techniques were successful in treating both problems. Many authors currently agree that limiting the responses considered to be examples of SIB among developmentally disabled individuals would be unwise at this time (Murphy & Wilson, 1985; Schroeder, Mulick, & Rojahn, 1980). Therefore, for the present chapter, we incorporate the aforementioned behaviors.

One further area deserves mention as related to defining SIB, namely, responses among normal infants and young children. Self-injury has been observed in normal infants and young children (Baumeister & Rollings, 1976; de Lissovoy, 1962) and from prevalence studies by Baumeister and Rollings (1976) and a summary by Schroeder, Mulick, & Rojahn (1980), a rate of 7 to 17% in normal infants is typical. When these behaviors occurred in otherwise normally developing young children, it usually occurred at around 7 or 8 months of age and tended to diminish by the age of 5 years. Unlike the SIB shown by mentally retarded individuals who self-injure, head-banging is generally the only injurious response displayed when normal infants and children are concerned. This behavior rarely results in physical damage (Murphy & Wilson, 1985).

Several characteristics distinguish head-banging in normal children from SIB displayed by other populations. According to de Lissovoy (1962), head-banging in normal infants tends to occur only in the child's bed. Moreover, Kravitz, Rosenthal, Teplitz, Murphy, and Lesser (1960) noted that 50% of a normal group of children identified by their mothers as head-bangers displayed the behavior for 15 minutes or less, whereas only 26% exhibited head-banging for an hour or longer. In addition, these infants were reported to emit 60 to 70 bangs per minute. Addi-

TABLE 1.1. Definitions of SIB and other similar or related behaviors.

| | |
|---|---|
| Self-injurious behavior (SIB): | |
| | *Tate & Barroff (1966)*—Behavior that produces physical injury to the individual's own body |
| | *Grossman (1973)*—To damage or disfigure a body part by one's own action |
| | *Matson (1989)*—A class of behaviors, often highly repetitive and rhythmic, that result in physical harm to the individual displaying the behavior |
| Suicidal gestures, self-neglect, self-destructive behavior, self-mutilation, and masochistic behavior: | |
| | *Schroeder et al. (1981)*—Self-inflicted damage where intentional or willful self-harm is evident |
| Stereotypy: | |
| | *Baumeister (1978)*—Highly consistent and repetitious motor or posturing responses that are excessive in rate, frequency, and/or amplitude and that do not appear to possess any adaptive significance. |

tionally of interest was the finding that 67% of this sample also engaged in body rocking.

In another study examining head banging in normal children (de Lissovoy, 1962), a significantly higher rate of ear infections were discovered in a group of normal-IQ head-bangers compared to a group of normal-IQ controls. Similar findings were reported in a study with mice (Harkness & Wagner, 1975). Potentially, this finding would have relevance for mentally retarded individuals who display SIB because mentally handicapped persons often display numerous health problems and also evince communication deficits that can impede identification of illness.

Although normal children sometimes engage in head-banging, severe SIB cases occur almost exclusively among mentally retarded persons. Because clinically significant cases are of interest here, they are the focus for the remainder of this chapter. Many of these persons display characteristics of autism or meet the full diagnostic criteria for autism (Murphy & Wilson, 1985). Further, approximately 5 to 15% of mentally handicapped and autistic populations have been reported to self-injure (Murphy & Wilson, 1985). For defining SIB, intelligence level would seem to provide an exclusion criterion or perhaps be important for delineating subgroups for treatment purposes, especially because there appear to be important differences between normal and mentally retarded individuals who injure themselves.

Thus far, we have reviewed several definitions of SIB and have contrasted this problem with other behavioral difficulties. Table 1.1

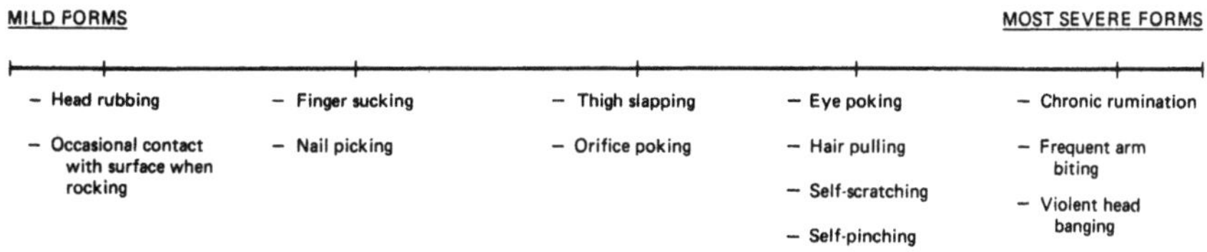


FIGURE 1.1. A continuum of self-injurious responses. Behaviors are located on the continuum according to severity of the response.

summarizes these definitions and provides a comparison with definitions of stereotypy and self-inflicted damage involving willful self-harm.

In order to settle on a working definition of SIB, it is necessary to highlight the heterogeneous nature of SIB responses. Examples of SIB reported in the literature represent a range of behaviors varying in severity, depending upon the rate and specific topography. The results of SIB form a continuum spanning from mild to life-threatening (Matson, 1989). Figure 1.1 depicts such a continuum with example behaviors located at points representing their potential dangerousness.

As a further method of illustrating a definition of SIB, a list of forms of the disorder seems appropriate. In their literature review of SIB treatment studies, Gorman-Smith and Matson (1985) provided a comprehensive list of SIBs. Among the behaviors described were head-hitting, head-banging, finger/hand-biting, eye-gouging, hair-pulling, nail-picking, and multiple self-injury. Operational definitions of these behaviors are provided in Table 1.2. As can be seen, these behaviors vary according to body part(s) involved, the specific motor acts required to perform the behavior, the potential for physical damage, and the seriousness of the damage that might be incurred.

In sum, defining SIB has not been easy. Definitions have lacked the specification of reinforcers maintaining the behavior, and no single treatment strategy is suggested by the term that would contrast the disorder from other problematic behaviors. Moreover, criteria for the systematic

TABLE 1.2. Operational definitions of SIB responses.

1. *Head-hitting*—forceful contact of the hand with any part of the head
2. *Head-banging*—forceful contact of the head with a stationary environmental object
3. *Finger/hand-biting*—closure of the upper and lower teeth on the flesh of the fingers or hand
4. *Eye-gouging*—any contact of any part of the hand within the ocular area
5. *Hair-pulling*—closure of the fingers and thumb on hair with a jerking motion away from the head
6. *Nail-picking*—nail-to-nail contact
7. *Multiple self-injury*—any of the preceding categories in combination

Source. From the Gorman-Smith and Matson (1985) Study (definitions adapted from Iwata et al., 1982)

inclusion or exclusion of behaviors do not currently exist (Schroeder, Mulick, & Rojahn, 1980). This chapter has summarized many of the existing controversies in the definition of SIB, including its relation to willfull self-damage, stereotypy, and behaviors with less directly damaging but potentially serious results.

Schroeder, Mulick, and Rojahn (1980) suggested future research where responses are classified according to their underlying parameters (e.g., frequency, intensity, duration, and sequence) and their interactions, (e.g., the combined impact of intensity and frequency). This type of research will be extremely important for improving current definitions of SIB, which are loose at best. At this stage, however, it is important to recognize that SIB may be defined in terms of a number of factors. A list of such factors is presented in Table 1.3. From this list of parameters, a more precise and comprehensive definition may emerge.

## Classification

Currently existing nosological systems for classifying SIB follow other areas of psychopathology, in that they may be initially based on commonsense hypotheses. Often, these systems, such as *DSM-III-R* (American Psychiatric Association, 1987), are popular and in use frequently (see Table 1.4). Also, as in other areas of psychopathology taxonomy, data-based systems also exist. A common theme in the behavioral classification literature is the idea that popular and data-based systems should become better integrated (Achenbach & Edelbrock, 1983).

This chapter describes both popular and empirically based taxonomies. In order to approach the aforementioned goal, however, some background literature on demographic characteristics correlated with SIB are discussed. Biological conditions associated with self-injury also are summarized.

TABLE 1.3. SIB definitional parameters.

1. Physical injury
2. Direct or indirect injury
3. Repetitiveness
4. Ritualistic nature
5. Frequency
6. Duration
7. Intensity
8. Increases with agitation
9. Response to treatment
10. Concern to caregivers
11. Body part involved
12. Motor movement required
13. Intelligence level of individual

TABLE 1.4. DSM-III-R diagnostic criteria/associated features.

Stereotypy/Habit Disorder
A. Intentional, repetitive, nonfunctional behaviors, such as hand-shaking or -waving, body-rocking, head-banging, mouthing of objects, nail-biting, picking at nose or skin
B. The disturbance either causes physical injury to the child or markedly interferes with normal activities (e.g., injury to head from head-banging; inability to fall asleep because of rocking)
C. Does not meet the criteria for either a pervasive developmental disorder or a tic disorder

Pervasive Developmental Disorders—Associated Features
In general, the younger the child and more severe the handicaps, the more associated features are likely to be present. They may include the following:
1. Abnormalities in the development of cognitive skills
2. Abnormalities of posture and motor behavior, such as stereotypies
3. Odd responses to sensory input
4. Abnormalities in eating, drinking, or sleeping
5. Abnormalities of mood
6. Self-injurious behavior (SIB)

## *Demographics and Populations That Display SIB*

An important step in classification is to examine the demographic characteristics of subjects in epidemiological studies and biological subgroups of mentally retarded individuals observed to self-injure. The value of this research for classification should not be underestimated because the identification of associated variables can provide hypotheses for both the cause and treatment of the problem. Also, early intervention becomes more efficient when the *potential* for developing the behavior is anticipated. A preventative focus may then become more realistic.

Epidemiological research involves the examination of a problem within specific populations. In addition to providing incidence data, these studies also examine demographic characteristics, such as age, gender, and intellectual or adaptive levels. Demographic studies have also examined the relation of SIB and other problem behaviors.

A variety of variables have been studied to discover factors that occur in association with SIB. This research has yielded some consistent information. For instance, one general finding appears to be that severely mentally retarded individuals are more likely to self-injure than those who have mild to moderate mental retardation (Ballinger, 1971; Bartak & Rutter, 1976; Maisto, Baumeister, & Maisto, 1978; Schroeder, Schroeder, Smith, & Dalldorf, 1978). Concerning etiology, these data suggest a CNS-damage hypothesis and/or the lack of skill and cognitive wherewithall to develop more adaptive responses. Persons exhibiting more severe levels of retardation are far more likely to display concomitant speech, motor, and social deficits. Schroeder et al. (1978) found that institutionalized SIB cases were more likely to have seizures and visual or language handicaps compared to those without SIB.

Findings also indicate that self-injury is most common in younger groups of mentally retarded children (Ballinger, 1971; Maisto, Baumeister, & Maisto, 1978; Schroeder et al., 1978). SIB may decrease with age in mentally retarded persons, a finding similar to that seen in normal children who bang their heads.

With regard to demographics, an important but unanswered question concerns sex differences in the incidence of SIB. According to the results of Barron and Sandman (1984), SIB occurs less often in females, and when it does occur, the effects are less serious. However, Schroeder et al. (1978) found no relation between gender of the individual and SIB. It is difficult then to draw any conclusions about this variable other than to suggest that the issue requires further study.

Another area receiving little attention but deserving considerable study is the degree to which other problem behaviors are correlated with SIB. For instance, one study reported that 55% of an institutionalized self-injurious group were found to display concomitant aggression (Griffin, Williams, Stark, Altmeyer, & Mason, 1986). It may be that among mentally retarded persons, the presence of self-injury acts as a marker that the person displays a large number of maladaptive behaviors. Alternatively, self-injury may be associated with milder problem constellations or with an absence of other behavioral difficulties. However, this question has not been systematically evaluated, except in the case of stereotypic behavior.

In an epidemiological study, Barron and Sandman (1984) attempted to delineate the association between SIB and stereotypy. Subjects in the study included 100 mentally retarded adolescents from a residential facility in California. These individuals were mainly from the profoundly mentally retarded range (86%). Other clients were from the severe level of mental retardation (14%). The total sample comprised four groups: (1) those who displayed both SIB and stereotyped behavior ($n$ = 22), (2) those who exhibited stereotypy only ($n$ = 40), (3) those who displayed SIB only ($n$ = 18), and (4) a randomly selected control group that displayed neither SIB nor stereotypy ($n$ = 20). Included in the study was a much broader range of SIB responses than those incorporated into other studies (e.g., Gorman-Smith & Matson, 1985; Rojahn, 1986) (see Table 1.5).

For the groups that displayed SIB, the mean frequency and severity of self-injurious responses were not significantly different for those who did and those who did not display associated stereotypy. An interesting discovery was that like other results described in Rojahn (1986), self-biting and head-banging were the most frequently displayed behaviors for the group of individuals exhibiting both self-injury and stereotypy. However, head-slapping and self-biting were the most frequent behaviors emitted by those who exhibited self-injury alone. This would appear to be a potentially important distinction between the groups. Both groups

TABLE 1.5. Behaviors from the Barron and Sandman (1984) study.

1. Threatens (verbal/gestural) self-abuse
2. Bites/chews/tears self
3. Hits (closed-fisted) head
4. Slaps (open-fisted) head
5. Hits/punches (closed fist) self, not on the head
6. Slaps/smacks (open fist) self, other than on the head
7. Snaps neck
8. Scratches self with hand or object
9. Puts inappropriate objects in own ears, nose, etc.
10. Pinches self
11. Pulls, tears, or twists own hair
12. Picks at own sores
13. Uses objects to hurt self (other than Items in 8 or 9)
14. Pulls own tubes (not defined)
15. Smothers self
16. Burns self
17. Cuts self
18. Attempts suicide
19. Pokes or gouges own eyes with fingers or objects
20. Bangs self (e.g., head) against objects (floor)
21. Voluntarily falls or throws self on wall, floor, objects, etc. (other than Item 19)
22. Other

frequently displayed self-biting but were differentiated on the basis of head-banging (SIB plus stereotypy) versus head-slapping (SIB alone). This finding suggests other differences between the groups, such as intelligence, response to treatment, or in terms of etiology. These hypotheses await further study.

Concluding comments made by Barron and Sandman (1984) attempted to link their results with previous work, although this was not done through statistical (e.g., cluster) analysis. Specifically, the authors stated that the majority of responses conformed to the subgroups "stereotyped SIB" (Napolitan, 1979). Antecedents of these behaviors cannot be reliably determined, leading to the hypothesis that motivation is "intrinsic" (Carr, 1977).

The Rojahn (1986) project also attempted to examine the link between SIB and stereotypy empirically. In Germany, 294 facilities serving 25,872 noninstitutionalized mentally retarded persons were studied. Here, it was found that the majority of individuals displaying SIB also exhibited stereotypy. The stereotypic behavior displayed by these individuals did not vary from control groups of non-SIB individuals except in the case of one stereotypic behavior. This behavior, self-restraint, occurred in 12% of the SIB subjects and 5% of controls. Moreover, cluster analysis showed this behavior to be significantly related to one SIB, namely, self-pinching. This is an interesting finding and suggests an association between the behavior categories, at least in some instances.

Biological subgroups of mentally retarded persons sometimes characteristically display SIB. For instance, research subjects have had such conditions as congenital rubella syndrome, Down syndrome, blindness, deafness, Rubinstein-Taybi syndrome, craniosynostosis, and cerebral palsy.

Lesch–Nyhan syndrome is a disorder of the metabolism of uric acid, the behavioral expression of which usually comprises mental retardation, spastic movements, and specifically, self-biting. Children with this disorder inflict severe injury through the characteristic biting and are physically noticeable by an absence of tissue about the lips. Untreated, some of these children have achieved the self-amputation of fingers (Nyhan, 1976).

Another serious condition is Cornelia de Lange syndrome, a disorder featuring low birth weight, mental and growth retardation, hirsutism, and characteristic facial features (Bryson, Skati, Nyhan, & Fish, 1971). Bryson et al. (1978) presented four cases of de Lange syndrome where multiple SIBs occurred and were unusually severe. Destructive responses included eye-picking that led to excoriation of the eyelids, face hitting resulting in open wounds, and biting the arms and tongue. In two earlier cases, Shear, Nyhan, Kirman, and Stern (1971) observed severe biting of the lips, similar to that seen in Lesch–Nyhan syndrome.

From the preceding discussion, it is apparent that SIB may accompany a variety of organic conditions and that the behaviors of some known subgroups are characteristically severe. Members of these subgroups display extreme SIBs (see Chapter 3, "Neurobiological Factors in Self-injurious Behaviors," this volume).

A biological model of causality would be insufficient at this time because little is known about potential biological variables in SIB. The previous discussion of epidemiological studies highlights the fact that no single variable occurs in all cases, and in regard to most variables, not even in a majority of cases. Persons displaying SIB represent a range of demographic variables. A minority possess identified biological syndromes that might explain the behavior's etiology.

From here, we describe several systems that have been used to classify SIB. The discussion is presented in two sections, based on the extent to which the systems have incorporated results from previous research. It should be obvious to the reader that classification is an extension of definition and should include the parameters described in Table 1.3 and also important demographic or biological factors.

## *Conceptually Based Classification Systems*

The most recent version of the *Diagnostic and Statistical Manual of Mental Disorders (DSM-III-R)* (American Psychiatric Association, 1987) provides a category called "Stereotypy/Habit Disorder" in the section on "Disorders Usually First Evident in Infancy, Childhood, or Adolescence." This category includes SIB. The criteria for the diagnosis of Stereotypy/Habit Disorder include "(a) intentional, repetitive, nonfunctional behaviors, such as hand-shaking or-waving, body rocking, head banging, mouthing of objects, nail biting, picking at nose or skin; (b) the disturbance either causes physical injury to the child or markedly interferes with normal activities, e.g., injury to head from head banging; inability to fall asleep because of constant rocking, (c) does not meet the criteria for either a Pervasive Developmental Disorder or a Tic Disorder" (American Psychiatric Association, 1987, p. 95).

Immediately evident is the authors' choice to combine stereotypy and SIB within a single category. In addition, the system implies that SIB is a subset of stereotypy. As is examined in detail later in this chapter, the relationship between SIB and stereotypy is definitely not clear-cut at this time (Schroeder, Mulick, & Rojahn, 1980). Of greater importance, the system does not provide for clear specification when behavior is physically damaging, a factor of great significance for those who come in contact with the person. Also problematic is that criterion excludes persons with pervasive developmental disorders (e.g., autistic persons) from being given the diagnosis. For communication purposes, the supplemental diagnosis would provide a good deal of additional information. SIB is discussed as an associated feature of pervasive developmental disorders but is not specified in the diagnosis. *DSM-III-R* does not provide a method for specifying when persons with pervasive developmental disorders exhibit SIB. This seems odd, given the research on this topic with persons displaying pervasive developmental disorders, such as autism. SIB among autistic persons is often severe and may limit residential or educational placement alternatives. This is one important reason for including its occurrence in classification systems for persons with autism.

Jones (1987) suggested a taxonomic system based on the frequency of SIB responses. This particular system is based on a hypothesis that SIB and stereotypy form an overlapping response class. The rationale for this contention included the finding that both categories of behavior have been successfully treated with similar treatments and that both behaviors are repetitive (Baumeister & Rollings, 1976; Matson, 1989).

Jones (1987) further suggested that it may be beneficial to divide those who self-injure into two subgroups, based on the frequency of the maladaptive response. The first category would include individuals who display injurious behaviors that are repetitive, with little variation, and performed at a relatively high rate (for instance more than 10 times an hour). This category of behaviors was labeled *stereotyped-self-injurious behavior* (*SSIB*). It was suggested that these responses be considered a subgroup of stereotyped behavior. Jones (1987) hypothesized that the other group of SIB, *self-aggression*, is performed at a much lower rate and possesses possible adaptive functions. Self-aggression would thus form a separate response class from stereotypy and SSIB.

Although the classification system proposed by Jones (1987) would provide researchers and therapists with valuable information concerning frequency of the response, several criticisms can be made. First, the author states that the system has not been tested empirically. In order for a classification system to provide valid decisions, it must be based on empirical categories. Second, the frequency of SIB often varies from one environment to another within a single individual (Schroeder, Mulick, & Rojahn, 1980). In addition, it would be difficult to determine the rate at which SIB should be considered "high."

Although the preceding frameworks may be important for guiding hypotheses, an important aspect in classification is to determine empirically the specific behaviors and parameters that might characterize other less obvious behavioral and demographic subgroups and to examine how different types of characteristics cluster within and among individuals across subgroups. Moreover, it is important to examine any other characteristics associated with the type and severity of the SIB response.

## *Empirically Based Classification Systems*

### Epidemiological Approaches

Epidemiological data has been used to develop classification systems for SIB. Here, researchers examine the topography of responses, including their rate, their frequency, and the specific acts as they occur in isolation and as they occur together to determine potential subgroups. Empirical approaches tend to be molecular, providing classification of factors within self-injury.

Schroeder, Mulick, and Rojahn (1980) described a system for classifying self-injurious responses using epidemiological data (Schroeder et al., 1976), and a review of 75 controlled research studies involving 140 subjects (Schroeder, Schroeder, Rojahn, & Mulick, 1980). In the Schroeder et al. (1978) project, 208 mentally retarded persons from a state facility displaying SIB were studied. In both studies, responses clustered in a similar manner.

In these analyses, the most frequently occurring response category was head-banging. Behaviors frequently occurring in combination with other responses were head-banging, self-biting, and self-scratching. The authors also reported that six behaviors were associated with direct injurious consequences, were more likely to be emitted in social settings, and were also associated with stereotyped behavior and other behavior problems. For this reason, the authors labeled this subgroup of behaviors "social SIB." These responses included head-banging, self-biting, self-scratching, gouging, pinching, and hair-pulling. Another subgroup was labeled "nonsocial SIB" because the consequences were less immediately obvious and less likely to be maintained by social reinforcement. Nonsocial responses were all consumatory behaviors and included stuffing orifices, mouthing, sucking, rumination, copophagy, aerophagia, and polydipsia.

According to Schroeder, Schroeder, Mulick, and Rojahn (1980), the classification system just described is comparable to that used by Berkson (1967) and by Foxx and Azrin (1973) where the labels "inner-directed" and "outer-directed" SIB were used. However, the term "nonsocial SIB" has less of an etiological connotation than the term "inner-directed SIB," and therefore would be preferred (Schroeder, Schroeder, Mulick, & Rojahn, 1980).

Another effort to classify SIB was described by Rojahn (1986). Subjects were examined on the topography of SIB, intensity, and frequency of self-injurious responses. A control group of non-self-injuring mentally retarded persons was also drawn, to account for possible selection biases. The most frequently occurring SIB was biting (45% of self-injurers), followed closely by head–body contact (44.7%). Other frequently occurring behaviors were scratching (42.2%), body–body contact (30.6%), head-to-object hitting (29.5%), pinching (19.3%), body-to-object hitting (16.9%), and fingers in body cavities (16.2%). Other behaviors occurred less often (<15%) and included pulling hair, pica, teeth grinding, extreme drinking (polydipsia) rumination, objects in cavities and air swallowing (aerophagia).

Results also indicated that most individuals displayed SIB from 2 or more topographies, whereas 24% displayed only 1 SIB. The most extreme case, in terms of variety of responses displayed, was an individual who exhibited 12 different types of SIB. The author also noted that there were significantly more individuals in the mild range of mental retardation who displayed only 1 self-injurious response as compared to those in the severe and profound range.

Results of the study showed no significant relations for type and number of SIB, unlike the study by Schroeder, Schroeder, Mulick, and Rojahn (1980). Similar to other studies (Maisto et al., 1978; Soule & O'Brien, 1974), however, the present authors found that females were less likely than males to engage in SIB. There were no significant sex differences in relation to the types of self-injury displayed. These results are in contrast to the Maisto et al. (1978) study, where females tended to exhibit self-biting and multiple injurious responses, whereas males were more likely to display headbanging and to exhibit an approximately equal split between singular and multiple responses. These results are consistent, however, with those of Smeets (1971) and of Schroeder et al. (1978), according to the authors.

### Treatment-Oriented Approach

One other empirical approach has emerged from the treatment literature. As is common in the behavioral literature, effective treatments are often developed before the problem is clearly understood. From the results of the treatment literature, causal hypotheses may be developed. It is not surprising that authors have suggested classifying SIB according to causal hypotheses because a recent focus of interest has been the identification of antecedent and consequent events associated with SIB.

A number of attempts have been made to examine variables that might control self-injury (Baumeister & Rollings, 1976; Carr, Newsom, & Binkoff, 1976; Iwata, 1987; Iwata, Dorsey, Slifer, Bauman, & Richman, 1982). This approach is potentially valuable for classification because an appropriate behavioral treatment procedure would be suggested by the motivational category assigned to the individual.

The general approach described by Carr (1977) is to determine environmental antecedents that consistently elicit the behavior. From here, a motivational hypothesis is selected that most closely corresponds to the antecedents that reliably precede displays of self-injury. Once a tentative hypothesis has been chosen, the therapist can then select a treatment strategy based on behavioral learning principles. For instance, a *self-stimulation* hypothesis would be selected when the environment is lacking in reinforcement. In this case, increasing the reinforcing value of the natural environment would be expected to reduce self-injury. Another motivational hypothesis, the *positive reinforcement* hypothesis, is suggested when social consequences follow exhibitions of self-injury. Here, the most appropriate treatment strategy would be one that removed social attention contingent on SIB. Finally, the *negative reinforcement* hypothesis is chosen when self-injury leads to the removal of demands or other unpleasant stimuli (Carr, 1977). Treatment approaches for this motivational category include lessening the aversiveness of the stimuli, positive reinforcement and/or punishment techniques, or an

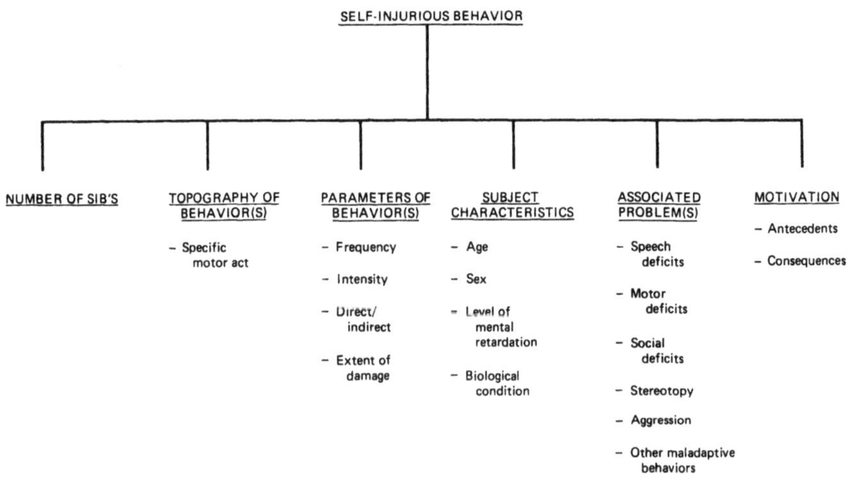


FIGURE 1.2. Classification variables in SIB.

extinction procedure that involves preventing escape from demands (Iwata, 1987).

That certain antecedents and consequences are associated with increases in SIB is a well-documented phenomenon (Baumeister & Rollings, 1976; Carr & McDowell, 1980; Iwata et al., 1982), and attempts at selecting effective treatment strategies based on hypothesized motivational factors have been successful (Repp, Felce, & Barton, 1988). Therefore, it is likely that this approach will be developed further (see Chapter 5, "Functional Analysis and Treatment of Self-injury," this volume).

In this section, we have described much of what is known about SIB as a background for examining classification systems. In Figure 1.2, we summarize the variables discussed. Evident is the fact that this is a very complex problem and that future research should attempt to take a more comprehensive look at the presenting problem. In addition, it is hoped that future researchers will carefully describe their subjects by including the parameters noted in Figure 1.2.

## Summary, Conclusions, and Future Directions

Work on the definition and classification of SIB is apparently just beginning (Jones, 1987; Rojahn, 1986; Schroeder, Schroeder, Mulick, & Rojahn, 1980). Efforts described in this chapter suggest a variety of directions to be followed. The primary emphasis has been on empirical approaches to definition and classification of SIB.

SIB denotes a category of responses where results range from very mild to life-threatening. The behavior may be directly or indirectly damaging to the person presenting the behavior. For most purposes, it may be wise to exclude normal children who display head-banging, through definitional criteria. Further, intellectual level appears to influence the severity of the problem, although why this is so is yet to be determined. Other demographic characteristics may also be important because preliminary data suggest more prevalent occurrence among youngsters and possibly among males.

SIB is similar to stereotypy in that it is repetitive and often responds in a like manner to behavioral procedures. In addition, stereotyped behavior may or may not cooccur with self-injury. However, the relation between the two is still unclear. Even less clear is the relation between SIB and other problematic behaviors, such as aggression. Some research has emerged examining the cooccurrence of SIBs. This line is important and warrants further attention.

The classification systems described in this chapter have included both those with empirical and those with popular support. Empirical studies have focused on two major areas: (1) the association between self-injury and stereotyped behavior (Barron & Sandman, 1984; Rojahn, 1986) and

(2) hypotheses concerning motivational variables (Baumeister & Rollings, 1976; Carr et al., 1976; Iwata, 1987; Iwata et al., 1982). The latter approach requires careful observation and is directly suggestive of effective interventions. Both research directions have been associated with emerging classification systems.

Further studies are needed to delineate the relationship between self-injurious and stereotyped behavior and whether these subgroups differ in terms of treatment efficacy/efficiency. Fortunately, an empirically sound foundation is being developed.

We now know that self-injury is a treatable problem. However, severe problems may warrant treatments designed specifically with regard to the frequency, duration, topograpy, and the number of SIBs displayed by the individual. Moreover, demographic characteristics may be helpful for determining those at risk for displaying the behavior at an early age. Further research will probably address these issues in greater detail and will be essential for understanding and treating this highly interesting and complex problem.

## *References*

Achenbach, T. M., & Edelbrock, C. S. (1983). Taxonomic issues in child psychopathology. In T. H. Ollendick & M. Hersen (Eds.), *Handbook of child psychopathology* (pp. 65–93). New York: Plenum Press.

American Psychiatric Association. (1987). *Diagnostic and statistical manual of mental disorders* (3rd Ed., rev.). Washington, DC: Author.

Ballinger, B. R. (1971). Minor self-injury. *British Journal of Psychiatry, 118*, 535–538.

Baroff, G. S. (1974). *Mental retardation: Nature, cause and management*. New York: Wiley.

Barron, B., & Sandman, C. A. (1984). Self-injurious behavior and stereotopy in an institutionalized mentally retarded population. *Applied Research in Mental Retardation, 5*, 499–511.

Bartak, L., & Rutter, H. (1976). Differences between mentally retarded and normally intelligent autistic children. *Journal of Autism and Childhood Schizophrenia, 6*, 109–120.

Baumeister, A. A. (1978). Origins and control of stereotyped movements. In C. E. Meyer (Ed.), Quality of life in severely and profoundly mentally retarded people: Research foundations for improvement. *AAMD Monograph, 3*.

Baumeister, A. A., & Rollings, J. P. (1976). Self-injurious behavior. In N. R. Ellis (Ed.), *International review of research in mental retardation*. New York: Academic Press.

Berkson, G. (1967). Abnormal stereotyped acts. In J. Zubin & H. Hunt (Eds.), *Comparative psychopathology*. New York: Grune & Stratton.

Bryson, Y., Sakati, N., Nyhan, W. L., & Fish, C. H. (1971). Self-mutilative behavior in the Cornelia de Lange syndrome. *American Journal of Mental Deficiency, 76*, 319–324.

Carr, E. (1977). The motivation of self-injurious behavior: A review of some hypotheses. *Psychological Bulletin, 84*, 800–816.

Carr, E. G., & McDowell (1980). Social control of self-injurious behavior of organic etiology. *Behavior Therapy, 11*, 402–409.

Carr, E. G., Newsom, C. D., & Binkoff, J. A. (1976). Stimulus control of self-destructive behavior in a psychotic child. *Journal of Abnormal Child Psychology, 4*, 139–153.

de Lissovoy, V. (1962). Head banging in early childhood. *Child Development, 33*, 43–56.

Foxx, R. M., & Azrin, N. H. (1973). The elimination of self-stimulatory behavior of autistic and retarded children by overcorrection. *Journal of Applied Behavior Analysis, 6*, 1–4.

Gorman-Smith, D., & Matson, J. L. (1985). A review of treatment research for self-injurious and stereotyped responding. *Journal of Mental Deficiency Research, 29*, 295–308.

Griffin, J. C., Williams, D. E., Stark, M. T., Altmeyer, B. K., & Mason, M. (1986). Self-injurious behavior: A state-wide prevalence survey of the extent and circumstances. *Applied Research in Mental Retardation, 7*, 105–116.

Grossman, H. J. (Ed.). (1973). *Manual on terminology and classification in mental retardation*. Washington: American Association on Mental Deficiency.

Gunter, P. L. (1984). Self-injurious behaviour: Characteristics, aetiology, and treatment. *The Exceptional Child, 31*, 91–98.

Harkness, J. E., & Wagner, J. E. (1975). Self-mutilation in mice associated with otitus media. *Laboratory Animal Science, 25*, 315–318.

Iwata, B. A. (1987). Negative reinforcement in applied behavior analysis: An emerging technology. *Journal of Applied Behavior Analysis, 20*, 361–378.

Iwata, B. A., Dorsey, M. F., Slifer, K. J., Bauman, K. E., & Richman, G. S. (1982). Toward a functional analysis of self-injury. *Analysis and Intervention in Developmental Disabilities, 2*, 3–20.

Jones, R. S. P. (1987). The relationship between stereotyped and self-injurious behaviour. *British Journal of Medical Psychology, 60*.

Kravitz, H., Rosenthal, V., Teplitz, Z., Murphy, J. B., & Lesser, R. E. (1960). A study of head-banging in infants and children. *Diseases of the Nervous System, 21*, 203–208.

Lang, P. T., & Melamed, B. G. (1969). Case report: Avoidance conditioning therapy of an infant with chronic ruminative vomiting. *Journal of Abnormal Psychology, 7*, 1–8.

Maisto, C. R., Baumeister, A. A., & Maisto, A. A. (1978). An analysis of the variables related to self-injurious behavior among institutionalized retarded persons. *Journal of Mental Deficiency Research, 22*, 27–35.

Matson, J. L. (1988). *Handbook of treatment approaches in childhood psychopathology*. New York: Plenum Press.

Matson, J. L. (1989). Self-injurious and stereotyped behavior. In T. H. Ollendick & M. Hersen (Eds.), *Handbook of child psychopathology* (2nd Ed.) (pp. 265–275). New York: Plenum Press.

Murphy, G., & Wilson, B. (Eds.). (1985). *Self-injurious behavior*. Birmingham, England: Birmingham Printers.

Napolitan, J. T. (1979). The classification of self-injurious behavior in mentally retarded children. *DAI, 40*, 1906.

Nyhan, W. L. (1976). Behavior in the Lesch-Nyhan syndrome. *Journal of Autism and Childhood Schizophrenia*, *6*, 235–252.

Repp, A. C., Felce, D., & Barton, L. E. (1988). Basing the treatment of stereotypic and self-injurious behaviors on hypotheses of their causes. *Journal of Applied Behavior Analysis*, *21*, 281–289.

Risley, T. (1968). The effects of punishing the autistic behaviors of a deviant child. *Journal of Applied Behavior Analysis*, *1*, 21–34.

Rojahn, J. (1986). Self-injurious and stereotypic behavior of noninstitutionalized mentally retarded people: Prevalence and classification. *American Journal of Mental Deficiency*, *91*, 268–276.

Schroeder, S. R., Mulick, J. A., & Rojahn, J. (1980). The definition, taxonomy, epidemiology and ecology of self-injurious behavior. *Journal of Autism and Developmental Disorders*, *10*, 417–432.

Schroeder, S. R., Schroeder, C. S., Rojahn, J., & Mulick, J. A. (1981). Self-injurious behavior: An analysis of behavior management techniques. In J. L. Matson & J. R. McCartney (Eds.), *Handbook of behavior modification with the mentally retarded*. New York: Plenum Press.

Schroeder, S. R., Schroeder, C. S., Smith, B., & Dalldorf (1978). Prevalence of self-injurious behavior in a large state facility for the retarded. *Journal of Autism and Childhood Schizophrenia*, *8*, 261–269.

Shear, C. S., Nyhan, W. L., Kirman, B. H., & Stern, J. (1971). Self-mutilative behavior as a feature of the de Lange syndrome. *Journal of Pediatrics*, *78*, 506.

Smeets, P. M. (1971). Some characteristics of mental defectives displaying self-mutilative behaviors. *Training School Bulletin*, *68*, 131.

Soule, D., & O'Brien, D. (1974). Self-injurious behavior in a state center for the retarded: Incidence. *Research and the Retarded*, *1*, 1–8.

Tate, B., & Barroff, G. (1966). Aversive control of self-injurious behavior in a psychotic boy. *Behaviour Research and Therapy*, *4*, 281–287.

Turner, S. M., Jacob, R. G., & Morrison, R. (1984). Somatoform and factitious disorders. In H. E. Adams & P. B. Sutker (Eds.), *Comprehensive handbook of psychopathology* (pp. 307–345). New York: Plenum Press.

# 2
# The Incidence and Prevalence of Self-injurious Behavior

WILLARD L. JOHNSON and ROBERT M. DAY

Of the events in the life of professionals working in the field of developmental disabilities, perhaps the most disturbing involve witnessing persons with handicaps inflicting injuries to themselves, through the display of such behaviors as self-biting and head-banging. For these professionals, and for researchers interested in the study of behavior problems, several important questions arise in regard to the extent of this phenomenon. At the most basic level is the question. How widespread is the problem of self-injurious behavior within developmentally delayed and other populations? Second, is the display of self-injurious behavior related to other characteristics? These questions are important for both theoretical and practical reasons. For example, an understanding of the relative rates of self-injury in persons who are not handicapped versus those who are mentally retarded is important information in our attempt to determine the extent to which self-injurious behavior may be a developmental phenomenon (Baumeister & Rollings, 1976). From a practical standpoint, statements regarding prevalence rates among various populations can be significant elements in justification for research into the understanding and treatment of self-injurious behavior.

In this chapter, we review the relevant literature on self-injurious behavior to determine the current state of our knowledge concerning the incidence and prevalence of self-injury and factors related to these incidence and prevalence figures. To the extent that this body of knowledge is found lacking, we suggest areas for further research.

In reviewing the literature pertinent to questions of the prevalence and incidence of self-injury, we found over 30 studies that appeared relevant to our questions. Unfortunately, there is no single accepted definition for the term *self-injurious behavior*. The definition that we used in deciding whether to reject or accept a report for inclusion in our analysis included the following elements: behavior of the individual directed against him- or herself; the behavior would be expected to cause pain and/or eventual tissue damage in an average person; and the behavior should be chronic or persistent, in the sense that it occurred repetitiously at some time rather than sporadically.

This definition was broad, in that it included behaviors such as rumination (Singh, 1981) and pica (Singh, 1983), in addition to the more traditionally included behaviors of self-striking, self-biting, head-banging, and so on. This was in keeping with the suggestion made by Schroeder, Schroeder, Rojahn, and Mulick (1980) that investigators should avoid prematurely limiting those behaviors included in the category of self-injurious behaviors without further taxonomic research. Specifically excluded from our definition, perhaps as much on the basis of tradition as sound research, were such suicidal behaviors as wrist-slashing, self-hanging, and anorexia. These behaviors appeared to be of a significantly different type than those of interest and were excluded for that reason.

## Critical Dimensions of Prevalence and Incidence Studies

Due to the different styles and perspectives of the researchers involved and because the reports containing relevant data were not necessarily conducted to answer the same questions, the available studies varied across a variety of dimensions important to the interpretation of the reported figures. Our review begins with a discussion of these dimensions.

### *Definition*

It is important to note that the various studies reviewed included differing types of self-injurious behavior. For example, Ressman and Butterworth (1952) studied mainly self-biting and chewing; Sallustro and Atwell (1978) considered nontantrum head-banging; while, Schroeder, Schroeder, Smith, and Dalldorf (1978) included a wide variety of behaviors, from head-banging to *coprophagy* (ingestion of feces) to *polydipsia* (excessive intake of fluids, often upsetting the body's electrolyte balance). In this review, we have listed the behaviors included in a study whenever the report involved a limited number of specific self-injurious behaviors, rather than employing a broad definition that included a variety of such responses.

A related issue involves the specification of time or frequency criteria that must have been met before a subject's behavior would be considered to have met the definition of being self-injurious. For example, Ballinger (1971) counted only those individuals displaying the behaviors of interest during the 1-month period preceding the study, while Singh (1977) considered those displaying self-injury at least once during a 6-month observation period.

## *Sampling Strategy*

When one considers studies of prevalence and incidence, it is important to consider the sampling strategies used. There are at least two significant aspects involved: (1) the description of the sample studied, and (2) the time period over which the data were collected.

### Description of Sample

In interpreting the results of the studies, it is important to consider the subject sample used in each study. None of the studies reviewed employed random samples drawn from a larger population. Rather, they generally involved collecting data on the entire population or clientele of one or more facillities or agencies. For example, Levy and Patrick (1928) surveyed mothers of children attending Better Baby Conferences in two small Minnesota communities. Lourie (1949) reported gathering his data from an "unselected clinic population" and from "private practice." Sallustro and Atwell (1978) questioned caregivers of healthy children between the ages of 3 months and 6 years who were brought to a Kaiser Pediatric Clinic. Only in the Sallustro and Atwell report were there details such as ethnic mix, socioeconomic status, and urban versus rural mix, suggesting that the sample probably was representative of the general population of nondelayed children. Several reports involved institutionalized populations. Comparison of findings among studies is facilitated when authors have included information on such variables as age, functioning level, and length of institutionalization of the institutional population surveyed, to permit comparisons with other institutions.

### Data Collection Time Period

According to Kiley and Lubin (1983),

> *Incidence* is the number of new cases which are manifest during a specific period of time. Incidence rates are the number of new cases of a disorder occurring in a population during a specified period of time relative to the number of persons at risk for the disorder in the same time period. (p. 544)
>
> *Prevalence* refers to the number of cases of a condition (whether old or new cases) that are present in a population at a designated time point. Prevalence rates are the number of cases relative to the total population from which the number of cases are ascertained. The total population, or denominator, includes all cases (i.e., the numerator), as well as all persons unaffected by the disorder. (p. 545)
>
> Incidence, prevalence, and duration are interrelated. Prevalence rates vary as a function of incidence and duration of the condition. In the hypothetical situation in which incidence and duration do not change, the prevalence will equal the incidence times the duration. (p. 545)

According to these definitions, most of the studies we reviewed would be considered investigations of prevalence rather than of incidence. In some cases, it was difficult to determine whether a study actually involved prevalence or incidence, as the procedures described fit neither of the preceding descriptions (e.g., Sallustro & Atwell, 1978). In such cases, we used our best judgment to classify the studies as either incidence or prevalence, based on the information provided in the article. In the tables that appear later in this chapter, we have noted our decision to classify each study as either incidence or prevalence; those cases for which we were unsure are denoted with a "?" following the word *incidence* or *prevalence* in the "Time period" column.)

Kiley and Lubin (1983) further noted that in the field of epidemiology, both prevalence and incidence are expressed as rates (i.e., rate/100, /1000, or/10,000, depending on sample size). The calculation of *prevalence* then requires figures representing the total number of individuals in the sample and the number of those who display self-injurious behavior at a given point in time. The length of this "point in time" varied among the studies reviewed here. Because a count of self-injurious individuals during an extended time period may include individuals who have discontinued displaying the behavior prior to the end of the sampling period, as well as individuals who begin displaying the behavior for the first time during the sampling period, it is important that sampling periods be as short as possible when prevalence data are the objective of the study.

The studies reviewed employed a variety of strategies in regard to sampling period. For example, Danford and Huber (1982) collected data over a 2-year period. Such a strategy could lead to significantly different results than, for example, the procedures employed by Shodell and Reiter (1968), who collected their data over 10 consecutive school days, or those of Ballinger (1971), who examined only those patients hospitalized on the day of the study but also considered the occurrence of self-injury during the preceding 1-month period. Other examples of strategies included distribution of questionnaires over a 10-month period (Green, 1967, 1968) and repeated surveys conducted in the fall of 1973, spring of 1975, and fall of 1976 (Schroeder et al., 1978).

## *Data Collection*

To determine how many members of a sample display self-injurious behavior, a number of different data collection techniques were used. Three of the most common methods were questionnaires completed by caregivers or professionals familiar with the subjects (e.g., de Lissovoy, 1961; Maisto, Baumeister, & Maisto, 1978; Ross, 1972; Sallustro & Atwell, 1978); interviews of caregivers (e.g., Kravitz, Rosenthal, Teplitz, Murphy, & Lesser 1960; Levy & Patrick, 1928); and direct observation (e.g., Kravitz et al., 1960; Shodell & Reiter, 1968). Some studies combined two or more of these methods (e.g., MacKay, McDonald, & Morrissey, 1974; Schroeder et al., 1978; Singh, 1977).

# Results

The following discussion is organized according to the questions outlined in the introduction. The rates reported herein are all expressed as prevalence or incidence per 100. Because the data reported in the various studies typically were not expressed as incidence or prevalence per 100 cases, we have taken the liberty of calculating such rates from the information provided in each of the articles. Tables 2.1, 2.2, and 2.3 contain summary information for nonhandicapped, psychiatrically impaired, and mentally retarded or developmentally delayed populations, respectively.

## *Gender*

Because the gender of a subject is a standard variable in epidemiological studies, it seemed important to examine gender as a variable potentially related to the display of self-injury. The following discussion is organized according to handicapping conditions.

### Nonhandicapped Subjects

Studies involving nonhandicapped subjects primarily were incidence rather than prevalence studies. Four studies contained actual incidence figures. All of these involved only children as subjects. Incidence of self-injurious behavior among males ranged from 3/100 cases (Levy & Patrick, 1928) to 22.3/100 cases (de Lissovoy, 1961). In virtually all of these studies, the incidence rates of self-injurious behavior among males were higher than those among females. Incidence rates of self-injury among females ranged from 1/100 cases (Kravitz et al., 1960) to 15.2/100 cases (de Lissovoy, 1961a, 1961b). Thus, the incidence rates of self-injurious behavior reported for males were between 1.5 (de Lissovoy, 1961; Levy & Patrick, 1928) and 3.5 times (Kravitz et al., 1960) as high as those reported for females.

### Psychiatrically Impaired Subjects

Four studies contained prevalence figures by gender for self-injury among psychiatric populations. For males, such figures ranged from 2.17 (Phillips & Alkan, 1961) to 37.5/100 cases (Green, 1967, 1968). For females, the prevalence of self-injurious behavior ranged from 4 (Ballinger, 1971) to 61.1/100 cases (Green, 1967, 1968). These figures indicate that the reported prevalence rates for self-injurious, psychiatrically impaired males range from .36 (Phillips & Alkan, 1961) to .93 (Ballinger, 1971)

TABLE 2.1. Studies of the prevalence and incidence of self-injurious behavior involving nonhandicapped subjects.

| Authors | Purpose | Data collection | Sampling strategy: Sample | Sampling strategy: Time period[a] | Definition or typograpy | Results/100 cases[b] |
|---|---|---|---|---|---|---|
| de Lissovoy, 1961 | Study of head-banging incidence in nonhospitalized infants | Mailed questionnaires to mothers | 368 normal, full-term babies born in an upstate NY hospital during 1958 | Unspecified; incidence | Nontantrum head-banging. | T = 15.2; M = 22.3 F = 15.2 |
| Kravitz & Boehem, 1971 | Study of rhythmic patterns in infancy | Group I—Observation Additional Group—Interview | Group I—140 randomly selected newborns, above 2500 gm, Apgar > 8 (excluded those with evidence of medical problems); additional group of 200 normal infants | Group I—from birth to onset of handsuck Additional group—monthly from 1 mo. to 1 yr. of age; incidence | Hand-suck<br>Lip-suck or -bite<br>Toe-suck<br>Head-banging<br>Teeth-grinding | I: T = 100<br>Additional: T = 93<br>Additional: T = 83.4<br>Additional T = 7<br>Additional T = 56 |
| Kravitz et al., 1960 | Study of head-banging in children and infants | Unspecified | 1168 children—Information from mothers in author's pediatric practice (white, middle & low income) & the mothers' friends. | Unspecified; incidence | Head-banging. | T = 3.6 (Ratio 3.5 M to 1 F) |

| | | | | | | |
|---|---|---|---|---|---|---|
| Levy & Patrick, 1928 | Study of relationship between parental fainting and headaches to SIB and other problems | Interview | Informants were mothers of children attending Better Baby Conferences in Mendota = 188 children & Aledo = 234 children | Unclear; incidenc | Head-banging or head-slapping. | Mendota: T = 2.6 (M = 3; F = 2)<br>Aledo: T = 3.8 (M = 6; F = 3) |
| Lourie, 1949 | Introduction to paper on related topic | Unspecified | Unspecified number—clinic population & private practice. | Unspecified; incidence | Rocking, swaying, & head-banging, | Clinic: T = 15–20<br>Private practice: T = 10 (Approx. 5% more M than F) |
| Sallustro & Atwell, 1978 | Study of prevalence of head-banging and other behaviors and their relationship to family factors and development | Questionnaire | 506 healthy children—Kaiser Pediatric Clinic, ages 3 mos.–6 yrs. representing wide range of ethnic, geographic, SES (details specified) | Questionnaires distributed Sept. 1975–June 1976; incidence? | Has child ever engaged in nontantrum headbanging? | T = 5.1 (Approximate ratio: 3 M to 1 F) |
| Shentoub & Soulairac, 1967, ated in Green, 1967 | Study of self-mutilation in infants | Not specified in secondary source | 300 infants—population of child care center in France | Each subject followed from age of 9 mos. to 6 yrs.; prevalence? | Self-mutilation (including bite, pinch, scratch, hit, hair-pull, and head-bang. | From graph—<br>9 mos. T = 16<br>12 mos. T = 11<br>18 mos. T = 16<br>2 yrs. T = 8<br>3 yrs. T = 5<br>4 yrs. T = 4<br>5 yrs. T = 0 |

[b] T = total; M = male; F = female.
[a] "?" After incidence or prevalence indicates difficulty classifying this study based on information in article.

TABLE 2.2. Studies of the prevalence and incidence of self-injurious behavior involving psychiatric subjects.

| Authors | Purpose | Data collection | Sampling strategy: Sample | Sampling strategy: Time period[a] | Definition or typograpy | Results/100 cases[b] |
|---|---|---|---|---|---|---|
| Ballinger, 1971 | Study of prevalence and nature of SIB | Unclear—"examined by writer and details obtained from ward staff." | All 584 patients in a psychiatric hospital in Scotland; diagnoses specified in results; ages above 10 yrs. (226 males; 358 females) | Included only patients in hospital on day of study; Included self-injury over preceding month; prevalence | Any painful or destructive act on own body; included rubbing & scratching when caused persistent & visible injury | Psychiatric hospital—T = 3 (M = 3; F = 4). |
| Green, 1967, 1968 | Study of incidence and nature of self-mutilation, including history of head-banging as an infant (1967); child abuse and self-destructive behavior (1968) | Reviewed records | 70 children—all those treated at child research center, diagnosed as schizophrenic & in residence for 6 mos; ages 5–12 yrs. (52 males; 18 females) | Archival review covering 10-yr. period; prevalence? | Self-mutilation = overtly painful or destructive act on own body | T = 40 (M = 32.7; F = 61.1) |

| | | | | | | |
|---|---|---|---|---|---|---|
| Maurice & Trudel, 1982 | Attempt to establish the prevalence of SIB and to measure some of the characteristics associated with it, in certain institutions. | Questionnaire completed during interview of caregivers. | 1385 psychotic residents of 3 different institutions in the Montreal area | Those who displayed SIB during 2-yr. period preceding the study; prevalence | Head-banging, hitting body, rubbing body part, scratching, pulling hair, eye gouging, biting self, pica, gouging, digging, insertion in body cavities, excessive masturbation, pinching self, other (vomiting, burning self, cutting self, self-choking, stopping blood circulation) | Psychotic group—T = 21.8 |
| Phillips & Alkan, 1961 | Study of number patients in facility displaying self-mutilation, and the types displayed | Referred by nurses; physical exam by authors | 2,816 patients—population of a large psychiatric hospital (1292 males; 1524 females) | Unspecified; prevalence? | Nonsuicidal self-mutilation including scratch, pick, dig, at skin; self-striking; swallow sharp objects; attempted genital removal | T = 4.29 (M = 2.17; F = 6.1) |
| Shodell & Reiter, 1968 | Study of relationship between incidence of head-banging & verbal ability | Parents and teachers observed and recorded | 58 schizophrenic children attending private special education program, but residing at home; 21 verbal & 38 nonverbal; ages 4–17 yrs. (48 males; 10 females) | Each child observed for a consecutive 10-day period, with extra days included when necessary due to absences; prevalence | Overtly painful or destructive act on own body, such as: head-banging, self-biting, pinching, self-scratching, hair-pulling, or self-hitting | T = 38 (M = 37.5; F = 40) |

[a] "?" After incidence or prevalence indicates difficulty classifying this study based on information in article.
[b] T = total; M = male; F = female.

TABLE 2.3. Studies of the prevalence and incidence of self-injurious behavior involving developmentally delayed subjects

| | | | Sampling strategy | | | |
|---|---|---|---|---|---|---|
| Authors | Purpose | Data collection | Sample | Time period[a] | Definition or typograpy | Results/100 cases[b] |
| Ballinger, 1971 | Study of prevalence and nature of SIB. | Unclear- "examined by writer and . . . details obtained from ward staff". | All 626 patients in hospital for the mentally subnormal in Scotland; all ages; IQ's 0–68 (343 males; 283 females). | Included only patients in hospital on day of study; Included self-injury over preceding month; Prevalence. | Any painful or destructive act on own body; included rubbing & scratching when caused persistent & visible injury. | Sub-normality hospital – T = 15 (M = 13; F = 17); |
| Barron & Sandman, 1984 | Study designed to examine similarities and differences between those who display SIB &/or stereotypy. | Structured staff interviews using checklist. | Mentally retarded clients of program in state MR facility; 9–26 yrs. (mean = 20.71); 14% severe; 84% profound; (males = 58; females = 42); info on length of institutionalization and diagnosis in article. | Unclear; staff interviews took place during a 2 mo. period; Prevalence. | Unclear, but included: slapping head, biting self, banging self, picking sores, scratching self, hitting head, voluntary falling. | T = 40 (M = 40; F = 40) |
| Danford & Huber, 1982 | Investigation of prevalence of pica, incidence, frequency, seasonality, types, and medical problems. | Staff interviews & observation. | Population of state MR facility; 11–88 yrs. (majority adults); (males = 560; females = 431), all levels of retardation. | Data collected over a 2 yr. period; Prevalence? | Nonfood pica = frequent consumption of nonfood items; | T = 16.7 |
| | | | | | Food pica = frequent consumption of food-related substances; | T = 5.4 |
| | | | | | Combined = both of above. | T = 3.7 |

| | | | | | | |
|---|---|---|---|---|---|---|
| Eyman & Call, 1977 | Study of prevalence of behavior problems, subject characteristics, & relationships among problem behaviors. | Caretaker ratings. | Retarded individuals served by 2 regional service centers in CA, by CO community and institutional services, and by Nevada Division of Mental Hygiene & Mental Retardation; all ages: Profound MR-Hospitalized = 191 Community (foster care, board & care, convalescent) = 89 Parent/Relative care = 42; Severe MR-Hospitalized = 63 Community = 90 Parent/Relative = 190 Mild/ Moderately MR-Hospitalized = 40 Community = 150 Parent/Relative = 772. | Individuals receiving services as of Je 30, 1975 – otherwise unspecified; Prevalence? | Physical damage to self. | Profoundly MR<br>Hospital-<13 yrs. T = 28, > = 13 yrs. T = 47<br>Community-<13 yrs. T = 17, > = 13 yrs. T = 20<br>Parent/Relative care-<13 yrs. T = 17, > = 13 yrs. T = 17<br>Community-T = 24<br>Severely MR<br>Hospital-<13 yrs. T = 44, > = 13 yrs. T = 38<br>Community-<13 yrs. T = 22, > = 13 T = 11<br>Parent/Relative care-<13 yrs. T = 14, > = 13 yrs. T = 11<br>Mild/Moderately MR<br>Hospital-<13 yrs. T = 35, > = 13 yrs. T = 15<br>Community-<13 yrs. T = 13, > = 13 yrs. T = 6<br>Parent/Relative care-<13 yrs. T = 8, > = 13 yrs. T = 5 |

TABLE 2.3. (Continued)

| | | | Sampling strategy | | | |
|---|---|---|---|---|---|---|
| Authors | Purpose | Data collection | Sample | Time period[a] | Definition or typograpy | Results/100 cases[b] |
| Griffin et al., 1984, 1986 | Survey conducted to determine the extent & circumstances of SIB among institutionalized MR individuals. | Forced choice questionnaire completed by psychologists & reviewed by interdisciplinary teams. | All of the 10549 residents of the 13 state MR facilities in Texas; mean age = 32.2 yrs.; (5,903 males; 4646 females); all functioning levels. | Individuals who had emitted SIB within previous 12 mos.; Prevalence. | Head hitting, head banging, orifice digging, arm hitting, throat gouging, eye gouging, biting, pica, mouthing, scratching, ruminating, trichotillomania, other. | T = 12.7 (M = 12.9; F = 12.5) |
| Griffin et al., 1987 | Study of extent, nature, and treatment of self-injurious behavior in public school population | Forced-choice questionnaire completed by teachers | All 2,663 special education students in one school district | Individuals who had emitted SIB within previous 12 mos.; prevalence | Repetitive or isolated acts toward self resulting in physical harm; or behavior typically considered self-injurious; or having received restraint or psychoactive medication for causing or attempting self-injury | T = 2.6 (ratio 1.46 M to 1 F) |

| | | | | | | |
|---|---|---|---|---|---|---|
| Hill & Bruininks, 1984 | Examination of maladaptive behavior | Staff interviews | Sample of 964 residents of 161 community-based residential MR facilities; & 997 residents, (289 new admissions, and 244 readmissions) of 75 state MR facilities; sampling procedure random within facilities, facilities chosen to provide proportionately valid representation of size and census regions | Not specified; prevalence? | Self-injurious behavior | Community T = 11.1<br>Residential—<br>residents T = 21.7<br>new admis T = 22<br>readmis T = 21.3 |
| Kravitz & Boehem, 1971 | Study of onset age of rhythmic patterns in infancy | Interview | 12 infants with cerebral palsy<br>22 infants with Down syndrome | Monthly from 1 mo. to 1 yr. of age; incidence | Hand-suck | CP group—T = 25<br>Down—T = 59 |
| | | | | | Lip-suck or -bite | CP group—T = .5<br>Down—T = .05 |
| | | | | | Toe-suck | CP group—T = .5<br>Down—T = .09 |
| | | | | | Head-banging | CP group—T = 17<br>Down—T = 14 |
| | | | | | Teeth-grinding | CP group—T = 0<br>Down—T = 0 |
| MacKay et al., 1974 | Survey of prevalence of self-mutilation and intensity, severity and types in cases of multiple self-abuse | Questionnaire; authors examined patients to confirm validity of intensity estimates | In-patient population of a British "sub-normality" hospital; 114 profound; 289 severe; 197 moderate | Based on 1 yr. observations—no further explanation provided; prevalence | Painful or destructive act committed against own body; includes head-banging; face-slapping; skin-picking; hair-pull; regurgitation, etc. | T = 19 (ratio 1.75 M to 1 F) |

TABLE 2.3. (Continued)

| | | | Sampling strategy | | | |
|---|---|---|---|---|---|---|
| Authors | Purpose | Data collection | Sample | Time period[a] | Definition or typograpy | Results/100 cases[b] |
| Maisto et al., 1978 | Study of prevalence of SIB, subject characteristics, & relationship to other problem behaviors | Checklist format questionnaire completed during interview of caregivers | Residents of a state MR facility; 10–70 yrs. (mean = 33.5); 5.2% mild; 8.7% moderate; 28.5% severe; 47.6% profound; (males = 725; females = 575); article includes info on length of institutionalization & diagnosis | Unspecified; prevalence | Self-injurious behavior, including head-bang, eye-gouge, hair-pull, bite, & scratch | T = 14 (M = 11; F = 17) |
| Maurice & Trudel, 1982 | Attempt to establish the prevalence of SIB and to measure some of the characteristics associated with it, in specific institutions | Questionnaire completed during interview of caregivers | 1249 mentally retarded residents of 3 different institutions in the Montreal area | Those who displayed SIB during 2-yr. period preceding the study; prevalence | Headbanging, hitting body, rubbing body part, scratching, pulling hair, eye gouging, biting self, pica, gouging, digging, insertion in body cavities, excessive masturbation, pinching self, other (vomiting, burning self, cutting self, self-choking, stopping blood circulation) | Mentally retarded group—T = 70.3 |

| | | | | | | |
|---|---|---|---|---|---|---|
| Mulick et al., 1986 | Study to determine prevalence of SIB in residential treatment centers | Checklist format questionnaire completed by teachers in residential units | All 102 residents of a facility for nonambulatory profoundly and severely MR adults; ages 21–68 (mean = 35 yrs.); 100% profound | Unspecified | Same as Rojahn et al., 1984; prevalence? | T = 54 some SIB; T = 12 SIB of high danger of injury with lasting damage |
| Reid et al., 1984 | Study of natural history of behavior problems | Staff & patient interviews, plus review of records | Sample of severely and profoundly retarded adults in a British hospital; 24–78 yrs. (mean = 41.3); (males = 37; females = 49); article contains info on diagnosis | Nurses' ratings for previous 1-wk. period; psychiatrist ratings for 20-min. interview period; prevalence | Self-injury | Nurse ratings—'75 T = 22 '81 T = 19; psychiatrist ratings—'75 T = 5 '81 T = 7 |
| | | | | | Pica | Psychiatrist ratings—'75 T = 3 '81 T = 2 |
| Ressman & Butterworth, 1952 | Study of acquired hypertrichosis (skin disease) | Unspecified in secondary source | Unspecified number—Population of a school for the feeble-minded | Unspecified in secondary source; prevalence? | Skin mutilation (mainly self-biting and -chewing) | T = 21. |

TABLE 2.3. (Continued)

| Authors | Purpose | Data collection | Sampling strategy: Sample | Sampling strategy: Time period[a] | Definition or typograpy | Results/100 cases[b] |
|---|---|---|---|---|---|---|
| Rojahn, 1984 | Study designed to investigate staff agreement on identification of SIB cases, determine prevalence of SIB, and investigate taxonomic classification of SIB | Checklist format questionnaire completed by direct-care staff | 91 mentally retarded residents from lowest-functioning wards of a German MR facility; 19–49 yrs. (females mean = 35 & males mean = 34); all estimated in severe or profound range; (males = 42; females = 49) | Behavior should have been observed in past 3 mos; prevalence | Behavior that causes physical damage to the person's own body, including head-to-object/object-to-head; body-to-object, body-to-body, biting, scratching, gouging, pinching, pulling hair, stuffing orifices, pica, mouthing & sucking, ruminative vomiting, coprophagy, aerophagy, polydipsia, other | T = 66 (M = 69; F = 61) |
| Rojahn, 1986 | Study to determine prevalence of SIB, to analyze for classification implications, & examine relationships with stereotypy | Checklist format questionnaire completed by staff familiar with individuals | Estimated 25, 827 individuals served by a private association for retarded citizens in Germany (community based) | Unclear, but subjects must have displayed one form of SIB during 14-day period preceding study; prevalence | Similar to Rojahn et al., 1984 | T = 1.7; (approx. ratio 1 M to 1 F) |

| | | | | | | |
|---|---|---|---|---|---|---|
| Ross, 1972 | Census survey re: relationship of levels of intelligence to physical disabilities, skills, & problem behaviors | Questionnaire | 11,139 mentally retarded residents in California state institutions; levels of retardation = 47% profound, 31% severe, 16% moderate, 7% mild; mean age = 23; (4683 male; 6466 female) | Data collected in 1970—otherwise unspecified; prevalence? | Self-destructive behavior (not further defined) | T = 23 |
| Schroeder et al., 1978 | Study of prevalence of SIB, subject characteristics, & relationship to other problem behaviors | Interview of social workers & ward staff | Population of state MR facility; 5–85 yrs.; (males = 633; females = 517); article includes info on functioning level, length of institutionalization, & associated problems | Unclear—surveys completed in fall 1973, spring 1975, fall 1976; prevalence? | Repetitive acts against self resulting in physical harm or tissue damage; i.e., head-bang, bite, scratch, gouge, pinch, pica, coprophagy, aerophagia, & polydipsia; severe = at least once per day and sometime caused bleeding, bruises, broken bones, or other tissue damage requiring medical staff intervention; mild = all other | Fall '73 T = 10 spring '75 T = 10 fall '76 T = 10 combined 3 yrs. ratio 1.08 M to 1 F |

TABLE 2.3. (Continued)

| Authors | Purpose | Data collection | Sampling strategy: Sample | Sampling strategy: Time period[a] | Definition or typograpy | Results/100 cases[b] |
|---|---|---|---|---|---|---|
| Singh, 1977 | Study of SIB prevalence | Initial screening by staff, followed by interview and observation | 368 patients on main campus of New Zealand MR hospital | Results pertain to self-injury during a 6-mo. period; prevalence | Self-inflicted behavior leading to lacerations, bruising, or abrasions; e.g., head-banging, face-slapping, gouging, rumination, hyperventilation-induced seizures | T = 22.8 (ratio 1.47 M to 1 F) |
| Smeets, 1971 | Study of number of subjects with self-mutilative behavior, their characteristics, & relationship to other aberrant behaviors | Unspecified | 400 residents of a private, residential school for MR & ED children & adults | Unspecified; prevalence? | Behavior that can cause direct physical damage to self and would be aversive to normal individuals; | T = 8.75 (approx. ratio 1.4 M to 1 F) |
| | | | | | severe = individuals who must be forcefully stopped; | T = 57 of self-mutilative (approx. ratio 1.2 F to 1 M) |
| | | | | | mild = those who will stop when told or warned | T = 43 of self-mutilative (approx. ratio 2.75 F to 1 M) |
| Soule & O'Brien 1974 | Survey of the SIB in a residential institution | Unspecified in secondary source | 966 residents of a state MR facility | Unspecified in secondary source; prevalence? | Self-injurious behavior such as biting & head-bang | T = 7.7 |
| Whitney, 1966 | Introduction to case report of SIB treatment | Unspecified | 950 residents—population of a mental retardation facility | Unspecified; prevalence? | Mutilated bodies to extent requiring restraint | T = 8.8 |

[a] "?" After incidence or prevalence indicates difficulty classifying this study based on information in article.
[b] T = total; M = male; F = female; CP = cerebral palsy.

times as high as those for similarly impaired women. Only one of these studies reported significance tests on these figures; Ballinger (1971) reported nonsignificant results for differences across gender in prevalence of self-injurious behavior among his psychiatrically impaired subjects.

### Mentally Retarded Subjects

There were six reports containing prevalence figures by gender for mentally retarded subjects. Prevalence figures for self-injurious behavior among males ranged from 11 (Maisto et al., 1978) to 69 (Rojahn, 1984). Thus, the reported prevalence rates for self-injurious behavior were between .76 (Ballinger, 1971; Maisto et al., 1978) and 1.5 (MacKay et al., 1974) times as high for males as females. Four other studies, although not reporting actual figures for males and females, did provide the ratio (or information enough to calculate a ratio) of self-injurious male to self-injurious female subjects. Among these studies, the ratios ranged from 1.1 (Rojahn, 1986) to 1.47 (Singh, 1977). Most investigations did not involve significance testing for the gender variable; however, those that did yielded mainly nonsignificance (e.g., Eyman & Call, 1977; Schroeder et al., 1978).

### Summary of Gender Variable

In those studies for which incidence and prevalence rates were reported by gender, results varied slightly between males and females. Among handicapped subjects (children), *incidence* rates for males were from 1.5 to 3.5 times as high as those for females. Similarly, for mentally retarded subjects, *prevalence* rates tended to be higher for males than for females, although there were some investigators who found slightly higher rates among females. Interestingly, among the psychiatrically impaired subjects, the *prevalence* rates of self-injurious behavior for females were all higher than those for males. To the extent that mental retardation represents arrested or delayed development and the display of self-injury is a manifestation of such delayed development (Baumeister & Rollings, 1976), the similarity in results between persons with mental retardation and nonhandicapped children might not be surprising. However, we are unable to offer a potential explanation for the opposite relationship between gender and self-injury among the psychiatric population.

## *Age*

As in the case of gender, age is a commonly investigated variable in incidence and prevalence studies, and it seemed appropriate to explore age in relation to self-injurious behavior. Again, the discussion is organized according to handicapping condition.

## Nonhandicapped Subjects

The studies of nonhandicapped subjects involved infants and children and generally did not include incidence or prevalence rates by age. Rather, most of these studies included information regarding the ages at onset of various behaviors that frequently would be considered self-injurious in older handicapped populations. For example, studies involving head-banging contained the following information about the age at onset: majority of cases began head-banging between 5 and 11 months, with the mean age of onset being 8.13 months (Kravitz et al., 1960) and 9.4 months (Sallustro & Atwell, 1978); the median age of onset of greater than 12 months (Kravitz & Boehem, 1971); and 61.4% of the male sample and 88.6% of the female sample before the age of 18 months (de Lissovoy, 1961). Kravitz and Boehem (1971) reported median ages of onset of 10 months or less for hand-sucking, lip-sucking or -biting, toe-sucking, and teeth-grinding.

In some cases, information regarding ages at which the subjects ceased to display these behaviors also was reported. For example, most subjects discontinued head-banging by the age of 25 months, but others continued well into their elementary school years (Kravitz et al., 1960). Similarly, Lourie (1949) reported that rocking, swaying, and head-banging generally lasted only 2.5 to 3 years, but that in some cases, such behaviors continued up to age 12 years.

## Psychiatrically Impaired Subjects

Only one study involving emotionally disturbed subjects reported prevalence rates of self-injury by age. Ballinger (1971) reported the following: ages 10 to 19 years, 50/100 cases (based only on four subjects in this age range in the sample); 20 to 29 years, 0/100 cases; 30 to 39 years, 2.4/100 cases; 40 to 49 years, 1.1/100 cases; 50 to 59 years, 3.1/100 cases; 60 to 69 years, 4.9/100 cases; and 70 years and above, 3.3/100 cases. No significance testing was reported for these data.

## Mentally Retarded Subjects

A few authors presented prevalence rates of self-injurious behavior among retarded subjects according to age groups. Among the lowest estimates were those of Eyman and Call (1977), who reported figures ranging from 8 to 22/100 cases for community-based subjects under 13 years of age and between 5 and 20 for those above that age. These figures varied, depending on level of retardation and whether residence was with relatives or in other community-based facilities. Rates among these subjects appeared to decrease or to remain constant as age increased within level of retardation. No significance testing was reported for age.

The estimates presented by Ballinger (1971) were comparable to those of Eyman and Call (1977), ranging from 9.1/100 cases for individuals between 50 and 59 years of age to 21.2/100 cases for those between 60 and 69 years. The range of prevalence rates in the Eyman and Call study did not show a linear progression across ages; rates sometimes increased and sometimes decreased as age increased. As with the Ballinger study, no significance testing was reported for age.

Obtained results of Danford and Huber (1982), which ranged from 12.3/100 cases for subjects 51 to 60 years of age to 38.5/100 cases for individuals 71 years and above, also varied in both directions as age increased. However, these authors reported a statistically significant decrease in the prevalence of self-injury as age increased among their subjects.

Eyman and Call (1977) also reported prevalence rates for an institutionalized sample. These rates were somewhat higher than those for the samples mentioned thus far, and ranged from 28 to 35/100 cases for those subjects 13 years of age and from 15 to 47/100 cases (depending on level of retardation) for those above that age.

Although not reporting prevalence rates by age groups, other investigators presented the results of significance testing involving the relationship between age and the prevalence of self-injury. Barron and Sandman (1984) reported no significant differences in age between groups that included self-injurious subjects and those groups that did not. Maisto et al. (1978) and Schroeder et al. (1978) reported just the opposite results, with the mean age of their self-injurious groups being lower those of their non-self-injurious groups.

### Summary of Age Variable

While there appears to be variation in the incidence and prevalence of self-injurious behavior across age groups, the data generally were inconclusive in regard to specific patterns. Incidence studies indicate that behaviors that would be labeled self-injurious among older populations are displayed by many nonhandicapped (or nondiagnosed) children, frequently appearing for the first time before the age of 18 months. Among nonhandicapped populations, such behaviors usually ceased during the preschool years. There were no incidence or prevalence studies involving nonhandicapped adults or adolescents. Presumably, if such behaviors occur at these ages, the individual is considered to have a psychiatric or developmental problem.

Only one study was found that reported prevalence rates for various age groups of psychiatrically impaired subjects. No clear pattern seemed apparent in the data from this study. As for mentally retarded subjects, a decrease in prevalence rates with increasing age was noted in many studies. However, examination of the data indicated that there was much variability in this pattern. It seems that any firm conclusions regarding age and prevalence rates would be premature at this time.

## Handicapping Conditions

The ideal study for examining the question of the relationship of handicapping conditions to the prevalence of self-injurious behavior would involve a broad definition and samples of individuals with the various handicaps of interest, as well as a sample of nonhandicapped individuals. Unfortunately, such a study has yet to be conducted. Therefore, we must review the results of several studies, each involving different samples, to attempt to answer our question. The articles reviewed included prevalence and incidence data for samples involving three handicapping conditions, as well as for samples of nonhandicapped individuals.

### Nonhandicapped Subjects

A total of seven studies of nonhandicapped persons was reviewed. Again, these generally involved only infants, although some did involve schoolaged children. The reported incidence rates ranged from 2.6/100 cases for head-banging or head-slapping (Levy & Patrick, 1928) to 100/100 cases for hand-sucking (Kravitz & Boehem, 1971). Examples of other incidence figures included 100/100 cases for lip-sucking or -biting, 83.4/100 cases for toe-sucking, and 56/100 cases for teeth-grinding (Kravitz & Boehem, 1971). While behaviors such as hand- and toe-sucking may not be considered self-injurious or otherwise abnormal in these young populations, it seems important to include these results here, as the same behaviors frequently are considered self-injurious when present in older handicapped children. Thus, the prevalence of these behaviors among infants may be important when developing theories of etiology for self-injury among older handicapped individuals.

Only one study involved a broad definition of self-injury, encompassing several different topographies (Shentoub & Soulairac, 1967, reported in Green, 1967). This study, involving prevalence rather than incidence, yielded rates varying from 0 to 16/100 cases for 9-month to 5-year-old infants.

### Psychiatrically Impaired Subjects

There were six studies that reported figures for prevalence of self-injurious behavior for mentally ill or emotionally disturbed subjects. Ballinger (1971), studying patients over 10 years of age in a Scottish psychiatric hospital, reported the lowest figure, 3/100 cases. At the other extreme were the figures of 40/100 cases and 38/100 cases reported by Green (1967, 1968) and by Shodell and Reiter (1968), in studies involving children diagnosed as schizophrenic.

### Mentally Retarded Subjects

Some 23 prevalence studies that involved mentally retarded subjects were located. Prevalcnce rates in these studies were reported in dramatic ranges, depending on the definition and sample. Among the lowest estimates were 1.7/100 cases among community-based individuals in Germany reported by Rojahn (1986); 2.1/100 reported by Ressman and Butterworth (1952), who investigated skin mutilation, mainly involving self-biting and chewing; 3.7/100 cases reported by Danford and Huber (1982), for individuals who displayed pica involving both food-related and nonfood items. At the other extreme, the highest prevalence estimates were 66/100 cases reported by Rojahn (1984), which involved severe and profoundly retarded, institutionalized subjects; 54/100 cases obtained by Mulick, Dura, Rasnake, and Callahan (1986), which also involved profoundly retarded subjects; and 44/100 cases reported by Eyman and Call (1977), for their sample of hospitalized, severely mentally retarded subjects.

### Other Subjects

Only one study was located that involved samples other than those reported previously herein. Kravitz and Boehem (1971) reported the following incidence figures for cerebral palsied infants: 25/100 cases for hand-sucking; 4.5/100 cases for lip-sucking or -biting; 4.5 cases/100 for toe-sucking; and 17/100 cases for head-banging.

### Summary of Handicapping Conditions Variable

Differences in prevalence and incidence rates for self-injurious behavior were found across the various handicapping conditions, ranging from the lowest among the nonhandicapped samples to the highest among the mentally retarded subjects. However, the results across the various samples were not without overlap. Among nonhandicapped subjects, incidence figures ranged from 2.6 to 100/100 cases, depending on the specific behavior studied. Prevalcnce figures involving a more traditional definition of self-injury ranged from 0 to 16/100. Prevalence rates among samples of psychiatrically impaired subjects ranged from 3 to 40/100 cases. Samples of mentally retarded subjects yielded prevalence figures ranging from 1.7 to 67/100 cases. Sources for the variation within types of handicapping conditions probably would be related to the aforementioned critical dimensions and to the following other characteristics.

## *Intelligence Level*

Another characteristic potentially related to incidence and prevalence rates of self-injurious behavior is that of intelligence or level of functioning. Of course, the comparison of rates for nonhandicapped and mentally retarded samples discussed previously was related to this analysis. However, not yet reviewed are the rates for the various levels of mental retardation.

### Profoundly Retarded Subjects

There were 10 studies that reported prevalence rates, or figures that could be converted to rates, for profoundly retarded subjects or profoundly and severely retarded subjects combined. Among the lower estimates were the 4 and 5/100 cases reported by Danford and Huber (1982), the 12/100 cases of Mulick et al. (1986), and the 14/100 cases of Schroeder et al. (1978). It is important to note that the first of these studies involved only food pica and combined food and nonfood pica; the second involved only severe self-injury, and the reported figure was for profoundly and severely retarded subjects combined; and the third estimate also was for profoundly and severely retarded subjects combined. The lowest estimates, which involved a broader definition and profoundly retarded subjects only, were the 17/100 cases reported by Eyman and Call (1977) for individuals 12 years old and under living in community-based facilities and for individuals of all ages living with parents or other relatives. At the other extreme were estimates of 74/100 cases by MacKay et al. (1974), 66/100 cases by Rojahn (1984), and 54/100 cases by Mulick et al. (1986). The last two figures were for profoundly and severely retarded subjects combined.

### Severely Retarded Subjects

Again, there were 10 studies that reported prevalence estimates for severely retarded subjects or for combined groups of profoundly and severely retarded subjects. The lowest of these were the 9, 5, and 2/100 cases reported by Danford and Huber (1982) for the various types of pica. Low estimates for studies involving broader-based definitions included 11/100 cases by Eyman and Call (1977) for individuals over the age of 12 years and living in community residences or with relatives, and 14/100 cases reported by the same authors for individuals 12 years and under living in community-based residences. Also relevant here are the estimates of 12/100 cases by Mulick et al. (1986) and the 14/100 cases by Schroeder et al. (1978). As mentioned previously, these last two figures are for combined groups that include both severely and profoundly retarded individuals.

Estimates ranged as high as the 44 and 38/100 cases reported by Eyman and Call (1977) for individuals living in institutions. Higher still were the 66 and 54/100 cases reported by Rojahn (1984) and Mulick et al. (1986), respectively, for combined groups of severely and profoundly retarded subjects.

### Moderately Retarded Subjects

Of the five reports involving moderately retarded subjects, the lowest prevalence rates were the figures of 3/100 cases reported by Maisto et al. (1978) and the 3/100 cases of Danford and Huber (1982). Again, the latter study involved pica only. The highest prevalence estimate for the moderately retarded group was the 35/100 cases reported by Eyman and Call (1977), which involved a combined mildly and moderately retarded group of institutionalized individuals 12 years old and under. The highest figure for a sample of only moderately retarded subjects was the 18/100 cases reported by Ross (1972).

### Mildly Retarded Subjects

There were five reports containing prevalence estimates for mildly retarded individuals, and the lowest were the estimates of 0/100 cases reported by Maisto et al. (1978) and Danford and Huber (1982). Again, the Danford and Huber study involved pica only. At the opposite extreme was the 35/100 cases mentioned previously, which involved a combined moderately and mildly retarded group (Eyman & Call, 1977). For mildly retarded subjects only, the highest estimate was the 13/100 cases reported by Ross (1972).

### Borderline Subjects

Two studies reported prevalence estimates for individuals between the mildly retarded and normal levels of intelligence. Ballinger (1971) reported 4/100 cases. Danford and Huber (1982) reported 11/100 cases of nonfood pica and no other pica among this group.

### Summary of Intelligence Level Variable

As with other variables, the ranges of prevalence estimates for the various levels of intelligence overlap. Despite the overlap in the ranges, it is apparent that the minimum and maximum estimates decreased as intelligence levels increased. If we ignore the studies involving only pica and those combining two levels of intelligence into one group, we obtain the following ranges: profoundly retarded = 17 to 74/100 cases; severely retarded = 11 to 44/100 cases; moderately retarded = 3 to 18/100 cases; mildly retarded = 0 to 13/100 cases; and borderline = 4/100 cases. These can be compared to the 0 to 16/100 cases reported earlier for nonhandicapped subjects. Thus, there does appear to be an inverse relationship between the incidence or prevalence of self-injury and level of functioning.

A number of studies have included statistical analyses related to this phenomenon and have reported significant differences across levels of intelligence (e.g., MacKay et al., 1974; Maisto et al., 1978; Schroeder et al., 1978). One exception to this general finding was a study of psychiatrically impaired subjects in which Green (1967) found no significant differences in intelligence scores between self-injurious and non-self-injurious groups. One other study of relevance is that of Sallustro and Atwell (1978); they found that the initial ages of holding the head erect and of walking without support were significantly higher among a group of infants who displayed head-banging than among the non-head-banging group (similar but statistically nonsignificant results were reported for 8 of 10 other developmental milestones).

In addition to the preceding studies, there were other studies that reported the percentage of their obtained samples of self-injurious subjects who fell into each of the various levels of intelligence (e.g., Griffin, Ricketts, Williams, Locke, Altmeyer, & Stark, 1987; Griffin, Williams, Stark, Altmeyer, & Mason, 1984, 1986; Maurice & Trudel, 1982; Singh, 1977). These studies generally contained greater numbers of self-injurious subjects as levels of intelligence decreased but did not provide the information necessary to calculate actual prevalence rates. Simply knowing that a given sample of self-injurious subjects contains more profoundly retarded than mildly retarded individuals is not very helpful, as it is possible that the population from which the sample was obtained contains correspondingly higher proportions of profoundly retarded subjects in general.

At least two possible explanations exist for the inverse relationship between the likelihood of self-injury and the level of functioning. If self-injury is a developmental phenomenon, then we would expect it to be more prevalent within populations of lower-functioning individuals. Seemingly arguing against this interpretation, however, is the disparity between incidence figures for nonhandicapped infants and toddlers (which are similar to prevalence figures for mildly retarded samples) and the prevalence figures reported for samples of profoundly and severely retarded individuals. A second potential explanation is that the lower-functioning individuals are likely to have a greater degree of brain damage and that this damage is responsible, at least in part, for the display of self-injury (Baumeister & Rollings, 1976).

## *Residential Setting*

It is possible to divide the handicapped subjects in the studies into those living in the community (e.g., with parents or relatives, in group homes) and those residing in institutions or residential schools. We felt that it would be interesting to examine the extent to which prevalence rate varied in relation to residential setting. In the following discussion, the groups are further divided into psychiatrically impaired and mentally retarded.

### Psychiatrically Impaired Subjects in Institutions

There were five studies that involved mentally ill or emotionally disturbed individuals residing in institutions or residential schools. Prevalence rates among these studies ranged from 3/100 cases (Ballinger, 1971) to 40/100 cases (Green, 1967, 1968).

### Psychiatrically Impaired Subjects in Community Residences

Only one study was located that involved mentally ill or emotionally disturbed subjects living in the community. Shodell and Reiter (1968) reported a prevalence rate of 38/100 cases for schizophrenic children living at home and attending private school.

### Mentally Retarded Subjects in Institutions

The vast majority (19) of the prevalence studies involved institutionalized mentally retarded subjects. The fact that prevalence estimates vary with level of functioning makes reviewing these studies difficult. To simplify this endeavor, we report the range in figures only for profoundly and mildly retarded samples, and only for those studies involving a definition of self-injurious behavior that includes a variety of topographies. Prevalence estimates involving institutionalized profoundly retarded subjects ranged from a low of 26/100 (Ross, 1972) to a high of 74/100 (MacKay et al., 1974). Estimates of prevalence levels among mildly retarded, institutionalized subjects ranged from 0/100 (Maisto et al., 1978) to 13/100 (Ross, 1972).

### Mentally Retarded Subjects in Community Residences

Of the prevalence studies reviewed, there were four that involved non-institutionalized mentally retarded subjects. Here, it is important again to recognize the variation across levels of functioning, and so, as in the previous section, we sought studies that reported separate figures for profoundly and mildly retarded subjects and that included multiple topographies in their definition of self-injurious behavior. Only the study by Eyman and Call (1977) even partially met these criteria. Estimates of prevalence in this study were 17 to 20/100 for profoundly retarded subjects, depending on age and whether they lived with relatives or in other community residences.

### Summary of Residential Placement Variable

Intuitively, one might expect a greater prevalence of self-injury among institutionalized than noninstitutionalized impaired individuals. Among psychiatrically impaired subjects, prevalence rates ranged from 3 to 40/100 cases for institutionalized subjects. The prevalence rate reported in one study involving noninstitutionalized subjects was 38/100 cases. With only one study of community-based subjects, it is difficult to make valid comparisons between institutionalized and noninstitutionalized psychiatrically impaired subjects. Prevalence rates for profoundly retarded subjects ranged from 26 to 74/100 cases for those in institutions, compared to 17 to 20/100 cases for those in a community living situation. For mildly retarded subjects, prevalence rates ranged from 0 to 13/100 cases for institutionalized subjects. There were no studies for prevalence of self-injurious behavior for those mildly retarded subjects living in the community.

Thus, for psychiatrically impaired and for mildly retarded subjects, there have not been enough studies to permit valid comparisons of prevalence rates for self-injurious behavior between institutionalized and noninstitutionalized individuals. For profoundly mentally retarded subjects, prevalence rates of self-injurious behavior are higher among those who are institutionalized than among those who are not. It is difficult, however, to know whether individuals are institutionalized due to their display of self-injurious behavior or the self-injurious behavior is displayed due to conditions within the institutions.

## *Other Factors*

In addition to the factors discussed previously, a number of authors, in studying the prevalence of self-injury, have explored a variety of other related factors. These other factors include frequency; severity; length of institutionalization; number of topographies; frequency of topographies; classification of topographies; relationship to other behaviors and handicaps; antecedents, motivation, and function; use of medication; and use of behavioral programs. The results of such investigations, most of which involved institutionalized populations of mentally retarded individuals, are briefly reviewed as follows.

### Frequency

Several authors reported information on the frequency with which their subjects displayed self-injurious behaviors (Barron & Sandman, 1984; Griffin et al., 1984, 1986, 1987; Maurice & Trudel, 1982; Singh, 1977). This information generally was based on estimates from interviews or questionnaires involving caregivers. Because each of the studies involved a different frequency categorization scheme, it is difficult to summarize the results of the various studies here. For the sake of example, we describe the results reported by Maurice and Trudel (1982). These authors found that of their self-injurious subjects, 56% displayed the behavior more than once daily, 17.1% more than once weekly, 10.3% more than once monthly, and 16.6% sometimes went more than a month without displaying the behavior.

### Severity

At least six reports included information on severity, or amount of physical damage resulting from the subjects' responses (Barron & Sandman, 1984; Griffin et al., 1986; Maisto et al., 1978; Maurice & Trudel, 1982; Schroeder et al., 1978; Singh, 1977). For example, Singh (1977) reported that of the self-injurious subjects in his survey, 25% displayed behavior resulting in severe tissue damage, 18% displayed behavior resulting in moderate damage, and 57% of the subjects sustained mild damage as a result of SIB.

Several authors examined the relationship of subject's gender to severity, with mixed results. Griffin et al. (1986) reported that a larger percentage of males than females engaged in repetitive self-injurious behavior without tissue damage. On the other hand, Maisto et al. (1978) reported that the severity of self-injury for females was less than that of males. Finally, Maurice and Trudel (1982) reported no significant differences between males and females related to severity. It is of some importance to note that the Griffin et al. and the Maisto et al. reports did not involve significance testing in regard to gender and severity.

### Length of Institutionalization

Two studies included length of institutionalization in their analyses. Maisto et al. (1978) reported that non-self-injurious residents had resided in the institution on an average of 4.8 years longer than self-injurious residents and that this differences was statistically significant. Schroeder et al. (1978) reported no significant difference in length of institutionalization between severely and mildly self-injurious subjects.

### Number of Topographies

Several studies reviewed included information regarding the number of forms or topographies of self-injurious behavior displayed by individual subjects (Barron & Sandman, 1984; Griffin et al., 1986; Maisto et al., 1978; Maurice & Trudel, 1982; Rojahn, 1984, 1986). While some authors have broken the number of topographies displayed into several groups, we examine just two categories, single topographies and multiple topographies, for summarization purposes. The following figures represent the percentages of subjects who were reported to display multiple forms of self-injurious responding: 58.4% (Griffin et al., 1986); 56.2% (Maurice & Trudel, 1982); 75% (Rojahn, 1984); and 76.1% (Rojahn, 1986). Thus, somewhere between one-half and three-quarters of self-injurious subjects were reported to display two or more forms of self-injury.

Other reports have included additional information related to the number of topographies. For example, Maisto et al. (1978), and Maurice and Trudel (1982) reported that females were significantly more likely to display multiple topographies than males. Rojahn (1986), and Maurice and Trudel (1986) reported a statistically significant inverse relationship between the number of topographies displayed and the level of mental retardation (i.e., more topographies positively related to more profound retardation). Similarly, Maurice and Trudel (1982) reported that mentally retarded subjects were significantly more likely to display multiple topographies than were psychotic subjects.

### Frequency of Topographies

Information on the most commonly appearing forms of self-injurious responding was provided in several of the reports (Griffin et al., 1984, 1986, 1987; Maisto et al., 1978; Maurice & Trudel, 1982; Rojahn, 1984; Singh, 1977). With the greatest frequency, head-banging (either against objects or with hands) was listed as the most common response (Maurice & Trudel, 1982; Rojahn, 1984; Singh, 1977). Biting appeared to be the next most common, appearing in several studies in either first or second place (Griffin et al., 1986; Maisto et al., 1978; Rojahn, 1984; Singh, 1977).

Two studies included summaries of frequency of topography by gender of subject (Maisto et al., 1978; Singh, 1977). One of these (Maisto et al., 1978) reported the results of significance testing involving these variables. For example, Maisto et al. (1978) found that self-biting of hand and hair-pulling were the first and second most frequent behaviors for females, whereas the most frequent response of males was self-hitting, with scratching and biting appearing in the second position.

### Classification of Topographies

Several years ago, Schroeder, Mulick, and Rojahn (1980) discussed the need for a classification scheme for self-injurious behavior that was based on empirical study and that involved the function of each topography of self-injury. Rojahn (1984, 1986) conducted several statistical analyses in an attempt to determine which topographies typically occurred together in subjects who displayed multiple forms of self-injurious behavior. For example, in the earlier study, Rojahn (1984) found significant correlations between various forms of self-hitting and other behaviors such as biting, scratching, gouging, pinching, and hair-pulling. He speculated that these behaviors form a class of self-injury that may serve a reinforcement function. Similarly, he reported significant correlations between such behaviors as mouthing and sucking, eating inedible objects, and coprophagy. He speculated that this group of behaviors may serve a nonsocial or self-stimulatory function for the subjects. Interestingly, Rojahn found that ruminative vomiting, which he originally grouped with the nonsocial responses, was correlated with several types of self-hitting (a supposedly social behavior). In his second study, Rojahn (1986) conducted a cluster analysis that yielded three groups of statistically related behaviors. These were identical to the groupings described earlier, with the exception that rumination and teeth-grinding appeared in a third group rather than being combined with either the social or the nonsocial groups originally envisioned by Schroeder et al. (1980) and by Rojahn (1984).

## Antecedents, Motivation, and Function

In the studies described in the previous section, Rojahn (1984, 1986) attempted to determine statistically related behaviors, to group them, and to speculate as to the possible function of these behaviors based on such groupings. A number of other prevalence studies have included procedures for eliciting (typically from reports of caregivers) the motivation for or function of self-injurious responding, or the antecedent situations that typically preceded the subject's self-injurious behaviors.

Maurice and Trudel (1982) offered the most detailed report of antecedent circumstances. These authors presented a long list of circumstances that caregivers could choose from as preceding a subject's self-injurious behavior. The list included both subject emotions, such as anger, and behaviors of others, such as contact by peer or reprimand. Maurice and Trudel (1982) reported that the most frequently reported antecedent circumstances were frustration, refusal, anger, and agitation. There also was a high percentage of cases in which the antecedent emotions and circumstances were reported as unidentified. These authors also found that 21% of their subjects were reported to display self-injury in specific settings, while the other 79% reportedly were likely to display the behavior in any location. Furthermore, it was reported that 54% of the self-injurious subjects displayed such behaviors only at specific times of the day, while the other 63% were likely to display self-injury at any time. Maisto et al. (1978) described "getting upset" and "wanting something" as the most frequently reported motivations for their subjects' self-injurious responding. Finally, Barron and Sandman (1984) noted that their female subjects were reported to have a higher number of antecedents for their self-injury than the males in their study.

From our perspective, the meaningfulness of such caregiver's reports without empirical validation is highly questionable. These reports may be of some potential value inasmuch as they provide information as to how caregivers may be viewing self-injurious behavior. Otherwise, it seems best to look to more observationally based studies for information on antecedents (e.g., Edelson, Taubman, & Lovaas, 1982; Iwata, Dorsey, Slifer, Bauman, & Richman, 1982). Further, it seems rather fruitless to speculate as to unobservable emotions such as anger and frustration, without employing operational definitions that allow empirical study of accompanying observable behaviors.

## Relationship to Other Behaviors and Handicaps

Some of the prevalence reports included information about the relationship of self-injury to other aberrant behaviors and to handicaps not discussed previously. For example, Barron and Sandman (1984) studied four groups of subjects, including those who displayed stereotypic and self-injurious behaviors, stereotypic behaviors only, self-injurious behaviors only, and neither stereotypic nor self-injurious behaviors. Among other findings, Barron and Sandman (1984) reported that there were no significant differences in the number and type of self-injurious behaviors between the group of self-injurious subjects who displayed stereotypic behavior and the group of subjects who did not. On the other hand, Maisto et al. (1978) reported that the body-rocking and hand-waving stereotypes were higher among self-injurious subjects, as was aggression toward others. Finally, Schroeder et al. (1978) reported no statistically significant differences between self-injurious and non-self-injurious subjects in regard to stereotypic and other misbehaviors. Schroeder et al. (1978) found differences between self-injurious and non-self-injurious subjects, with the former group displaying significantly more visual, receptive language, and expressive language disorders. Maisto et al. (1978) reported higher rates of eye-gouging among blind subjects, and they reported that their young self-injurious subjects suffered from significantly more physical disabilities than did other subjects.

## Use of Medication

Medication has been used as one approach in the attempt to control self-injury, especially among institutionalized population. A number of prevalence studies have included figures on the percentage of self-injurious subjects taking medication. Griffin et al. (1986) presented the smallest percentage, with 32% of their subjects on medication (or a combination of medication and physical restraint). Rojahn (1986) and Maisto et al. (1978) reported the figures of 40% and 61%, respectively. Finally, Schroeder et al. (1978) reported that 47% of those self-injurious subjects not involved in behaviorally based programs for reduction of self-injury received neuroleptic medication.

## Use of Behavioral Programs

The responses of caregivers to subjects' self-injury (typically involving behavior management approaches) were included in a number of the prevalence surveys. For example, Griffin et al. (1986) reported that 33.1% of their self-injurious subjects were on formal programs based on positive reinforcement and 6.8% were on aversive programs that also included a positive reinforcement component. Barron and Sandman (1984) noted that caregivers reported that the most common measure used to control self-injury involved verbal/gestural instructions, that extinction was used significantly more for stereotypic behavior than for self-injury, and that time-out and over-correction were used significantly more for self-injury than for stereotypy. Maurice and Trudel (1982) reported that only 5.5% of their self-injurious subjects were involved in a formal program of reducing the behavior, but that 75% of such programs were behavioral in nature. Finally, with regard to reducing self-injury, Schroeder et al. (1978) reported a statistically significant advantage for those subjects who were involved in a behavior modification program versus those with no such involvement.

## Summary and Conclusions

Knowledge regarding the incidence and prevalence of self-injurious behavior among various populations is important for both theoretical and practical reasons. For agencies approving and funding research related to self-injury, information regarding the prevalence of such behavior can be a critical factor in their planning and decision making. For researchers attempting to gain an understanding of self-injury in regard to etiology or treatment, knowledge of differential rates across various populations, as well as possible relationships between self-injury and other variables, can be very helpful.

Over 30 incidence and prevalence studies were reviewed to determine which of the following characteristics were predictive of self-injurious behavior: gender, age, handicapping condition, level of intelligence, and residential placement. Although differences in such dimensions as definition, sampling strategy, and data collection made comparisons and summarization difficult, it was possible to draw a number of tentative conclusions. For example, it can be concluded that (a) incidence rates for nonhandicapped and prevalence rates for mentally retarded individuals tend to be higher for males than for females, while the opposite is true among psychiatrically impaired populations; (b) self-injury rarely appears in nonhandicapped individuals beyond infancy and preschool years; (c) drawing firm conclusions related to age and prevalence rates among mentally retarded or psychiatric populations is difficult; (d) rates of incidence or prevalence are lowest for nonhandicapped infants and children, highest for mentally retarded individuals of all ages, and intermediate for psychiatrically impaired samples; (e) an inverse relationship is noted between the prevalence of self-injury and level of intelligence; and there do appear to be higher rates of self-injury among those profoundly retarded individuals who are institutionalized than those who are not.

These results suggest a number of fruitful areas for future research. For example, why does self-injurious behavior tend to disappear in nonhandicapped populations after the preschool years and yet continue in the mentally retarded population? Could a difference in parental reactions/discipline for handicapped versus nonhandicapped children account for this fact? Further, why are the rates of self-injury higher among institutionalized profoundly retarded individuals than among similar individuals living in the community? Do profoundly retarded individuals tend to develop self-injurious responding after institutionalization, or is self-injurious behavior one of the original reasons for admission?

In regard to future areas of research related to the incidence and prevalence of self-injurious behavior, we believe that further studies of handicapped school-aged children are needed. In addition, further research involving handicapped and nonhandicapped infants and preschool populations is needed. Earlier studies involving infants and preschoolers generally have highly idiosyncratic samples and only address limited forms of self-injurious behaviors. We suggest that there is a need for empirical research in these areas, which involves both incidence and prevalence studies, employing standardized methods, and including a more comprehensive definition of self-injury, as well as reliably establishing logical sampling methods and appropriate data-collection time periods.

*Acknowledgments.* Preparation of this paper was supported in part by the U.S. Department of Education, Office of Special Education, Grant #G00-83-02980 "Innovative Programs for Severely Handicapped Children: Kansas Self-Injurious Behavior Project." We gratefully acknowledge the assistance of Joe Spradlin, Jeff Wells, and Chuck Spellman for their help in preparation of this paper.

## *References*

Ballinger, B. R. (1971). Minor self-injury. *British Journal of Psychiatry*, *118*, 535–538.

Barron, J. L., & Sandman, C. A. (1984). Self-injurious behavior and stereotypy in an institutionalized mentally retarded population. *Applied Research in Mental Retardation*, *5*, 499–511.

Baumeister, A. A., & Rollings, J. P. (1976). Self-injurious behavior. In N. R. Ellis (Ed.), *International review of research in mental retardation* (Vol. 1, pp. 1–34). New York: Academic Press.

Danford, D. E., & Huber, A. M. (1982). Pica among mentally retarded adults. *American Journal of Mental Deficiency*, *87*, 141–146.

de Lissovoy, V. (1961). Head banging in early childhood. *The Journal of Pediatrics*, *58*, 803–805.

Edelson, S. M., Taubman, M. T., & Lovaas, O. I. (1982). Some social contexts of self-destructive behavior. *Journal of Abnormal Child Psychology*, *11*, 299–312.

Eyman, R. K., & Call, T. (1977). Maladaptive behavior and community placement of mentally retarded persons. *American Journal of Mental Deficiency*, *82*, 137–144.

Green, A. A. (1967). Self-mutilation in schizophrenic children. *Archives of General Psychiatry*, *17*, 234–244.

Green, A. (1968). Self-destructive behavior in physically abused schizophrenic children. *Archives of General Psychiatry*, *19*, 171–179.

Griffin, J. C., Ricketts, R. W., Williams, D. E., Locke, B. J., Altmeyer, B. K., & Stark, M. T. (1987). A community survey of self-injurious behavior among developmentally disabled children and adolescents. *Hospital and Community Psychiatry*, *38*, 959–963.

Griffin, J. C., Williams, D. E., Stark, M. T., Altmeyer, B. K., & Mason, M. (1984). Self-injurious behavior: A statewide prevalence survey, assessment of severe cases, and follow-up of aversive programs. In J. C. Griffin, M. T. Stark, D. E., Williams, B. K. Altmeyer, & H. K. Griffin (Eds.), *Advances in the treatment of self-injurious behavior* (pp. 1–25). Austin, TX: Department of Health and Human Services.

Griffin, J. C., Williams, D. E., Stark, M. T., Altmeyer, B. K., & Mason, M. (1986). Self-injurious behavior: A statewide prevalence survey of the extent and circumstances. *Applied Research in Mental Retardation*, *7*, 105–116.

Hill, B. K., & Bruininks, R. H. (1984). Maladaptive behavior of mentally retarded individuals in residential facilities. *American Journal of Mental Deficiency*, *88*, 380–387.

Iwata, B. A., Dorsey, M. F., Slifer, K. J., Bauman, K. E., & Richman, G. S. (1982). Toward a functional analysis of self-injury. *Analysis and Intervention in Developmental Disabilities*, *2*, 3–20.

Kiley, M., & Lubin, R. (1983). Epidemiological methods. In J. L. Matson & J. A. Mulich (Eds.), *Handbook of mental retardation* (pp. 541–556). New York: Pergamon Press.

Kravitz, H., & Boehem, J. J. (1971). Rhythmic habit patterns in infancy: Their sequence, age of onset, and frequency. *Child Development*, *42*, 399–413.

Kravitz, H., Rosenthal, V., Teplitz, Z., Murphy, J. B., & Lesser, R. E. (1960). A study of head-banging in infants and children. *Diseases of the Nervous System*, *21*, 203–208.

Levy, D. M., & Patrick, H. T. (1928). Relation of infantile convulsions, head banging and breath-holding to fainting and headaches in the parents. *Archives of Neurology and Psychiatry*, *19*, 865–887.

Lourie, R. S. (1949). The role of rhythmic patterns in childhood. *American Journal of Psychiatry*, *105*, 653–660.

MacKay, D., McDonald, G., & Morrissey, M. (1974). Self-mutilation in the mentally subnormal. *Journal of Psychological Research in Mental Subnormality*, *1*, 25–31.

Maisto, C. R., Baumeister, A. A., & Maisto, A. A. (1978). An analysis of variables related to self-injurious behavior among institutionalized retarded person. *Journal of Mental Deficiency Research*, *22*, 27.

Maurice, P., & Trudel, G. (1982). Self-injurious behavior prevalence and relationship to environmental events. In J. H. Hollis & E. Meyers (Eds.), *Life-threatening behavior: Analysis and intervention* (pp. 81–275). Washington, DC: American Association on Mental Deficiency.

Mulick, J. A., Dura, J. R., Rasnake, K., & Callahan, C. (1986, August). *Prevalence of SIB in institutionalized nonambulatory profoundly retarded people.* Poster presented at the 94th annual convention of the American Psychological Association, Washington, DC.

Phillips, R. H., & Alkan, M. (1961). Some aspects of self-mutilation in the general population of a large psychiatric hospital. *Psychiatric Quarterly*, *35*, 421–423.

Reid, A. H., Ballinger, B. R., Heather, B. B. & Melvin, S. J. (1984). The natural history of behavioural symptoms among severely and profoundly mentally retarded patients. *British Journal of Psychiatry*, *145*, 289–293.

Ressman, A. C., & Butterworth, T. (1952). Localized acquired hypertrichosis. *Archives of Dermatology and Syphilis*, *65*, 418–423.

Rojahn, J. (1984). Self-injurious behavior in institutionalized, severely/profoundly retarded adults: Prevalence data and staff agreement. *Journal of Behavioral Assessment*, *8*, 13–27.

Rojahn, J. (1986). Self-injurious and stereotypic behavior of noninstitutionalized mentally retarded people: Prevalence and classification. *American Journal of Mental Deficiency*, *91*, 268–276.

Ross, R. T. (1972). Behavioral correlates of levels of intelligence. *American Journal of Mental Deficiency*, *76*, 545–549.

Sallustro, F., & Atwell, C. W. (1978). Body rocking, head banging, and head rolling in normal children. *Journal of Pediatrics*, *93*, 704–708.

Schroeder, S. R., Mulick, J. A., & Rojahn, J. (1980). The definition, taxonomy, epidemiology, and ecology of self-injurious behavior. *Journal of Autism and Developmental Disorders*, *10*, 417–432.

Schroeder, S. R., Schroeder, C. S., Rojahn, J., & Mulick, J. A. (1980). Self-injurious behavior: An analysis of behavior management techniques. In J. L. Matson & J. R. McCartney (Eds.), *Handbook of behavior modification with the mentally retarded* (pp. 61–115). New York: Plenum Press.

Schroeder, S. R., Schroeder, C. S., Smith, B., & Dalldorf, J. (1978). Prevalence of self-injurious behaviors in a large state facility for the retarded: A three-year follow-up study. *Journal of Autism and Childhood Schizophrenia*, *8*, 261–269.

Shentoub, S., & Soulairac, A. (1967). L'enfant automutilateur. Reported in A. A. Green, *Archives of General Psychiatry*, *17*, 234–244.

Shodell, M. J., & Reiter, H. (1968). Self-mutilative behavior in verbal and nonverbal schizophrenic children. *Archives of General Psychiatry*, *19*, 453–455.

Singh, N. N. (1977). Prevalence of self-injury in institutionalized retarded children. *New Zealand Medical Journal*, 325–326.

Singh, N. N. (1981). Rumination. In N. R. Ellis (Ed.), *International review of research in mental retardation* (Vol. 10, pp. 139–182). New York: Academic Press.

Singh, N. N. (1983). Behavioral treatment of pica in mentally retarded persons. *Psychiatric Aspects of Mental Retardation Reviews*, *2*, 33–36.

Smeets, P. M. (1971). Some characteristics of mental defectives displaying self-mutilative behaviors. *Training School Bulletin*, *68*, 131–135.

Soule, B., & O'Brien, D. (1974). Self-injurious behavior in a state center for the retarded: Incidence. *Research and the Retarded, Spring*, 1–8.

Whitney, L. R. (1966). The effect of operant conditioning on the self-destructive behavior of retarded children. In *Exploring Progress in Maternal and Child Health Nursing Practice, ANA, 1965, Regional conference #3*. New York: Appleton-Century-Crofts.

# Part 2
# Etiology and Assessment

# 3
# Neurobiological Factors in Self-injurious Behavior

JAMES C. HARRIS

## Introduction

Self-injurious behavior is a relatively infrequent problem in the general population but a serious one, particularly when it occurs in severely retarded and psychiatrically disturbed individuals. The term *self-injurious behavior* or *SIB* is used when referring to the mentally retarded population, and the term *deliberate self-harm syndrome* or *DSH* (Pattison & Kahan, 1983) has been proposed to describe self-aggression in emotionally disturbed individuals. SIB is one of the least understood and most difficult behavioral problems to treat in the developmentally disabled population. It is characterized by multiple episodes of physically self-damaging acts of low lethality, although the cumulative effect of this behavior may be life-threatening.

Self-injury may occur in conjunction with severe mental disorders or as a feature of several rare syndromes (the Lesch–Nyhan syndrome, the Cornelia de Lange syndrome, fragile X syndrome, Riley–Day and Rett syndrome); however, it most often occurs sporadically in association with severe to profound mental retardation or pervasive developmental disorder. It is also associated with severe language handicap, visual impairment, and seizure disorders. The occurrence of one of these conditions in a mentally retarded person increases the risk of SIB. In the severely retarded, it is commonly associated with stereotypic behavior, such as body rocking and head-banging. It is the major behavioral problem that results in the failure of community placement for the mentally retarded (Griffith et al., 1987).

Until recently, the primary emphasis in studies of self-injury has focused on environmental determinants; there are substantial data on the effects of environmental contingencies on SIB. Behavior modification treatment procedures have been the most commonly used forms of treatment of SIB (Bachman, 1972; Frankel & Simmons, 1976; Johnson & Baumeister, 1978; Maisto, Baumeister, & Maisto, 1978; Picker, Poling, & Parker, 1979; Russo, Carr, & Lovaas, 1980; Schroeder, Schroeder,

Smith, & Dalldorf, 1978). However, behavioral treatment techniques may not be successful in reducing self-injury, or even if they are initially effective, they may not maintain the improvement in behavior. Carr (1977) has convincingly argued that self-injury is multiply determined. Neurobiological factors must be considered as well as environmental ones.

This has led to more careful consideration of the possible biological bases for self-injury, its association with organic brain conditions, and how biological factors relate to treatment approaches. Knowledge about the possible biological mechanisms involved in self-injury might be employed in conjunction with other treatment procedures for more effective treatment and to reduce the considerable cost involved in both initial treatment and generalization of treatment into a home or community setting.

This chapter reviews the prevalence of self-injury in normal and deviant populations and discusses its association with psychiatric, neurologic, and developmental diagnoses. Several models for self-injurious behavior are reviewed that may be pertinent to this condition. These include models of psychosocial deprivation (e.g., isolation rearing carried out in early life), stress-induced analgesia, administration of drugs that affect neurotransmitter systems, surgical procedures that affect sensory input (e.g., forelimb deafferentation), certain mental retardation syndromes with a high prevalence of self-injury, and pervasive developmental disorder and other conditions associated with deficits in attachment behavior, sensory processing, and social communication.

## Prevalence

Stereotypy and self-injury may occur both in the normally intelligent child and in the mentally retarded population; head-banging is the most common presentation (Abe, Oda, & Amatomi, 1984). De Lissovoy (1962) found the onset of head-banging in children averaged about 8 months of age and disappeared in the normally intelligent group by 36 months of age. Other stereotyped movements, such as rocking, occurred in early life before the onset of head-banging. In two other investigations involving nearly 2000 children, the incidence of head-banging was 3.6–6.5%; males predominated over females, 3.5 to 1 (Kravitz, Vin Rosenthal, Teplitz, Murphy, & Lesser, 1960). Ordinarily, the behavior ceased to occur after 32 months of age. Kravitz et al. (1960) found self-injury in about 20% of the siblings of head-bangers in their sample, suggesting a familial pattern. The most common factor preceding the onset of head-banging was the eruption of central and lateral incisors. In another study of 15 head-bangers who were compared to matched controls, the only statistically significant factor differentiating the two groups was that the head-bangers had a higher incidence of otitis media (Lissovoy, 1963).

In the developmentally disabled, Griffin et al. (1987) have documented the prevalence of SIB among 2663 mentally retarded, autistic, or multiply handicapped children and adolescents in a large community metropolitan school district. They found that 69 cases (2.6%) demonstrated SIB during the 12 months chosen for the survey; 59% were male and 41% were female. The majority of this population (83%) were severely or profoundly retarded. The mean age was 10.2 years, and the frequency of occurrence for the majority (72%) was daily. For those ages 14 years of age or above, the community prevalence was lower, a factor the authors attribute to residential placements for older individuals. The most common symptoms were hand-biting, head-hitting, and head-banging. Only one third were in documented treatment programs. In this community sample, 8.7% of those with symptoms were receiving medications. Medical and psychiatric diagnoses were not provided for this population.

In contrast, SIB has been reported in 10–17% of institutionalized retarded individuals (Baumeister & Rollings, 1976; Schroeder, et al., 1978); the lower the IQ, the higher the prevalence rate. Over a 3-year period, Schroeder, et al. (1978) found in institutional settings that cases occurred most frequently in younger children who also had associated severe language handicaps, visual impairments, or seizure disorders and who tested in the profoundly retarded range of mental retardation. Other investigators, such as Smeets (1971), had come to the same conclusions that severe mental retardation accompanied by physiologic abnormalities led to a higher risk for the individual to develop SIB in early childhood.

Besides the occurrence of SIB in a heterogeneous group of severely or profoundly mentally retarded individuals, SIB is also seen associated in several specific medical syndromes which, although associated with mental retardation, show a range in degree of mental retardation. These are the Lesch–Nyhan syndrome, where hand-biting occurs in all cases, Rett syndrome where hand–mouth stereotypies with tissue involvement occur in essentially all cases, the fragile-X syndrome where hand-biting was reported in 74% of 37 cases reported (Hagerman et al., 1986), the Cornelia de Lange syndrome, the Riley–Day syndrome, and congential insensitivity to pain where self-injury is common, and although usually accidental, may come under operant control. The high frequency of self-injury suggests that this behavior is sufficiently characteristic in these disorders to be designated as a behavioral phenotype (Nyhan, 1972). In addition, in developmental disorders, such as pervasive developmental disorder, SIB is often associated, particularly in lower-functioning individuals.

TABLE 3.1. Stereotypy/habit disorder.

| | |
|---|---|
| 1. | Intentional, repetitive, nonfunctional behaviors, such as hand-shaking or waving, body-rocking, head-banging, mouthing of objects, nail-biting, picking at nose or skin |
| 2. | The disturbance either causes physical injury to the child or markedly interferes with normal activities (e.g. injury to head from head-banging; inability to fall asleep because of constant rocking) |
| 3. | Does not meet the criteria for either a pervasive developmental disorder or tic disorder |

## Diagnostic Considerations

Descriptions of self-injury are commonly listed according to their topography, (e.g., hand-biting, head-hitting, and head-banging). This descriptive approach has received acknowledgment in the psychiatric diagnostic system (American Psychiatric Association, 1987, *DSM-III-R*) in current use in the United States, where self-injury is classified as "Stereotypy/Habit Disorder" on the Axis I descriptive syndrome axis (See Table 3.1 for criteria for stereotypy/habit disorder, based on *DSM-III-R*). Self-injury accompanying the Axis II category, pervasive developmental disorder, is considered as an aspect of that condition, but the stereotypy/habit disorder designation is not also used when pervasive developmental disorder is diagnosed.

The essential features of stereotypy/habit disorder are intentional and repetitive behaviors that are nonfunctional and may include body-rocking, head-banging, face-slapping, hand-biting, skin-licking or -scratching, teeth-grinding (bruxism), bodily manipulations (e.g., incessant nose-picking, hair-pulling, eye- and anus-gouging), noncommunicative and repetitive vocalizations, breath-holding, hyperventilation, and swallowing air (aerophagia). This diagnosis is only given when the disturbance either causes physical injury to the child or markedly interferes with normal activities. How to judge intentionality is a major issue. By definition, a *stereotypy* is a meaningless behavior. Hamilton (1985) defines it as a repetitive, non-goal-directed action, which is carried out in a uniform way. Although it may come under environmental control and become functional in the environment, ascribing intentionality is problematic in this definition. Some self-injury, such as in the Lesch–Nyhan syndrome seems not to be a learned behavior and has been described as a behavioral phenotype (Harris, 1987); once initiated, there may be a role for environmental contingencies in its maintenance. It is common for children with this disorder to insist on being restrained because they are unable to control their self-injury, their expressed intention being not to harm themselves.

On the other hand, the term *deliberate self-harm syndrome* (DSH) (Pattison & Kahan, 1983) has been applied to individuals with psychiatric disorders who intend to harm themselves. (See Table 3.2 for criteria for

TABLE 3.2. Deliberate self-harm syndrome.

1. A sudden, irresistible impulse to harm oneself physically
2. A psychological experience of existing in an intolerable, uncontrollable situation from which one cannot escape
3. Mounting anxiety, agitation, and anger in response to the perceived situation
4. Perceptual and cognitive constriction, resulting in a narrowed perspective of the situation and of alternatives to action
5. Self-inflicted destruction or alteration of body tissues done in a private setting
6. A rapid, temporary feeling of relief following the act of self-harm

DSH, based on Pattison & Kahan). Pattison and Kahan suggested that this term be introduced into the psychiatric nomenclature to describe other forms of deliberate self-harm, such as those associated with alcohol and other drug abuse; with feelings of worthlessness, hopelessness, and helplessness; and with vegetative signs of depression. However, in DSH, the individual intends self-harm and ordinarily uses a specific means to carry out the action (e.g., a weapon such as a knife). These individuals who may be diagnosed with personality disorders or may be intoxicated at the time of the behavior generally do not have the intention of dying. They may injure themselves as a way of dealing with and perhaps reducing extreme anxiety. Their clinical course is characterized by many episodes of physically self-damaging acts that are of low lethality. The question about motivation in the deliberate self-harm syndrome is an interesting one, because in the psychiatrically disturbed population, these individuals often state that they are deliberately trying to hurt themselves to reduce "tension," in contrast to those with the SIB syndrome who are often nonverbal and cannot offer verbal reports. Deliberate self-harm has only been described in verbal individuals. A major issue in the assessment of self-injury is to establish whether the behavior has meaning to the individual and is intentional or whether it is a true stereotypy that in some mentally subnormal individuals has come under operant control or may be an extension of self-stimulation, or the result of a concurrent mental illness.

The DSH and the SIB syndromes are both diagnostic designations that need to be considered phenomenologically as potentially distinct and distinguishable according to their associated diagnoses. The psychiatric diagnosis in children and adolescents that is most commonly used with SIB is the Axis II diagnosis of pervasive developmental disorder—autism. However, self-injury may also be associated with affective disorder, psychosis (Green, 1967), or disruptive behavior disorders, such as oppositional disorder and conduct disorder. The Axis III diagnoses that are most often associated with self-injury are the Lesch–Nyhan syndrome, the Cornelia de Lange syndrome, congenital insensitivity to pain, fragile-X syndrome, Rett syndrome, and specific diagnostic etiologies of blindness, such as retrolental fibroplasia. The focus of this review is mental retardation and developmental disorders, so DSH is not addressed further.

## Conditions Associated with Self-injury (Behavioral Phenotypes)

### *Pervasive Developmental Disorder*

Pervasive developmental disorders have commonly been associated with self-injurious behavior. In the first edition of *DSM-III*, a syndrome referred to as "childhood onset pervasive developmental disorder" included self-injury among its diagnostic characteristics. Although this condition is no longer specifically included in the classification system, self-injury is a major consideration in individuals with pervasive developmental disorders and, in fact, these conditions may account for the majority of mentally retarded subjects with severe self-injury. There is no specific topography of self-injury in this population; head-banging, face-biting, and other forms of SIB are seen.

Bartak and Rutter (1976) compared a group of autistic children with IQs below 70 and above 70 on nonverbal scales. The two groups differed in their pattern of symptoms, although they were similar in terms of the primary diagnostic considerations. However, the low IQ and high IQ groups differed substantially, in that the lower-IQ group had statistically significantly more self-injury and stereotypies.

In working with autistic individuals, one must take into account the characteristics of the developmental disorder itself when applying behavioral principles. Neuroanatomical changes in the hippocampus, septal nuclei, selected nuclei in the amygdala and neocerebellar cortex were reported in one well-documented case, and cerebellar abnormalities were found in 18 cases (Bauman & Kemper, 1985; Courchesne, Yeung-Courchesne, Press, Hesselink, & Jernigan, 1988). In addition, Ornitz (1974) has suggested that there are problems in sensory modulation and motility based on his neurophysiologic studies. The social deficits in this disorder may relate to disturbances in sensory modulation. These neurobiological changes may lead to a disruption of adaptive, integrative, and motivated behavior. Complex behavioral interactions require communication skills, thc ability to apply past experiences to current ones, a sense of self in relation to others, the adaptive use of imitation, and the capacity to make choices. Perhaps as a consequence of these deficits, certain behavioral symptoms result. These are characterized by a qualitative impairment in the development of reciprocal social interaction, impairment in the development of verbal and nonverbal communication skills, and impaired use of the imagination. This is associated with a markedly restricted repertoire of activities and interests, which include stereotyped and repetitive movements. Their behavior is deviant from the norm rather than delayed.

In planning a program in dealing with self-injury in this population, it is important to first take into account the impairment in reciprocal social interactions and in the development of social attachment. It is also important to work out strategies to get the child's attention. This was done in a study using water mist and a loud statement. Jenson, Rovner, Cameron, Petersen, & Kesler (1985) applied behavioral approaches to SIB in autistic individuals. These authors used a fine water mist combined with a loud statement, followed by verbal praise. The child responded to the therapy, although the mechanism of the response is unclear. Getting the child's attention is extremely important because these are children who often do not spontaneously respond to language communication or initiate social interaction. Their lack of social awareness and the failure to establish attachment is a major factor in choosing therapeutic strategies, such as time-out from positive reinforcement. The autistic child may not demonstrate proximity-seeking behavior, and social interaction may not be rewarding. Their impairments in communication and imaginative skills are important to consider in program planning. Lower-functioning autistic children, especially, do not spontaneously initiate social communication or respond to nonverbal cues, such as a frown from an adult or other gestures that ordinarily signal to terminate an activity. The stereotypies that these children demonstrate may be used as reinforcers in working with the child.

The serotonin system, the dopamine system, and the endogenous opiate systems have been reported to be involved in autism, and based on neurotransmitter hypotheses, a variety of psychoactive drugs have been utilized in treatment. However, improvement following psychopharmacological intervention for their SIB has been inconsistent, and reported changes are in symptom reduction. Campbell et al. (1982) have shown changes in behavior and learning in a placebo-controlled study of 33 autistic children using haloperidol, an agent that effectively blocks the dopamine system. Despite these clinical changes in behavior with a dopamine-blocking agent, central and peripheral dopamine turnover has not been found to be significantly altered in autism (Minderaa, Anderson, Volkmar, Akkerhuis, & Cohen, 1989), indicating that more sophisticated means are needed to demonstrate neurotransmitter involvement.

An extensive multicenter drug treatment trial (Ritvo, Freeman, Geller & Yuwiler, 1983) for the treatment of autism was carried out using fenfluramine, an agent affecting the serotonin system. The rationale for using this agent was that the brain serotonin system may be involved in the modulation of sensory input, which may be important in autism (Geller, Ritvo, Freeman, & Yuwiler, 1982). Serotonin has also been implicated in signal processing in the brainstem, where modulation of sensory input, activity level, attention, and sleep cycle regulation take place. Although initial reports were positive in regard to response to fenfluramine, this has not been demonstrated to be a specific treatment for autism. However, evaluation of serotonergic mechanisms in autism is ongoing, as demonstrated by recent neuroendocrine challenge studies, which suggest that central serotonergic responsivity is decreased in this disorder (McBride et al., 1989). More recently, nalterxone, an opiate antagonist, has been utilized in treatment. A preliminary report by Campbell et al. (1989) found improvement in withdrawn behavior, verbalization, and stereotypies using this medication but no clear-cut change in self-aggressiveness. They suggest that some children may become more responsive to other nonpharmacological interventions when naltrexone is used. They note that symptomatic improvement is greater with haloperidol (Campbell, personal communication) than with naltrexone. Because there are interactions among the various neurotransmitter systems, it is currently unclear whether there is one specific system involved in this condition or whether the interaction between systems is the primary consideration.

## *Lesch–Nyhan Syndrome*

The Lesch–Nyhan syndrome (Lesch & Nyhan, 1964; Nyhan, 1976) is an inborn error of purine metabolism in which self-injury is a major behavioral manifestation. (Table 3.3 lists characteristics of the syndrome). The disorder is X-chromosome linked and therefore only affects males. The primary product of the abnormal gene in this disorder is a variate enzyme, hypoxanthine phosphoribosyltransferase (HPRT) (Sweetman & Nyhan, 1972). This enzyme is normally present in each cell in the body, and its presence is highest in the brain. Its absence prevents the normal metabolism of hypoxanthine, resulting in excessive uric acid production and manifestations of gout, without specific drug treatment (i.e., allopurinol). The full syndrome requires virtual absence of the enzyme. Other syndromes with partial HPRT deficiency are associated with gout without the neurological and behavioral symptoms. Hypoxanthine accumulates in the cerebrospinal fluid (CSP), but uric acid does not because it is not produced in the brain and does not cross the blood–brain barrier from the blood.

TABLE 3.3. Lesch–Nyhan syndrome.

1. Mental retardation
2. Spastic cerebral palsy
3. Compulsive self-injury
4. Dsyarthric speech
5. Choreoathetosis
6. Torsion dystonia

There are a variety of abnormalities in this syndrome not related to increases in uric acid in body fluids. The onset of self-injury may be as early as 1 year or—rarely—as late as the teens. Children demonstrate self-mutilation initially through self-biting, which is intense and causes tissue damage often leading to amputation of fingers and loss of tissue around the lips (Mizuno & Yugari, 1974). With increasing age, they also may self-mutilate by picking the skin with their fingers. The biting often results in extraction of primary teeth, and severe SIB may lead to institutional placement. In type, the behavior is different from that seen in other mental retardation syndromes of self-injury where self-hitting and head-banging are the most common presentations. The self-injury occurs although all sensory modalities, including the pain sense, are intact. The SIB requires that the patient be restrained. Despite their dystonias, when restraints are removed, the patient may appear terrified and quickly and accurately place a hand in the mouth. The child may ask for restraints to prevent elbow movement. When restraints are placed, the child may appear relaxed and more good humored (Nyhan, 1976). Their dysarthric speech may result in interpersonal communication problems; however, the higher-functioning children can express themselves and participate in their treatment. Hemiballismic arm movements can also create difficulty because the raised arm is sometimes interpreted as a threatening gesture by others and is socially reinforced.

Understanding the molecular disorder has led to effective drug treatment for those aspects of a disease that are related to uric acid accumulation and subsequent arthritic tophi, renal stones, and neuropathy. However, reduction in uric acid has not influenced the neurological and behavioral aspects. In fact, some children have been treated from birth for the elevation in uric acid and have behavioral and neurological symptoms despite never having high levels of uric acid.

Because it is a condition where self-injury has been described as a behavioral phenotype in that it is uniquely present in all cases, the Lesch–Nyhan syndrome has been investigated as a potential biological model for self-biting. Both anatomical and neurochemical studies have been undertaken in this condition. Turning first to neuropathological studies, no appreciable morphological abnormality in any part of the brain, including the basal ganglia, where changes might be expected, given the motor symptoms, has been demonstrated. Watts et al. (1982) reported no abnormality with detailed histopathology and electron microscopy of 13 brain regions in one case studied.

A second alternative is that biochemical alterations might be involved and might underlie the behavioral abnormality. This possibility might be assessed in three ways: (1) direct measurement of neurotransmitters in brain tissue, (2) measurement of neurotransmitters and their metabolites in CSF, and (3) clinical response to neurotransmitter precursor treatment. Lloyd et al. (1981) have directly examined different brain regions postmortem for indices of dopamine, norepinephrine, serotonin, gamma-aminobutyric acid (GABA) and acetylcholine function in basal ganglia and other brain areas from three patients (ages 13, 14, and 27) who died with Lesch–Nyhan syndrome. Lloyd's group compared the pathological material from patients with age-matched control subjects without neurological disease. They found that all three patients with Lesch–Nyhan syndrome had very low HPRT levels (less than 1% in striatal tissue and 1% to 2% of control in the thalamus). The finding that the phosphoribosyl transferase for adenine, another amino purine, was normal in these patients demonstrated that there was no general deficit in purine metabolism. The basal ganglia may be particularly vulnerable to damage in the absence of HPRT during the developmental period when dopamine terminals are proliferating into the striatum. This brain region lacks the capacity to synthesize needed protein at a time when purine nucleotides are needed for protein synthesis. The absence of the enzyme prevents the saving or salvage of nucleotides needed for neuronal growth. The consequence may be a reduction in arborization of these dopamine neurons (Baumeister & Frye, 1985). This was demonstrated in the Lesch–Nyhan syndrome by a general deficit in dopamine areas of the brain containing dopamine neurons. Low dopamine levels and decreased homovanillic acid, its main metabolites, as well as low levels of the synthesizing enzymes, dopamine decarboxylase, esterase, and hydroxylase, were noted in terminal-rich dopamine areas, including the caudate nucleus, putamen, and nucleus accumbens. There was a functional loss of 65% to 90% of the nigrostriatal and mesolimbic dopamine terminals. The cell body region where these fibers originate, the substantia nigra, had normal dopamine levels. There was then a decrease in dopamine levels in the terminal areas, but the cell bodies of origin were preserved. Therefore, the neurochemical changes in this disorder may be related to functional abnormalities, perhaps resulting from a diminution of arborization or branching out of dopamine terminals and dendrites rather than cell loss with dopaminergic supersensitivity. Impaired protein synthesis during times of rapid brain growth could inhibit axonal growth and branching of nigrostriatal neurons. There was also a decrease in striatal cholinergic function, but norepinephrine, serotonin, and GABA from representative areas were normal.

In regard to blood and CSF measurements of neurotransmitters and their metabolites, several authors have found changes in the Lesch–Nyhan syndrome. Serum dopamine β-hydroxylase has been reported to be altered in these patients, and low levels of homovanillic acid (HVA) were observed in the CSF of one case of Lesch–Nyhan syndrome. The major serotonin metabolite, 5-hydroxy indoleactic acid, has also been reported to be decreased. CSF levels of HVA have also been reported to be decreased in comparison to controls.

A third approach to study of neurotransmitters is the use of precursor treatment. There are reports that the administration of the serotonin precursor 5-hydroxytrytophan, both with and without a peripheral decarboxylase inhibitor leads to beneficial effects in the Lesch–Nyhan syndrome (Mizuno & Yugari, 1975). This response would be consistent with a lower level of serotonin in brain regions despite the changes noted by Lloyd and coworkers (1981) in the brain areas that they studied. Nyhan (1976; Nyhan, Johnson, Kaufman, & Jones, 1980) suggests temporary improvement with the administration of a serotonin precursor. However, long-term improvement has not been demonstrated with a serotonin precursor.

Kopin (1981) finds it tempting to speculate that a diazepam binding site may be involved in producing some of the behavioral manifestations of the Lesch–Nyhan syndrome. He suggests that future studies of interactions between neurotransmitters and modulators that regulate brain function might have an impact on developing a rational approach to chemotherapy. In a disorder such as Lesch–Nyhan syndrome, these fundamental mechanisms should continue to be studied.

In regard to treatment, behavioral techniques using operant conditioning approaches have limited effectiveness in Lesch–Nyhan syndrome. However, Nyhan (1976) notes that extinction procedures do have some selective success in reducing self-injury. The biting response rate does differ in some cases when an adult is present, and contingent withdrawal of attention, but not contingent shock, has reduced self-biting, suggesting that self-injury in the Lesch–Nyhan syndrome may become sensitive to environmental–social contingencies. Contingent electric finger shock with response prevention increased self-injury in five cases studied; however, time-out plus reinforcement of non-SIB led to substantial reduction in a controlled setting (Anderson, Dancis, Albert, 1978; Anderson, Hermann, Alpert, Dancis, 1975; 1977). Generalization outside the experimental setting is problematic (Nyhan, 1976) and patients under stress may revert to previous behavior. Behavioral techniques alone have not proved to be an adequate general treatment.

Watts et al. (1982) noted that because SIB commonly responds to aversive techniques and Lesch–Nyhan cases proved insensitive, then abnormality in neurotransmitters such as serotonin, which also may be involved in aggressive behavior (Gilbert, Spellacy, & Watts, 1979), and punishment-learning, requires consideration. Drug treatments using diazepam, haloperidol, clomipramine, L-dopa, and pimozide (Watts, et al., 1982) have not been successful. Watts suggested an imbalance in dopamine/serotonin systems or dopamine in interaction with another neurotransmitter system. The use of a mixed $D_1/D_2$ antagonist, which predominantly affects the $D_1$ system, such as fluphenazine, requires exploration, following Goldstein's (Goldstein, Anderson, Reuben, Dancis

1985) findings that $D_1$ or mixed $D_1/D_2$ dopamine agonists lead to self-biting in monkeys who previously had nigrostriatal lesions. He postulates that HPRT deficiency results in abnormal nucleotide regulation of the dopamine system. There is a report of improvement in self-injury in one patient with fluphenazine; however, three other patients seen by another investigator did not improve. Nyhan recently completed a bone-marrow transplant in one adult subject. Although the procedure was successful and blood cell lines did contain HPRT, no change in behavior was demonstrated.

Future treatment studies may need to address subgroups of Lesch–Nyhan syndrome and take into account the existence of a variety of mutations in the HPRT gene structure. Why partial HPRT deficiency does not lead to neurological and behavioral symptoms remains unclear. Finally, it is advisable to study combined drug and behavioral treatment. An emphasis on parent training is of particular importance to ensure drug compliance and for generalization of treatment effects. As in other inborn errors of metabolism, continuous family support is essential.

Continuing genetic investigations using restriction enzyme analysis may further clarify the specific genetic abnormality in the full Lesch–Nyhan syndrome. Findings from Lloyd et al.'s (1981) study can now be investigated in vivo, using positron emission tomography (PET) to evaluate the dopamine supersensitivity hypothesis. Identification of dopamine receptors in the caudate and putamen is now feasible. A PET scan has been carried out on two cases of Lesch–Nyhan syndrome to investigate dopamine receptor $D_1/D_2$ dopamine function. The authors found a ratio of $D_1:D_2$ receptors of 1:1 rather than the expected 3:1 ratio (Gjedde, Wong, Harris, Dannals, Ravert 1986). Interactions of dopamine systems require further study. Two-deoxyglucose metabolism using the PET scanner may also provide additional knowledge regarding the site or sites of brain dysfunction related to the self-injury.

## *Cornelia de Lange Syndrome*

This syndrome was first identified by Cornelia de Lange in 1933 (de Lange, 1933) in two infants with abnormally small heads (brachycephaly), enlargement (hypertrophy) of the brows and lashes, small hands and feet, short limbs (micromelia), delayed dentition and webbing (syndactylism) of the feet. By 1970, 248 patients had been identified with this syndrome (Berg, McCreary, Ridler, & Smith, 1970). This rare disorder, with an incidence of 1:30,000 to 1:50,000 livebirths, has been associated with genetic abnormalities and severe mental retardation. Although chromosomal abnormality has been suggested, no specific genetic or biological basis for this disorder has been clearly demonstrated. Self-injury in this population includes face-hitting, face-picking, and lip-biting, but no one specific pattern has been found, nor is the behavior as intense as in Lesch–Nyhan syndrome (Shear, Nyhan, Kirman, & Stern, 1971; Singh & Pulman, 1979). In a review of 64 cases, Hawley, Jackson, and Kurnit (1985) found frequent tantrum behavior but do not indicate how often it was associated with self-injury. The self-injury may be treated by operant procedures, but no specific treatment series of Cornelia de Lange patients has been reported. In several cases, onset of SIB coincided with eruptions of teeth. There is one case report (Fellow & Tennstedt, 1986) when insensitivity to pain was found, but other reports have not shown this finding. The relationship of self-injury to tantrums and biological factors related to delayed tooth eruption, chewing behavior, and pain sensitivity requires further evaluation. Furthermore, Greenberg and Coleman (1973) have reported low serotonin levels in whole blood in contrast to controls in 7/7 males and 2/4 females ranging in age from 10 to 30 years with the disorder, another finding that requires replication. The relationship of serotonin levels and self-injury requires continuing assessment.

## *Congenital Insensitivity to Pain/Familial Dysautonomia*

Congenital insensitivity to pain has been associated with self-injury. With congenital insensitivity to pain, the self-injury may be accidental and not follow the syndrome pattern suggested previously. In this condition, the following criteria are required for diagnosis: (1) pain sensation should be absent from birth; (2) the entire body should be affected; (3) all other sensory modalities should be intact or minimally impaired and the deep tendon reflexes present. This condition has been reported as an autosomal recessive disorder. Mental retardation is seen in approximately one third of reported cases, and skeletal injuries commonly occur. Thrush (1973) reports chewing of the fingers and tongue in one child in a report of four children in the same family with this disorder. Another child had a behavior disorder and took unnecessary risks leading to self-injury. Dehen, Amsallem, Colas-Linhart, and Cambier (1986) have reported that spontaneously elevated nociceptive (pain) threshold levels were markedly diminished after naloxone injections in four patients with insensitivity to pain. Although CSF beta-endorphin either was not elevated or was only slightly elevated in these patients, their clinical response to opioid antagonists suggests a possible treatment in identified children with this disorder. By restoring the pain response with naloxone, accidental self-injury would be expected to be reduced.

In two studies of patients with congenital insensitivity to pain, endogenous opiates have been strongly implicated. In one study, administration of naloxone dramatically reduced the pain threshold by 67%, as measured by the nociceptive flexion reflex (Dehen, Willer, Boureau, & Cambier, 1977). The second study failed to replicate the antagonist effect but noted elevated opioid levels in the CSF (Manfredi, Bini, Cruccu, Accornero, Berardelli, & Medolago, 1981).

## Riley–Day Syndrome

The Riley–Day syndrome (Riley, Day, Greeley & Langford 1949) or familial dysautonomia is an identified autosomal recessive disorder with an estimated incidence of 1:10,000 to 1:20,000, which has been identified in over 200 families. Patients with Riley–Day syndrome have distinctive physical features and both neurological and physiologic abnormalities; the most pertinent to self-injury are those associated with abnormal sensory nerves, nerve fibers, and autonomic nerve plexuses. Taste perception and discrimination are markedly deficient, and pain perception is reduced or absent (Riley, Day, Greeley, & Langford, 1949). Studies of Riley–Day syndrome have shown decreases in dopamine-β-hydroxylase, the enzyme that converts dopamine to norepinephrine. This suggests that investigation of the dopamine system might be profitable in this disorder.

## Rett Syndrome

Rett syndrome (Rett, 1966) is an infantile dementia found only in females and characterized by progressive loss of cognitive function and ability to communicate, seizures, respiratory disturbance, apraxia of hand movements, ataxia, and characteristic hand-wringing and hand-to-mouth behavior. Although Rett described this condition in 1966, it was not until 17 years later, when Hagberg described a progressive syndrome of autism, dementia, ataxia and loss of purposeful hand movements in girls, that the term *Rett syndrome* became widely known. This condition has been widely recognized, and international conferences have been held for the past several years.

The diagnosis of Rett syndrome is based on a particularly characteristic neurodevelopmental phenotype. A system for staging the progress of the condition is as follows (Naidu, Murphy, Moser, & Rett, 1986): In stage one, a general slowing of development is noted, particularly in motor abilities. Developmental delays themselves are insidious at onset, and the symptoms are vague. The girls are hypotonic. In the second stage, loss of

TABLE 3.4. Diagnostic criteria for Rett syndrome.

1. Female sex
2. Normal pre/perinatal period with normal development in the first 6–18 months of life
3. Normal head circumference at birth, with deceleration of head growth between 6 months and 4 years
4. Early behavioral social and psychomotor regression, with evolving communication dysfunction and dementia
5. Loss of purposeful hand skills between ages 1 and 4 years
6. Hand wringing/clapping/washing stereotypies between ages 1 and 4 years
7. Gait apraxia and truncal apraxia/ataxia between ages 1 and 4 years

acquired abilities is identified. It is during this stage that characteristic hand-wringing and hand-to-mouth movements begin. These stereotyped behaviors are important diagnostic clues and consist of constant hand-wringing or hand-washing and hand-to-mouth behavior to the exclusion of other types of hand use. During this phase of deterioration, autisticlike features have been described, along with hyperventilation, clumsy movements, and seizures. The autisticlike behaviors are probably related to a developing encephalopathy, and the child may be misdiagnosed as having a pervasive developmental disorder. When autism is considered in girls, Rett syndrome must be ruled out. This stage is followed by a third stage, where there is a plateau in symptomatology with no further loss of skills. The girls subsequently appear less autistic, but seizures are common, as is severe mental retardation and gait apraxia/ataxia. During the fourth stage, motor deterioration is noted, with decreasing mobility, spasticity, scoliosis, muscle wasting, and vasomotor disturbances; social response and eye contact is improved. This is an important syndrome to recognize in girls, as the hand-to-mouth movement may be reduced, but not eliminated, by behavioral intervention (Iwata, Pace, Willis, Gamache, & Hyman, 1986). Differential reinforcement procedures combined with response interruption techniques has been used to reduce hand-to-mouth behavior. Because of reported involvement of the dopamine system reported from postmortem brain tissue of a patient with Rett syndrome and increased CSF neurotransmitter metabolites (Riederer et al., 1985), PET was carried out in a 25-year-old woman with Rett syndrome to assess $D_2$ dopamine receptor binding in the corpus striatum (Harris, Wong, Wagner, Rett, & Naidu, 1986). Unlike Huntington disease, there was no reduction in the volume of the basal ganglia. Abnormalities were not identified in $D_2$ receptor binding. Future studies of the dopamine system in this disorder should address $D_1$ receptor binding because these receptors have been linked to self-biting in neonatal rats (Breese et al., 1984).

## *Fragile-X Syndrome*

The fragile-X syndrome is associated with self-biting, as well as autisticlike symptoms. It is the most common familial form of mental retardation. The prevalence is as high as 1:1000. Among males, 25–50% of all cases of X-linked mental retardation is caused by the fragile-X syndrome. Because it is X-linked, unlike Down syndrome, it is carried from one generation to the next. It has been found in all races, including blacks, whites, Asians, and Australian aborigines.

The classical clinical features are macroorchidism, large and prominent ears, and a narrow face. Approximately 80% of adult males have one or more of these features. However, the individual features are not pathognomonic for fragile-X and may be seen in other conditions and in normal individuals. Among the features, macroorchidism is seen in 70 to 90% of adult males. Sutherland (1985), in reviewing 22 reports, have found this characteristic in 87% of postpubertal males, but in only 21% of prepubertal males.

Large or prominent ears are a useful but nonspecific sign. Approximately 50% of males have an ear length that is two standard deviations or more above the mean of the general population. Another 30% will have normal sized but prominent ears, protruding more than 30% out from the side of the head. The ear itself is well-formed, but the antihelical fold may be poorly developed. In the prepubertal patient, the ear findings may be the only physical feature. Ears are only occasionally low-set. The third feature, a long and narrow face, is seen more commonly in the postpubertal group. One study found that only one fourth of subjects had a face length that was more than two standard deviations above the mean.

To account for these physical findings, it has been suggested that a connective tissue abnormality may be involved. This would be consistent with reports of hyperextensibility of finger joints and double-jointed thumbs. Furthermore, biopsies of the testicle have shown an increased interstitial volume with excessive connective tissue. Fertility is normal. Other physical features are seen in less than 60% of the males with this condition but are also probably related to connective tissue problems. The height of adult males tends to be reduced; 26% of 87 men were below the fifth percentile. Other associated features include seizure disorder in 20% and a diffusely abnormal EEG in 50%.

Multiple studies of retarded individuals in institutions have been carried out with fragile-X syndrome. If all individuals in an institution for the retarded are screened, the percentage with fragile-X varies from 1.6% to 6.2%. However, if only those individuals at high risk, with features such as macroorchidism, are studied, then up to one third of males in institutional settings have been identified as having the fragile-X syndrome. Using the other features, including long ears and hand changes, the yield may go up to 50%. In screening prepubertal individuals, Kahkonen (Kahkonen, Leisti, Thoden, Autio, 1986) found cytogenetic abnormalities in 4% of 240 mildly retarded boys, but only one was positive for the fragile-X syndrome.

The behavioral features and the cognitive profile are features that are useful in identifying higher-functioning individuals. Behavioral features are helpful in diagnosis, especially for prepubertal males who may not show the classical physical features. There is a range of behavioral problems, from difficulties in social communication with strangers to pervasive developmental disorder—autism, and periodic violent outbursts of behavior. Although many boys with the fragile-X syndrome can be sociable, 77 to 90% have been reported to have poor eye contact by history. Other characteristics include hand-flapping noted in 66% of 50 males, hand-biting in 74%, and unusual hand mannerisms in 88%. Largo and Schinzel (1985) found one or more of the following features in 12 of 13 boys studied: poor eye contact, movement stereotypies, or social isolation. Although these features are autisticlike, most males with the fragile-X syndrome do not have a pervasive lack of relatedness to caregivers, so they do not meet the *DSM-III* criteria for autism. Males with fragile-X syndrome can be happy, likable, and friendly. Consequently, there has been controversy regarding a relationship between this disorder and autism. Currently, pervasive developmental disorder—not otherwise specified, rather than classic autism, would be the more common diagnosis. As indicated, the older category, childhood-onset pervasive developmental disorder, includes oddities in motor movement, abnormalities of speech, self-mutilation, and hyper- or hyposensitivities to sensory stimuli among its characteristics. A diagnosis of autism has been reported in 5% to 15% of males with the fragile-X syndrome; these estimates depend on the criterion used for autism. It should be noted that hand-flapping, hand-biting, perseverative speech, and poor eye contact in a child who is overactive and mentally retarded or learning disabled suggest evaluation for the fragile-X syndrome.

Attention deficit and hyperactivity are commonly seen in younger subjects with fragile-X syndrome. Fryns, Jacobs, Kleczkowska & Van Den Berghe (1984) found attentional problems in 21 study patients who underwent a psychological profile. These authors noted that the hyperactivity disappeared after puberty. Hagerman (Hagerman, Jackson, Levitas, Rimland, & Braden, 1986), using the Connors Rating Scales in 37 males ages 4 to 11 years, found that 73% of boys had a score of more than 2 standard deviations above the mean for hyperactivity. All subjects had concentration difficulties.

Speech and language abnormalities are characteristic, including delays in language development. Although the IQ may be in the normal range, there are associated learning disabilities. Heterozygous females may be completely unaffected; however, there are reports of severe mental retardation in female subjects, and deviant behaviors were noted.

Furthermore, problems in visuomotor integration, as demonstrated in poor handwriting, motor delays, delays in sitting and walking, and hypotonicity, have been noted. The difficulties in sensory integration have been evident in early infancy and may be associated with histories of irritability, tantrums, problems with molding (arching or pulling away), and evidence of tactile defensiveness. Repetitive hand mannerisms that are seen may increase when the child is upset, angry, or frightened. Characteristics seen in autistic children, such as spinning, are also noted. These autisticlike behaviors may relate to problems in sensory integration, a feature of autistic subjects as well. Reiss (1988) has recently reported reductions in the size of the cerebellar vermis in this disorder similar to those previously reported in autism. No specific neurotransmitter abnormalities have been identified in the fragile-X syndrome.

### *Self-injury Syndrome in the Severely and Profoundly Retarded*

Self-injury occurs in a heterogeneous group of individuals diagnosed as severely to profoundly mentally retarded. Although the identification of specific syndromes where self-injury is associated may provide a more productive focus for research, these specific syndromes account for only a very small percentage of self-injury episodes in the retarded. Because self-injury may result from abnormalities in neurotransmitters necessary for basic brain functioning, this larger population requires continued evaluation. As indicated in the discussions of the various syndromes, catecholamine, indoleamine, and opioid neurotransmitter systems have been implicated in these conditions. Biochemical investigation in this larger population may also provide new knowledge as to the mechanisms of self-injury.

## Models of Self-injury

### *Isolation Rearing*

Nonhuman primates show considerable self-directed behavior, such as scratching and self-grooming. Other types of self-directed behavior are pathological and typically are seen in animals who experience privation or deprivation early in life, especially rearing apart (the deprivation syndrome). Self-directed behaviors include: (1) self-clasping—using hands or feet to grasp legs, arms, chest, or head; (2) self-orality—involving digit sucking; (3) self-aggression—consisting of biting, slapping, or hitting body parts; (4) rock/sway—back and forth; (5) saluting—which involves raising a hand to the ipsilateral eye, like a salute, occasionally with the thumb pressure against the eye ball. These behaviors may be seen in combination, such as self-clasp with rocking. They have been noted (1) with fear or frustration, (2) when activities are thwarted or escape prevented, (3) during apparent dissatisfaction, and (4) when an animal could not adapt to a new situation. Isolation results in limitation of motor activity, lack of parent and peer contact, impaired learning of social skills, and altered affective state.

These forms of self-stimulation and self-mutilation may be sequelae of isolation during sensitive developmental periods. Anderson and Chamove (1980) compared animals who received restricted rearing experience with a control group of feral and group-reared animals. At 5 years of age, the restriction-reared monkeys showed four times more self-aggression than social aggression, while the control monkeys were never observed to be self-aggressive. Self-biting occurred in social contexts, such as displacement by a more dominant monkey during social aggression, and when startled by sudden movement of others. Self-biting was noted at less than 3 months, frequently in the context of digit sucking. Goosen and Ribbens (1980) reported self-aggression in individually housed, wild-born, stumptailed macaques which decreased in frequency with social pairings. These behaviors are reported in animals raised in captivity, as opposed to feral animals transferred to a zoo. They have been noted in such diverse species as opossums, jackals, hyenas, marmosets, squirrel monkeys, and long-tail monkeys (Meyer-Holzapfel, 1968).

Closer to humans is the substantial research that has been conducted with rhesus macaques (Jones & Barraclough, 1978). Isolation-reared males showed self-biting in 50% of the observed sessions, and isolation-reared females in 35%, but nondeprived animals showed virtually no self-injury (Sackett, 1968). An important aspect of the effects of isolation on the pathogenesis of self-injury is that the aberrant behavior may be increased when the organism is placed in a new environment or confronted with stress or novel stimuli (Hutt & Hutt, 1968). The effects of isolated rearing on self-stimulation and self-injury in humans has been suggested by reports of children reared in severely deprived and isolated situations (Davis, 1940, 1946; Freedman & Brown, 1968).

The factors that related to the development of self-injury subsequent to isolation are found more often in the early developmental periods. For example, in one study, two groups of animals were reared under conditions that were identical with respect to physical restriction but differed in terms of the amount of visual stimuli (i.e., one group was housed outside and in view of other animals and activities). The visually isolated animals demonstrated greater stereotyped behavior (Mason, 1968). Mason provides two suggestions for the effects of developmental isolation on behavior: (1) the filial response or contact-seeking behavior with the mother to establish attachment, which reduces arousal, and (2) exploratory behavior through social and motor play, to increase stimulation or arousal. He suggests that behavior such as a rocking stereotypy may be a self-provision of passive movement stimulation ordinarily received from the parent and notes that infant monkeys raised with a mobile surrogate do not show rocking, while those raised with a stationary surrogate do rock, indicating the importance of movement stimulation.

Subsequently (Mason & Capitanio, 1988), he has reported that experience with an animate surrogate (dog) leads to both attachment and increased environmental responsiveness. With regard to increased arousal, Mason suggests that primates who are deprived of general environmental stimulation have a motivational disturbance and become overwhelmed and hyperexcitable in new and novel situations. They are fearful, or extremely aggressive; males may be sexually inadequate, and females maternally inadequate.

The most severe forms of self-injury occur in animals who are the most agitated, and self-injury may lead to reduced agitation. This could be a homeostatic mechanism elicited in severely socially deprived environments (Jones, 1982). Another means of reducing arousal is autogrooming or *allogrooming*. Allogrooming leads to reduced arousal, and because an isolated animal has no companion, it may groom itself, resulting in stereotypy and perhaps self-injury. Goosen found some self-injury preceded by allogrooming. Finally, self-injury may occur when fighting behavior is prevented. Stereotypy and self-injury might reduce other more aversive stimulation or indicate loss of control in a new and novel situation. Early experiences may result in behavioral sensitization and may predispose to recurrence when there is exposure to a situation analogous to the original one. It has been hypothesized that children may have similar responses, beginning with stereotypies that may extend to self-injury. The arousal-increasing and arousal-decreasing hypotheses are of interest, although the evidence for them may be subject to a variety of interpretations. Additional research on rearing in physical and social isolation and studies on early infant stimulation and early attachment are needed for a better understanding of the biological factors involved in self-injury related to deprivation of early experience.

## *Neuromaturational Processes in Development*

Neuromaturational changes may also be important in the occurrence of stereotypies. Other authors have suggested that the development of the cerebellum was of importance in relation to the emergence of self-stimulation, a finding of interest, given the recent demonstration of cerebellum abnormalities in some autistic children (Courchesne, Yeung-Courchesne, Press, Hesselink, & Jernigan, 1988). Furthermore, the onset of self-biting during a particular stage of development suggests a relationship to neuromaturational changes. For example, Iriki, Shuicki, and Nakamura (1988) have reported that different regions of the frontal lobe in a rodent are responsible for sucking and chewing. Chewing is a developmental acquisition that requires synaptic reorganization, which ordinarily takes place around the time that teeth erupt. The transition from finger-sucking to biting may be a consequence of the maturational acquisition and exercise of chewing. Stimulation of the vestibular system by rocking, spinning, or other forms of body movement has been shown to influence motor development of normal and developmentally delayed children (Clark, Kreutzberg, & Chee, 1977) and may be a factor in children with abnormalities in this brain region. From these studies, stereotypy and self-injury might be a mentally subnormal individual's attempt at providing neurologically based self-stimulation. This stimulation may be not only reinforcing but also necessary for neuronal development.

## Opioid and Nonopioid Stress-Induced Analgesia (SIA)

The identification of endogenous peptides with similar structure and function to morphine (Snyder, 1977) has opened new avenues for research on pain and pain-related behavior. Three genetically distinct families of opioid peptides have been identified in the central nervous system: β-endorphin/corticotrophins, enkephalins, and dynorphin/neoendorphins. The localization of their binding sites indicates that these peptides play an important role in the control of pain (Kuhar, Pert, & Snyder, 1973; Murrin, Coyle, & Kuhar, 1980). Infusions into the periaqueductal gray matter have been shown to decrease pain responsiveness (Hosobuchi, 1981). Increases in opioid peptide production and inhibition in pain responsiveness may accompany acutely stressful states, leading to insensitivity to pain, so-called stress-induced analgesia (SIA) in animals (Madden, Akil, Patrick, & Barchas, 1977) and in humans (Willer, Dekers, & Cambier, 1981). Such effects are partially reversible with naloxone, an opiate antagonist, the administration of which has been associated with an increase in pain-perception threshold (Buchsbaum, Davis, & Bunny, 1977). The administration of an enkephalinase inhibitor has been shown to potentiate SIA; this effect has also been blocked by naloxone. Both central and peripheral opioid mechanisms have been suggested for SIA (Kelly, 1982; Lewis, Tordoff, Sherman, & Liebeskind, 1982). In addition, anatomical studies by Stuckey, Marra, Minor, and Insel (1989) have found decreased binding of mμ opiate receptors in rat brain following inescapable shock.

The discovery of opioid receptors has led to investigations into opioid self-administration. Opiate receptors are densely distributed in brain regions associated with self-stimulatory behavior in animals, and opioid substances have been shown to have reinforcing properties for self-stimulation (Olds & Fobes, 1981). Animal studies with rhesus minkeys and rats have demonstrated that microinfusions of opioids (methionine enkephalin, morphine) into the ventral tegmentum, substantia nigra, or nucleus accumbens facilitate self-stimulation, in some instances, in a dose-related manner. Animals will bar-press for the delivery of enkephalin (Belluzzi & Stein, 1977), demonstrating its reinforcing properties. These findings regarding the opiate system have led to several hypotheses in regard to self-injury. First repeated occurrence of SIB might lead to opioid-mediated SIA, which may be associated with elevated levels of endogenous opioid peptides that inhibit pain. Second, it is possible that some individuals might engage in SIB as a means of self-administering opioid peptides. These hypotheses have been tested indirectly by administering naloxone or naltrexone and have been reported in a series of individual case reports (Bernstein, Hughes, Mitchell, & Thompson, 1987; Davidson, (Kleene, Carroll, & Rockowitz, 1983; Richardson & Zaleski, 1983); four subjects who were chronically self-injurious were described, and three of these showed at least temporary decreases in SIB in association with the administration of the antagonists. The method of administration was intravenous, by slow intravenous drip, or orally, and results were attributed either to acute effects on opiate systems or receptor downregulation. The authors suggest that naloxone or naltrexone effects might have been due to either (1) reducing the pain threshold, therefore intensifying the normally painful effects of SIB, or (2) extinguishing the reinforcing effects of SIB. However, other authors (Szymanski, Kedesdy, Sulkes, & Cutler, 1987) found no effects of naltrexone on SIB in two cases in a double-blind, placebo-controlled study utilizing a within-subject design.

The opiate system is not the only neurotransmitter system involved in SIA. Animal studies showed that footshock stress produced potent analgesia in the rat; prolonged intermittent footshock elicits analgesia medicated by opioid peptides, but brief continuous shock produces nonopioid analgesia, as does the cold water swim test. Nonopioid SIA may involve histamine $H_2$ receptors (Gogas & Hough, 1988). Furthermore, estrogen has been implicated in the modulation of SIA (Ryan & Maier, 1988). Therefore, in addition to neuronal opiate-induced analgesia, there are other categories of SIA, including neuronal nonopiate, humoral opiate, and humoral nonopiate forms. Furthermore, there are interactions among these neurotransmitter systems. For example, the dopamine system has been investigated in intracranial self-stimulation studies, and ascending dopaminergic fibers from the ventral tegmental area (VTA) have been implicated in "brain reward circuitry" (Olds & Fobes, 1981). Opioid peptides and dopamine are closely related to one another and found in similar brain regions. Enkephalins might influence self-stimulation indirectly via dopamine neurons, which are thought to be presynaptically inhibited by enkephalin (Mülder, Wardeh, Hogenboom, Frandhuyzen, 1984; Pallard, Llorens, Schwartz, Gross, & Dray, 1978). Morphine alters the turnover of dopamine in the brain (Lal, 1975) and dopaminergic manipulations alter morphine analgesia. Intrastriatal enkephalins have been found to stimulate dopamine synthesis in the caudate nucleus by an action on opiate receptors localized on dopamine nerve terminals. Substantia nigra lesions have been shown to result in 40 to 50% reductions in opiate receptor density. These findings suggest that pharmacological studies must take into account the type of SIA, as well as interactions among neurotransmitter systems, when planning pharmacotherapy.

The identification of specific neurotransmitter abnormalities such as these in patients who exhibit SIB could provide evidence related to both etiology and an experimental basis for future pharmacological intervention.

## *Altered Anatomy and Physiological State*

Numerous surgical procedures have resulted in self-injury in animals, including lesions in the temporal lobe in macaques (Kluver & Bucy, 1939) and lesions in the spinal cord (bilateral cervicothoracic dorsal rhizotomy from C5 to T2) (Busbaur, 1974), sciatic nerve section, and sectioning of the middle of the lateral funiculus (Jones & Barraclough, 1978). A primary consideration is whether the surgery results in the complete elimination of sensory input (anesthesia) or alters input (paresthesia), possibly associated with constant irritation. Taub (Taub, Perrella, Barro, 1973; Taub, 1976) found self-injury in sensory deafferentated monkeys whose sensory pathways have been disrupted, which suggests sensory isloation as a mechanism.

Other investigators have studied paresthesia in animals. For example, Innovar, a drug causing local irritation, has resulted in self-injury in animals. One possible explanation for these stereotypies and self-injury is that arousal is increased by local irritation and that stereotypies reduce arousal. Stereotypies and self-injury have been frequently noted under conditions of increased arousal, suggesting (1) neurophysiological arousal causes increased stereotypies and self-injury, and (2) specific motor activity related to stereotyped and self-injurious behavior reduces arousal.

## *Drug-Induced Changes in Physiological State*

Although drugs or surgical lesions involving the spinal cord or affecting the peripheral nervous system may lead to self-injury, centrally acting drugs that increase stereotypies and lead to self-injury in animals also may provide important information on mechanisms. These substances include alcohol (Charmove & Harlow, 1970), caffeine (Mueller, Saboda, Palmour, & Nyhan, 1982; Peters, 1967), methylxanthine (Lloyd & Stone, 1981) clonidine (Bhattacharya, Jaiswal, Mukhopadhyay, & Diafia, 1988; Katsuragi, Ushijima, & Furukawa, 1984; Mueller & Nyhan, 1982(a); pemoline (Mueller & Nyhan, 1982(b); Mueller, Hollingsworth, & Petit, 1986), and amphetamine (Randrup & Munkvad, 1967). Rylander (1971) has studied the relationship of amphetamine administration to stereotypies in humans in amphetamine addicts who show stereotyped movements. Amphetamine-induced stereotypies in animals are used to test neuroleptic drugs. High-dose pemoline has similar effects to amphetamine on self-injury and is blocked by the dopamine antagonist, haloperidol. Low-dose pemoline has similar effects on adult and weaning rats and results in intermittent SIB and stereotypy; however, Mueller et al. (1986) suggest that although they occur together, there are distinct mechanisms for self-injury and stereotypy. However, O'Neill (1982) found that isolation-induced SIB and stereotypy were not different in their response to a drug treatment with imipramine. She investigated eight rhesus monkeys and found a decrease in SIB duration and frequency of stereotypy, with an increase in self-clasp, self-stimulation, and self-grooming with medication.

Rats and rabbits who were underfed and then received long-term administration of very high doses of caffeine or theophylline (methylpurine derivatives) eventually developed self-mutilating behavior. The ability of these purine derivatives to produce self-injury in animals is of interest. Purine derivatives are released from cells and influence neuronal activity as presynaptic modulators of neurotransmitter release, and as regulators of receptor sensitivity (Kopin, 1981). Most of the purines affecting the central nervous system are related to adenine or guanine. Behavioral stimulants, such as caffeine or theophylline, do bind to adenosine receptors. Hypoxanthine interferes with the binding of diazepam to its receptor. Because caffeine also inhibits the binding of diazepam to its receptors, Kopin (1981) suggested that a diazepam binding site may be involved in producing some of the behavioral manifestations of self-biting. He suggests that future studies of interactions between neurotransmitters and modulators that regulate brain function might have impact on developing a rational approach to chemotherapy.

Endogenous peptides, such as ACTH, also may produce stereotypies. Intraventricularly administered $ACTH_{1-24}$ in rats has been shown to produce excessive grooming (Gispen, Wiegant, Greven, & de Wied, 1976; Jolles, Rompa-Barendregt, & Gispen, 1979), and the dopaminergic system has been linked to the effects of ACTH on grooming (Cools, Wiegant, & Gispen, 1978). It is suggested that excessive grooming is a response that serves to decrease arousal of the organism following activation of the ACTH system (Delius, Craig, & Chaudoir, 1976; Jolles et al., 1979). The response to the particular stimulus continues until the stimulus condition is altered. Once avoidance responding has stabilized, the pituitary–adrenal response to a previously arousing stimulus is attenuated (Hennessey & Levine, 1979). An inhibitory feedback effect upon adrenocortical activity is exerted by the execution of species-specific behavior that either removes the external excitatory stimulus (escape, avoidance behavior, etc.), or mitigates the internal state (e.g., arousal stereotypy). A retarded individual in an environment that makes excessive demands in novel situations where there is uncertainty and conflict may have an appropriate behavioral response to these situations (avoidance or escape). Under such conditions, stereotypies may serve as an effective means to reduce the level of arousal. Under these circumstances, self-injury may be present as an extreme form of stereotyped behavior when the individual is stressed and highly aroused. Ordinarily, pain suppresses behavior; however, as previously described, SIA may occur, leading to a decrease in pain perception in these circumstances.

## *Effects of Surgical and Neurotoxic Lesions in the Developmental Period*

Another approach to self-injury is through administration of neurotoxins during the developmental period, followed by subsequent pharmacological challenge. Using this approach, a relationship between dopaminergic supersensitivity and self-injury has been demonstrated in experimental animals (Breese et al., 1984). Rats were given injections of 6-hydroxydopamine (6-OHDA) at 5 days of age to unilaterally denervate basal ganglia regions. These brain regions developed supersensitive dopamine receptors. Self-biting was seen in the lesioned animals when they were challenged as adults with a dopamine agonist; however, untreated adult rats did not show this behavior after being given the agonist. Similar studies in monkeys were carried out by Goldstein (Goldstein, Anderson, Reuben & Dancis, 1985) to investigate the striatal dopamine regulation of motor activity. Goldstein studied the effects of dopamine agonists on monkeys who had unilateral denervated nigrostriatal systems for 10–14 months. L-dopa and apomorphine, dopamine agonists, elicited self-biting of the digits of the fingers contralateral to the lesion. This effect was blocked by a $D_1$ dopamine antagonist (SCH 23390) and by fluphenazine, a $D_1/D_2$ antagonist, but was not blocked by a pure $D_2$ antagonist. The self-injury was elicited by dopamine agonists, the effects of which are predominantly on the $D_1$ receptor and were blocked by a $D_1$ antagonist, suggesting a potential $D_1$ antagonist drug treatment for the self-injury.

Ungerstedt (1971) produced unilateral destruction of a dopamine pathway in the nigrostriatal system, resulting in postsynaptic supersensitivity following 6-hydroxydopamine injections, and also reported self-injury. Another investigation involving the nigrostriatal system in self-biting was carried out by Baumeister and Frye (1983). Their work focuses on the mediation of dopamine-related stereotypy through striatal nigral GABA pathways. They injected muscimol, a GABA agonist, which mimics the activity of GABA, into the substantia nigra in rats. When gnawing was prevented, self-biting was demonstrated in 42%, 69%, and 36% of animals when 10, 30, or 100 mg of the substance was injected. The administration of saline did not lead to self-biting. Bicuculline, a GABA antagonist, did not prevent this effect. Behaviors noted were stereotyped sniffing and head-nodding. Here, the administration of GABA agonist into the substantia nigra led to self-biting. In each instance, biting behavior was produced by damage to the nigrostriatal system. The mechanism is unclear, and both studies require replication.

The emphasis in these studies of the effects of injury during the developmental period on later behavior is of considerable importance and may potentially suggest new approaches to treatment.

## Summary

1. Self-injury is seen in children less than 3 years of age and most commonly in the severely and profoundly retarded whose mental ages are in this range. This suggests the potential importance of neuromaturational factors and perhaps also disrupted brain development.
2. Environmental experiences during sensitive phases of development have been implicated in self-injury in animals. Isolation, particularly from social contact, with subsequent impairment in social skills, is one of the best-documented examples of an environmental intervention occurring during a sensitive period.
3. Self-injury may follow increased arousal, leading to frustration and rage. Some forms of self-injury may involve exaggerations of the grooming mechanism, and others relate to averted fighting behavior.
4. Self-injury has been specifically associated with pervasive developmental disorder and several mental retardation syndromes. This raises the question of whether self-injury is a learned response, the result of deviant development, or an ethologically derived pattern of behavior elicited in stressful circumstances. Involvement of catecholamine, indoleamine, and opioid neurotransmitter systems or their interaction has been proposed; however, no specific interaction leading to self-injury has been demonstrated.
5. A variety of centrally acting psychotropic drugs have been implicated in eliciting stereotypy and self-injury, including subcutaneous amphetamine and intermittent dosages of pemoline. These effects may be antagonized by dopamine antagonists. Other drugs produce paresthesias and provide a peripheral stimulus for arousal, perhaps leading to stereotypy, and possibly self-injury.
6. Stereotypy and self-injury can result from surgery or administration of neurotoxins early in development and anatomical lesions, such as sensory deafferentation, may result in self-injury.
7. SIA may be a factor in eliciting or maintaining self-injury. Whether subjects stimulate to facilitate sensory input or to self-administer endogenous opioids is an open question, as is the issue of whether SIA is a secondary consequence of the behavior. Studies of SIA are complicated because there are both opioid and nonopioid forms of SIA.

From a ncurobiological perspective, SIB is multiply determined and involves maturational factors, physiological state, past experience, social context, and novel environmental settings, which vary among individuals. In both human and animal studies, one must take into account the form of the self-injury, considering a severe form with sudden onset and a less severe form following stereotypy with regularly repeated injury. The social context must be considered because past social isolation lends vulnerability for future injury when stressed. In pervasive developmental disorder, where there is deviant social development, the deficiency in bonding may enhance vulnerability because of lack of response to social reinforcement. The role of depression and learned helplessness also should be considered. The physiological state of the organism must be taken into account. A state of agitation may accompany emotional lability, as a temperamental factor, as an aspect of a mental disorder, or as a consequence of environmental variables. Both surgical and neurochemical interventions show that abnormal neurological conditions, particularly those affecting sensory input, result in stereotypy and sometimes self-injury. Mentally subnormal individuals often have neurological abnormalities involving sensory systems, and excessive agitation and SIB may occur when conditions are perceived as confusing or threatening.

## References

Abe, K., Oda, N., & Amatomi, M. (1984). Natural history and predictive significance of head banging, headrolling, and breath holding spells. *Developmental Medicine and Child Neurology*, *26*, 644–648.

American Psychiatric Association. (1987). *Diagnostic and statistical manual of mental disorders* (3rd ed. rev.). Washington, DC: Author.

Anderson, J. R., & Chamove, A. S. (1980). Self-aggression and social aggression in laboratory reared macaques. *Journal of Abnormal Psychology*, *89*, 539–550.

Anderson, L., Dancis, J., & Alpert, M. (1978). Behavioral contingencies and self-mutilation in Lesch–Nyhan disease. *Journal of Consulting and Clinical Psychology*, *3*, 529–536.

Anderson, L., Dancis, J., Alpert, M., & Herman, L. (1977). Punishment learning and self-mutilation in Lesch–Nyhan disease. *Nature*, *265*, 461–463.

Anderson, L. T., Hermann, L., Alpert, M., & Dancis, T. (1975). Elimination of self-mutilation in Lesch–Nyhan disease. *Pediatric Research*, *9*, 257.

Bachman, J. A. (1972). Self-injurious behavior: A behavioral analysis. *Journal of Abnormal Psychology*, *80*, 211–224.

Baroff, G. S., & Tate, B. S. (1968). The use of aversive stimulation in the treatment of chronic self-injurious behavior. *Journal of American Academy of Child Psychiatry*, *7*, 454–460.

Bartak, L., & Rutter, M. (1976). Differences between mentally retarded and normally intelligent autistic children. *Journal of Autism and Childhood Schizophrenia*, *6*, 109–120.

Bauman M., & kemper, T. L. (1985). Histoanatomical observations of the brain in early infantile autism. *Neurology*, *35*, 866–874.

Baumeister, A. A., & Frye, G. D. (1985). The biochemical basis of the behavioral disorder in the Lesch–Nyhan syndrome. *Neuroscience & Biobehavioral Reviews*, *9*, 169–178.

Baumeister, A. A., Frye, G. D., & Moore, L. L. (1987). An investigation of the role played by the superior colliculus and ventromedial thalamus in self-injurious behavior produced by intranigral microinjection of muscimol. *Pharmacology, Biochemistry, and Behavior*, *26*, 187–189.

Baumeister, A., & Rollings, J. P. (1976). Self-injurious behavior. *International Review of Research in Mental Retardation*, *8*, 1–34.

Belluzzi, J. D., & Stein, L. (1977). Enkephalin may mediate euphoria and drive-reduction reward. *Nature*, *266*, 556–558.

Berg, J. M., McCreary, B. D., Ridler, M. A. C., & Smith, G. F. (1970). *The de Lange syndrome*. Oxford: Pergamon Press.

Bernstein, G. A., Hughes, J. R., Mitchell, J. E., & Thompson, T. (1987). Effects of narcotic antagnoists on self-injurious behavior: A single case study. *Journal of the American Academy of Child and Adolescent Psychiatry*, *26*, 886–889.

Bhattacharya, S. K., Jaiswal, A. K., Mukhopadhyay, M., & Datla, K. P. (1988). Clonidine-induced automutilation in mice as a laboratory model for clinical self-injurious. *Journal of Psychiatric Research*, *22*, 43–50.

Breese, G. R., Baumeister, A. A., McCown, T. J., Emerick, S. G., Frye, G. D., Crotty, K., & Mueller, R. A. (1984). Behavioral differences between neonatal and adult 6-hydroxy-dopamine-treated rats to dopamine agonists: Relevance to neurological symptoms in clinical syndromes with reduced brain dopamine. *Journal of Pharmacology and Experimental Therapeutics*, *231*, 343–354.

Buchsbaum, M. S., Davis, G. C., & Bunny, W. G. (1977). Naloxone alters pain perception and somatosensory evoked potentials in normal subjects. *Nature*, *267*, 620–622.

Busbaur, A. I (1974). Effects of central lesion on disorders produced by dorsal rhizotomy in rats. *Experimental Neurology*, *42*, 490–501.

Campbell, M. (Personal communication). AACP meeting, 1990.

Campbell, M., Anderson, L. T., Small. A. M., Perry, R., Green, W. H., & Caplan, R. (1982). The effects of haloperidol on learning and behavior in autistic children. *Journal of Autism and Developmental Disorders*, *12*, 167–75.

Campbell, M., Overall, J. E., Small, A. M., Sokol, M. S., Spencer, E. K., & Adams, P. (1989). Naltrexone in autistic children: An acute open dose range tolerance trial. *Journal of the American Academy of Child and Adolescent Psychiatry*, *28*, 200–206.

Carr, E. G. (1977). The motivation of self-injurious behavior: A review of some hypotheses. *Psychological Bulletin*, *84*, 800–816.

Cataldo, M. F., & Harris, J. C. (1982). The biological basis for self-injury in the mentally retarded. *Analysis and Intervention in Developmental Disabilities*, *2*, 21–39.

Charmove, A. S., & Harlow, H. F. (1970). Exaggeration of self-aggression following alcohol ingestion in rhesus monkeys. *Journal of Abnormal Psychology*, *75*, 207–209.

Clark, D. L., Kreutzberg, J. R., & Chee, F. K. W. (1977). Vestibular stimulation influence on motor development in infants. *Science*, *196*, 1228–1229.

Cools, A. R., Wicgant, U. M., & Gispen, W. H. (1978). Distinct dopaminergic systems in ACTH induced grooming. *European Journal of Pharmacology*, *50*, 265–68.

Courchesne, E., Yeung-Courchesne, R., Press, G. A., Hesselink, J. R., & Jernigan, T. L. (1988). Hypoplasia of cerebellar vermal lobules VI and VII in infantile autism. *New England Journal of Medicine*. *318*, 1349–1354.

Davidson, P. W., Kleene, B. M., Carroll, M., & Rockowitz, R. J. (1983). Effects of naloxone on self injurious behavior: A case study. *Applied Research in Mental Retardation*, *4*, 1–4.

Davis, K. (1940). Extreme isolation of a child. *American Journal of Sociology*, *45*, 554–565.

Davis, K. (1946). Final note on a case of extreme isolation. *American Journal of Sociology*, *52*, 432–437.

Dehen, H., Amsallem, B., Colas-Linhart, N., & Cambier, J. (1986). Cerebrospinal fluid beta endorphin in congenital insensitivity to pain. *Review of Neurology (Paris)*, *142*, 541–544.

Dehen, H., Willer, J. C., Boureau, F., & Cambier, J. (1977). Congenital insensitivity to pain, and endogenous morphine-like substances. *Lancet*, *2*, 293–294.

De Lange, C. (1933). Sur un type nouveau de degeneration (Typus Amstelodamensis). *Archives de Medicine des Enfants*, *36*, 713–719.

De Lissovoy, V. (1962). Head-baning in early childhood. *Child Development*, *33*, 43–56.

De Lissovoy, V. (1963). Head-banging in early childhood. A suggested cause. *Journal of Genetic Psychology*, *102*, 109–114.

Delius, J. D., Craig, B., & Chaudoir, C. (1976). Adrenocorticotropic hormone. Glucose displacement activities in pigeon. *Zeitschrift fur Tierpsychologie*, *40*, 183–193.

Fellow, P., & Tennstedt, A. (1986). Cornelia de Lange syndrome with analgesia. *Psychiatry Neurology Medicine and Psychology*, *38*, 33–38.

Frankel, F., & Simmons, J. Q. (1976). Self-injurious behavior in schizophrenic and retarded children. *American Journal of Mental Deficiency*, *80*, 512–522.

Freedman, D. A., & Brown, S. L. (1968). On the role of coenesthetic stimulation in the development of psychic structure. *Psychoanalytic Quarterly*, *37*, 418–438.

Fryns, J. P., Jacobs, J., Kleczkowska, A., & Van Den Berghe, H. (1984). The psychological profile of fragile X syndrome. *Clinical Genetics*, *25*, 131–34.

Geller, E., Ritvo, E. R., Freeman, B. J., & Yuwiler, A. (1982). Preliminary observations on the effect of fenfluramine on blood serotonin and symptoms in three autistic boys. *New England Journal of Medicine*, *307*, 165–169.

Gilbert, S., Spellacy, E., & Watts, R. W. E. (1979). Problems in the behavioral treatment of self-injury in the Lesch–Nyhan syndrome. *Developmental Medicine and Child Neurology*, *21*, 795–800.

Gispen, W. H., Wiegant, V. M., Greven, H. M., & de Wied, D. (1976). The induction of excessive grooming in the rat by intraventricular application of peptides derived from ACTH: Structure–activity studies. *Life Sciences*, *17*, 645–652.

Gjedde, A., Wong, D. F., Harris, J., Dannals, R. F., & Ravert, H. T. (1986). Quantification of D1 and D2 dopamine receptors in Lesch–Nyhan syndrome as measured by positron tomography. *Society for Neuroscience Abstracts*, *12*, 486.

Gogas, K. R., & Hough, L. B. (1988). H2 receptor mediated stress induced analgesia is dependent on neither pituitary nor adrenal activation. *Pharmacology, Biochemistry, and Behavior*, *30*, 791–794.

Goldstein, M., Anderson, L. T., Reuben, R., & Dancis, J. (1985). Self-mutilation in Lesch–Nyhan disease is caused by dopaminergic denervation. *Lancet*, *1*, 338–339.

Goosen, C., & Ribbens, L. G. (1980). Autoaggression and tactile communication in pairs of adult stump tailed macaques. *Behavior*, *73*, 155–174.

Green, A. H. (1967). Self mutilation in schizophrenic children. *Archives of General Psychiatry*, *17*, 234–244.
Greenberg, A., & Coleman, M. (1973). Depressed whole blood serotonin levels associated with behavioral abnomalities in the de Lange syndrome. *Pediatrics*, *51*, 720–724.
Griffin, J. C., Ricketts, R. W., Williams, D. E., Locke, B. J., Altmeyer, B. K., & Stark, M. T. (1987). A community survey of self-injurious behavior among developmentally disabled children and adolescents. *Hospital and Community Psychiatry*, *38*, 959–963.
Hagerman, R. J., Jackson, A. W., Levitas, A., Rimland, B., & Braden, M. (1986). An analysis of autism in fifty males with fragile X syndrome. *American Journal of Medical Genetics*, *23*, 359–374.
Hamilton, M. (1985). *Fish's clinical psychopathology: Signs and symptoms in psychiatry*. Bristol: John Wright & Sons.
Harris, J. C. (1987). Behavioral phenotypes in mental retardation syndromes. In R. Barrett & J. Matson (Eds.), *Advances in developmental disorders* (Vol. 1), pp. 77–106. New York: JAI Press.
Harris, J. C., Wong, D. F., Wagner, H. N., Rett, A., & Naidu, S. (1986). Positron emission tomographic study of $D_2$ dopamine receptor binding and CSF biogenic animal metabolites in Rett syndrome. *Americal Journal of Medical Genetics*, *24*, 201–210.
Hawley, P. P., Jackson, L. G., & Kurnit, D. M. (1985). Sixty four patients with Brackman de Lange syndrome: A survey. *American Journal of Medical Genetics*, *20*, 453–459.
Hennessey, J. W., & Levine, S. (1979). Stress, arousal, and the pituitary adrenal system: A psychoendocrine hypothesis. In J. M. Strague & A. N. Epstein (Eds.), *Progress in psychobiology and physiological psychology* (Vol. 8). New York: Academic Press.
Hosobuchi, Y. (1981). Periaqueductal gray simulation in humans produces analgesia accompanied by elevation of beta-endorphin and ACTH in ventricular CSF. *Modern Problems in Pharmacopsychiatry*, *17*, 109–122.
Hutt, C., & Hutt, S. J. (1968). Stereotypes and their relation to arousal: A study of autistic children. In S. J. Hutt & C. Hutt (Eds.), *Behavior studies in psychiatry*. London: Pergamon.
Iriki, A., Shuicki, N., & Nakamura, Y. (1988). Feeding behavior in mammals: Corticobulbar projection is reorganized during conversion from sucking to chewing. *Developmental Brain Research*, *44*, 189–196.
Iwata, B. A., Pace, G. M., Willis, K. D., Gamache, T. B., & Hyman, S. L. (1986). Operant studies of self-injurious hand biting in the Rett syndrome. *American Journal of Medical Genetics*, *24*, 157–166.
Jenson, W.R., Rovner, L., Cameron, S., Petersen, B. P., & Kesler, J. (1985). Reduction of self-injurious behavior in an autistic girl using a multifaceted treatment program. *Journal of Behavior Therapy & Experimental Psychiatry*, *16*, 77–80.
Johnson, W., & Baumeister, A. (1978). A self-injurious behavior: A review and analysis of methodological details of published studies. *Behavior Modification*, *2*, 465–484.
Jolles, J., Rompa-Barendregt, J., & Gispen, W. H. (1979). ACTH-induced excessive grooming in the rat: The influence of environmental and motivational factors. *Hormones and Behavior*, *12*, 60–72.

Jones, I. H., & Barraclough, B. M. (1978). Auto-mutilation in animals and its relevance to self-injury in man. *Acta Psychiatrica Scandinavia*, *58*, 40–47.

Jones, I. H. (1982). Self-injury: Toward a biological basis. *Perspectives in Biology and Medicine*, *26*, 137–150.

Kahkonen, M., Leisti, J., Thoden, C. J., & Autio, S. (1986). Frequency of rare. Fragile sites among mentally subnormal school children. *Clin Genetics*, 30: 234–238.

Katsuragi, T. I., Ushijima & Furukawa, T. (1984). The clonidine-induced self-injurious behavior of mice involves purinergic mechanisms. *Pharmacology Biochemistry & Behavior*, *20*, 943–946.

Kelly, D. D. (1982). The role of endorphins in stress-induced agalgesia. *Annals of the New York Academy of Science*, *398*, 260–271.

Kluver, H., & Bucy, A. S. (1939). Preliminary analysis of functions of the temporal lobe in monkeys. *Archives of Neurology and Psychiatry*, *42*, 978–1000.

Kopin, I. J. (1981). Neurotransmitters and the Lesch–Nyhan syndrome. *The New England Journal of Medicine*, *305*, 1148–1150.

Kravitz, H., Vin Rosenthal, Y., Teplitz, Z., Murphy, I., & Lesser, R. (1960). A study of headbanging in infants and children. *Diseases of the Nervous System*, *21*, 203–208.

Kuhar, M. J., Pert, C. B., & Snyder, S. H. (1973). Regional distribution of opiate receptor binding in the monkey and human brain. *Nature*, *245*, 447–450.

Largo, R. H., & Schinzel, A. (1985). Developmental and behavioral disturbances in 13 boys with fragile X syndrome. *European Journal of Pediatrics*, *143*, 269–75.

Lal, H. (1975). Narcotic dependence, narcotic action, and dopamine receptors. *Life Sciences*, *17*, 483–496.

Lesch, M., & Nyhan, W. L. (1964). A familial disorder of uric acid metabolism and central nervous system function. *American Journal of Medicine*, *36*, 561–570.

Lewis, J. W., Tordoff, M. G., Sherman, J. E., & Liebeskind, J. C. (1982). Adrenal medullary enkephalin-like peptides may mediate opioid stress analgesia. *Science*, *217*, 557–559.

Lloyd, H. G. E., & Stone, T. W. (1981). Chronic methylxanthine treatment in rats: A comparison of wistar and fischer 344 strains. *Pharmacology, Biochemistry Behavior*, *14*, 827–830.

Lloyd, K. G., Hornykiewicz, O., Davidson, L., Shanak, K., Farley, I., Goldstein, M., & Shibuya, M. (1981). Biochemical evidence of dysfunction of brain neurotransmitters in the Lesch–Nyhan syndrome. *The New England Journal of Medicine*, *305*, 1106–1111.

Madden, J., Akil, H., Patrick, R. L., & Barchas, J. D. (1977). Stress-induced parallel changes in central opioid levels and pain responsiveness in the rat. *Nature*, *265*, 358–60.

Maisto, C. R., Baumeister, A. A., & Maisto, A. A. (1978). An analysis of variables related to self-injurious behavior among institutionalized retarded persons. *Journal of Mental Deficiency Research*, *22*, 27–36.

Manfredi, M., Bini, G., Cruccu, G., Accornero, N., Berardelli, A., & Medolago, L. (1981). Congenital absence of pain. *Archives of Neurology*, *38*, 507–511.

Margolin, D. I., & Moon, B. H. (1979). Naloxone blockade of apomorphine-induced stereotyped behavior. *Journal of the Neurological Sciences*, *43*, 13–17.

Mason, W. A., (1968). Early social deprivation in nonhuman primates: Implications for human behavior. In D. C. Glass (Ed.), *Environmental influences* (pp. 70–101). New York: Rockefeller University Press.
Mason, W. A., & Capitanio, J. P. (1988). Formation and experssion of filial attachment in rhesus monkeys raised with living and inanimate mother substitutes. *Developmental Psychobiology*, *21*, 401–430.
McBride, P. A., Anderson, G. N., Hertzig, M. E., Sweeney, J. A., Kream, J., Chone, D. J., & Mann, J. J. (1989). Serotonergic responsivity in male young adults with autistic disorder: Results of a pilot study. *Archives of General Psychiatry*, *46*, 213–221.
Meyer-Holzapfel, M. (1968). Abnormal behavior in zoo animals. In F. W. Fox. (Ed.), *Abnormal behavior in animals*, (pp. 476–503). Philadelphia: W. B. Saunders.
Minderaa, R. B., Anderson, G. M., Volkmar, F. R., Akkerhuis, G. W., & Cohen, D. J. (1989). Neurochemical study of dopamine functioning in autistic and normal subjects. *Journal of the American Academy of Child and Adolescent Psychiatry*, *28*, 190–194.
Mizuno, T. & Yugari, Y. (1974). Self-mutilation in the Lesch–Nyhan syndrome. *Lancet*, *1*, 761.
Mizuno, T. & Yugari, Y. (1975). Prophylactic effect of L-5 hydroxytryptophan on self-mutilation in the Lesch–Nyhan syndrome. *Neuropaediatrie*, *6*, 13–23.
Mueller, K., Hollingsworth, & Petit, H. (1986). Repeated pemoline produces self-injurious behavior in adult and weanling rats. *Pharmacology Biochemistry & Behavior*, *25*, 933–938.
Mueller, K., & Nyhan, W. L. (1982a). Clonidine potentiates drug induced self-injurious behavior in rats. *Pharmacology Biochemistry & Behavior*, *18*, 891–894.
Mueller, K., & Nyhan, W. L. (1982b). Pharamacologic control of pemoline induced self-injurious behavior in rats. *Pharmacology Biochemistry & Behavior*, *16*, 957–963.
Mueller, K., Saboda, R., Palmour, & Nyhan, W. L. (1982). Self-injurious behavior produced in rats by daily caffeine and continuous amphetamine. *Pharmacology Biochemistry & Behavior*, *17*, 613–617.
Mülder, A. H., Wardeh, G., Hogenboom, F., & Frankhuyzen, A. L. (1984). Kappa and delta opiate receptor agonists differentially inhibit striatal dopamine and acetylcholine release. *Nature*, *308*, 278–280.
Murrin, L. C., Coyle, J. T., & Kuhar, M. J. (1980). Striatal opiate receptors: Pre and postsynaptic localization. *Life Sciences*, *27*, 1175–1183.
Naidu, S., Murphy, M., Moser, H. W., & Rett, A. (1986). Rett syndrome: Natural history in 70 cases. *American Journal of Medical Genetics*, *24*, 61–72.
Nyhan, W. L. (1972). Behavioral phenotypes in organic genetic disease. (1971). *Pediatric Research*, *6*, 1–9.
Nyhan, W. L. (1976). Behavior in the Lesch–Nyhan syndrome. *Journal of Autism and Childhood Schizophrenia*, *6*, 235–252.
Nyhan, W. L., Johnson, H. G., Kaufman, I. A., & Jones, K. L. (1980). Serotonergic approaches to the modification of behavior in the Lesch–Nyhan syndrome. *Applied Research in Mental Retardation*, *1*, 25–40.
Olds, M. E., & Fobes, J. L. (1981). The central basis of motivation: Intracranial self-stimulation studies. *Annual Review of Psychology*, *32*, 523–594.

O'Neil, M. N. (1982). *Effects of an anti-depressant drug given to isolate primates who display self-injurious behaviors: A comparative study. Unpublished doctoral dissertation.* University of Wisconsin, Madison.

Ornitz, E. M. (1974). The modulation of sensory input and motor output in autistic children. *Journal of Autism and Childhood Schizophrenia, 4,* 197–215.

Pallard, H., Llorens, J., Schwartz, J. C., Gros, C., & Dray, F. (1978). Localization of opiate receptors and enkephalins in the rat striatum with relation to the nigrostriatal dopaminergic system: lesion studies. *Brain Research, 151,* 392–398.

Pattison, E. M., & Kahan, J. (1983). The deliberate self-harm syndrome. *American Journal of Psychiatry, 140,* 867–872.

Peters, J. M. (1967). Caffeine induced hemorrhagic automutilation. *Archives Internationales de Pharmaco-dynamie et de Therapy, 169,* 139–146.

Picker, M., Poling, A., & Parker, A. (1979). A review of children's self-injurious behavior. *The Psychological Record, 29,* 435–452.

Randrup, A., & Munkvad, I. (1967). Stereotyped activities produced by amphetamines in several animal species and man. *Psychopharmacologia, 11,* 300–310.

Reiss, A. L. (1988). Cerebellar hyperplasia and autism. *New England Journal of Medicine, 319,* 1152–1153.

Rett, A. (1966). Über ein eigneartiges hirnatrophisches syndrom bei hyperammonamie im kindersaltger. *Wein Med Wochenschr., 116,* 723–726.

Richardson, J. S., & Zaleski, W. A. (1983). Naloxone and self-mutilation. *Biological Psychiatry, 18,* 99–101.

Riederer, P., Brucke, T., Kienzl, E., Schnecker, K., Schay, V., Kruzik, P., Killian W., & Rett, A. (1985). Neurochemistry of Rett syndrome. *Brain and Development, 7,* 351–60.

Riley, C. M., Day, R. L., Greeley, D. M., & Langford, W. S. (1949). Central autonomic dysfunction with defective lacrimation. *Pediatrics, 3,* 468–478.

Ritvo, E. R., Freeman, B. J., Geller, E., & Yuwiler, A. (1983) Effects of fenfluramine on 14 autistic outpatients. *Journal of the American Academy of Child Psychiatry, 22,* 549–558.

Russo, D. C., Carr, E. G., & Lovaas, O. I. (1980). Self-injury in pediatric populations. In J. Ferguson & C. B. Taylor (Eds.), *Comprehensive handbook of behavioral medicine* (Vol. 3, pp. 23–41). New York: Spectrum Publications.

Ryan, S. M., & Maier, S. F. (1988). The estrous cycle and estrogen modulate stress induced analgesia. *Behavioral Neuroscience, 102,* 371–380.

Rylander, G. (1971). Stereotypy in man following amphetamine abuse. In S. B. de Baker (Ed.), *The correlation of adverse effects in man with observations in animals.* Series No. 220, (pp. 28–31). Amsterdam: Excepta Medica, International Congress.

Sackett, G. P. (1968). Abnormal behavior in laboratory reared rhesus monkey. In F. W. Fox (Ed.). *Abnormal behaviour in animals* (293–374). Philadephia: W. B. Saunders.

Schroeder, S. R., Schroeder, C. S., Smith, R., & Dalldorf, J. (1978). Prevalence of self-injurious behaviors in a large state facility for the retarded: A three-year follow-up study. *Journal of Autism and Childhood Schizophrenia, 8,* 261–269.

Shear, C. S., Nyhan, W. L., Kirman, B. H., & Stern, J. (1971). Self-mutilative behavior as a feature of the de Lange syndrome. *Journal of Pediatrics, 78,* 506–509.

Singh, N. N., & Pulman, R. M. (1979). Self injury in the de Lange syndrome. *Journal of Mental Deficiency Research*, *23*, 79–84.

Smeets, P. M. (1971). Some characteristics of mental defectives displaying self mutilative behaviors. *Training School Bulletin. (Vineland)*, *68*, 131–135.

Snyder, S. H. (1977). Opiate receptors in the brain. *New England Journal of Medicine*, *296*, 266–271.

Stuckey, J., Marra, S., Minor, T., & Insel, T. R. (1989). Changes in mu opiate receptors following inescapable shock, *Brain Research*, *476*, 167–169.

Sutherland, G. R. (1985). Heritable fragile sites on human chromosomes: XII. Population cytogenetics. *Annals of Human Genetics*, *49*, 153–161.

Sweetman, L., & Nyhan, W. L. (1972). Further studies of the enzyme composition of mutant cells. *Archives of Internal Medicine*, *130*, 214–220.

Szymanski, L., Kedesdy, J., Sulkes, S., & Cutler, A. (1987). Naltrexone in treatment of self injurious behavior: A clinical study. *Research in Developmental Disabilites*, *8*, 179–190.

Taub, E. (1976). Movement in nonhuman primates deprived of somatosensory feedback. In J. F. Keogh (Ed.), *Exercise and sports sciences reviews* (Vol. 4, pp. 335–376). Santa Barbana, CA: Journal Publishing Affiliates.

Taub, E., Perrella, P. N., & Barro, G. (1973). Behavioral development following forelimb deafferentation on the day of birth in monkeys with and without blinding. *Science*, *81*, 959–60.

Thrush, D. C. (1973). Congenital insensitivity to pain: A clinical, genetic, and neurophysiological study of four children from the same family. *Brain*, *96*, 369–386.

Ungerstedt, U. (1971). Postsynaptic supersensitivity after 6-hydroxydopamine induced degeneration of the nigra-striatal dopamine system. *Acta Physiology Scandanavia (Suppl).*, *367*, 69–93.

Watts, R. W. E., Spellacvy, E., Gibbs, D. A., Allsop, J., McKeran, R. O., & Slavin, G. E. (1982). Clinical, postmortem, biochemical, and therapeutic observations in Lesch–Nyhan syndrome. *Quarterly Journal of Medicine*, *5*, 73–78.

Willer, J. P., Dekers, & A. Cambier, J. (1981). Stress induced analgesia in humans: Endogenous opioids and naloxone reversible suppression of pain reflexes. *Science*, *212*, 689–691.

# 4 Psychophysiology and Issues of Anxiety and Arousal

RAYMOND G. ROMANCZYK, STEPHANIE LOCKSHIN, and JULIA O'CONNOR

It is only in recent years that self-injurious behavior has been viewed as a complex behavior pattern that under certain circumstances may have specific functional value. Because the behavior pattern appears so paradoxical and contrary to very basic characteristics of the behavior of organisms (i.e., that they tend to avoid painful stimuli), we must examine very carefully the controlling variables for self-injurious behavior as well as the many subtypes of self-injurious behavior. However there is also a danger in oversimplifying the understanding of self-injurious behavior. To label it as functional and purposeful provides a perspective superior to viewing it simply as a psychotic behavior but also lends itself to a simplistic and naïve understanding as well. That is, self-injurious behavior represents a classification of behavior, and therefore, one cannot assume that the causal and maintaining factors are (1) similar across individuals, (2) consistent for the same individual at different points in time, and (3) similar for different topographies of self-injurious behavior both within and across individuals.

Self-injurious behavior in the form that produces delayed long-term consequences is familiar to everyone. This involves health-risk behavior such as cigarette smoking, excessive alcohol consumption, overeating, and poor exercise habits. In such instances, however, we are able to recognize a certain cost–benefit balance to the self-injurious behavior. We understand and often agree with the evaluation that an athlete makes with respect to the pain and suffering produced by long strenuous workouts, in that it balances the benefits that accrue with respect to performance increases. In like manner, the pleasure that a cigarette smoker obtains provides us with an understanding, although not an endorsement, of the perpetuation of cigarette smoking even in the face of knowledge concerning its detrimental health consequences. Thus, the degree to which we are able to perceive the cost–benefit balance of a particular behavior allows us to engage in some degree of empathy and understanding that the self-injurious behavior is not a psychotic or irrational act.

The second form of self-injurious behavior, that of acute self-mutilation, is often more difficult to understand, but again, its rationale can often be articulated by the individual. An example is very minor self-mutilation (such as various cosmetic changes, practiced in various cultures), which is often seen as quite appropriate within, but not necessarily across, cultures. Further, various religious practices that promote or condone high levels of self-inflicted pain, and at times mutilation, are often also associated with endorsement within a particular religious group although not necessarily outside that group. One often sees such self-injurious behavior in individuals labeled as "schizophrenic" or "psychotic" where there appears to be acute episodes of self-cutting, burning, self-blinding, or self-amputation in response to strong stressors. In such instances, even when individuals can articulate their particular perception of a cost–benefit balance of their behavior, we typically strongly disagree with their analysis to the extent that it provides further evidence for their psychotic ideation and behavior.

The third form of self-injurious behavior, that of stereotyped, repetitive and rhythmic responses that produce either immediate or delayed injury, such as head-banging, face-slapping, self-kicking, biting, scratching, is the focus of the current chapter and is primarily associated with individuals having developmental disabilities. It is also, although not exclusively so, associated with individuals with poor communication skills. A review of the treatment literature indicates a remarkable array of topography of self-injurious behavior, as well as a seemingly unlimited number and variety of treatment techniques and approaches. Indeed the treatment of self-injurious behavior became quite controversial during the 1980s and has served as a focus for various debates concerning more general issues on treatment and educational services for individuals with developmental disabilities. Unfortunately, due to the extreme difficulty in conducting well-controlled research on self-injurious behavior, given that paramount emphasis must be given to the safety of the individual, after several decades of research, with over 500 published reports, it is still difficult to interpret the basic and applied literature, and it is not possible to state unequivocally the superiority of one treatment approach over another. Further, the difficulty of long-term treatment maintenance is severe, and there are very few published studies of long-term effectiveness. The difficulty of long-term treatment maintenance has often been conceptualized as primarily a problem in generalization. However, it has also been proposed that the difficulty of long-term maintenance is associated with poor analysis of etiological and maintaining factors such that current treatment approaches are often incomplete and therefore set the stage for reacquisition of the behavior pattern.

In this context, it is important to review the various major etiological models. They each are quite complex and have been reviewed extensively elsewhere (Romanczyk, in press). However, a brief review is merited in order to place into context the importance of physiological assessment of the anxiety/arousal components of self-injurious behavior. There are five major etiological models at present, which are reviewed with respect to their basic conceptualization, as well as supporting research. These five models are as follows: (1) psychodynamic, (2) biological, (3) sensory stimulation, (4) behavioral, and (5) complex behavioral (operant–respondent).

## Psychodynamic Model

The psychodynamic model is extremely rich in clinical description and presents a fascinating conceptual structure. It focuses on the delicate interplay of forces between the id, ego, and superego. Within the model, there are two primary submodels. The first relies heavily on the process of ego development and is characterized by the writings of Karl Menninger and Anna Freud. The speculation is that ego boundaries have been poorly formed, so that in the attempt to differentiate self from environment, the pain of self-directed aggression is utilized. Similarly, in extreme instances of anxiety caused by guilt associated with aggressive impulses toward primary figures such as the mother, or guilt concerning transgression of boundaries set by the superego, self-injurious behavior may be utilized as a form of anxiety reduction. Similar to the preceding cost–benefit analysis, Menninger (1935) has labeled this process of anxiety reduction as "bargaining" with the self, and that even when gross bodily harm results from this attempt at reduction of anxiety, it is nevertheless a healing process and thus positive, albeit in a very limited context.

The second submodel does not rely upon ego development per se and has been articulated by Cain (1961). He distinguishes between *auto-aggression* and *self-aggression*. Auto-aggression does not require a developed ego and thus he views it in the context of a primitive outburst that requires no appeal to superego functioning.

The descriptions by most psychoanalytic writers of clinical cases are very rich in subjective interpretations but lacking in objective measurement and analysis. However, a central theme in most of these writings is the anxiety or tension that precipitates such self-injurious behavior. The specific behavior is often abstracted, and great significance is paid to symbolic aspects. Thus, treatment emphasis is focused almost entirely at the perceived source of the anxiety and tension rather than at the specific topography and symptomatology of the self-injurious behavior.

This theoretical model has not proven to be of use with the developmentally disabled for the purpose of the treatment of self-injurious behavior, although it has produced some interesting phenomenological descriptions of self-mutilation that is associated with individuals with psychotic disorders. However, in these instances, the behavior is typically not repetitive in nature and is better conceptualized as acute episodes in response to high degrees of stress. Further, even within this limited description, there remain other etiological and therapeutic models that represent a significant improvement over the psychodynamic model, but acknowledgment is given to the emphasis placed upon arousal/anxiety.

## Biological Model

The identification of specific syndromes and illnesses in which self-injurious behavior is observed has been used as strong support for the biological model of self-injurious behavior (Harris, Chapter 3, this volume). In particular, the Lesch-Nyhan syndrome has generated a great deal of interest and research. It is an X-linked genetic disorder in which a specific enzyme is lacking, which normally is used to metabolize purine, and thus results in high uric acid levels. Individuals who have Lesch-Nyhan syndrome typically have severe to mild mental retardation and their self-injurious behavior is often in the form of biting the lips, tongue, and fingers. Cataldo and Harris (1982) have described several specific hypotheses that arise from the research literature: (1) because uric acid is an irritant, its presence in the saliva may stimulate self-injurious behavior focused on the mouth region; (2) when depleted, serotonin, an endogenous neurotransmitter, can produce increased aggression, which, when self-directed, is termed *self-injurious behavior*; (3) another endogenous neurotransmitter, dopamine, which is important in regulating motor activity, may serve to stimulate self-injurious behavior. (This is an interesting hypothesis, as purine is related to dopamine production.) While these are quite logical hypotheses, unfortunately, as Cataldo and Harris (1982) present, none have had strong experimental support.

The endogenous opioid peptides have also received great interest (see following discussion). One of the more frequently mentioned groups of endogenous opioid peptides are the endorphins. It is hypothesized that these neurochemicals (which serve a pain-reducing function) may produce addictivelike behavior. (The "runners' high" that marathon runners experience may be associated with the endogenous opioid peptides.) It may be that self-injurious behavior serves to release endorphins and thus the individual is able to tolerate higher and higher intensities and frequencies of self-injurious behavior, as the behavior itself serves to attenuate pain through the endorphin mechanism. This hypothesis does not have direct support, but it does raise important questions with respect to factors that may serve to maintain self-injurious behavior, which are discussed later.

Physical problems and ailments that can cause irritation, pain, and discomfort are also of importance to the biological model. For instance, dermatitis and skin lacerations can serve to both elicit and maintain so-called vicious-circle self-injurious behavior, a phenomenon that most people are familiar with. In its simplest form, scratching makes the itch feel better, even though scratching serves to produce further irritation, which produces more inflammation and itching, thus leading to more scratching. This pattern is well illustrated in a study by Carr and McDowell (1980) with respect to the treatment of self-injurious behavior prompted by dermatitis, which also had significant social reinforcement maintaining factors, which in turn was the focus of treatment.

With respect to common ailments, otitis media has also been implicated in self-injurious behavior. It is a form of middle-ear infection that can be extremely painful and can result in permanent damage and hearing loss. Common earaches (otitis externa) are less serious and are associated with simple activities such as bathing, swimming, and not cleaning the ear properly. However, otitis media is a very painful form of earache and does appear to be related in some cases to self-injurious behavior. It is possible that the self-injurious behavior may serve to attenuate the pain produced by the ear infection, as in the *gate model of pain*, in which the production of intense stimulation or pain in one part of the body attenuates pain from a second source. This is a common form of pain control often observed in individuals in the dentist chair, where they squeeze the handles of the chair or even press their fingernails into their palm in an effort to attenuate the pain occurring in the teeth. Such a process is probably not a common phenomenon with respect to the production of self-injurious behavior, but it may be significant for some individuals (Romanczyk, in press), and it is important in research both with humans (DeLissovoy, 1963) and in infrahumans (e.g., mice; Harkness & Wagner, 1975).

The biological model has clearly stimulated pharmacological treatment of self-injurious behavior. There are several excellent reviews of this area (Farber, 1987; Lapierre & Reesal, 1986; Singh & Millichamp, 1984), and at present, it must be stated that there is not strong evidence for the efficacy of pharmacological treatment of self-injurious behavior. While this does not imply that there are not isolated instances of positive effects, when one critically analyzes the specificity of effect and the frequency with which effects cannot be replicated, it is clear that the impact is limited and that the use of pharmacology is not proportionate to the controlled research reports of its efficacy. However, this lack of strong pharmacological effect should not detract from attempts to understand basic mechanisms that contribute to the etiology and maintenance of self-injurious behavior. The interaction of various mechanisms and factors such as stress-induced analgesia is most likely the source of the persistence of self-injurious behavior and the diversity of topography and pattern.

## Sensory Stimulation

The third model, sensory stimulation, is related to both the biological model and the behavioral model. Romanczyk (in press), Romanczyk, Kistner, and Plienis (1982), and Baumeister and Rollings (1976) have argued that self-injurious behavior and self-stimulatory behavior may be related, and that the distinction between them can be a function of intensity or external effect, rather than etiological and motivating conditions. (This does not imply a direct equivalence, as self-stimulatory behavior, for example, is typically much less sensitive to social attention than self-injurious behavior. As always, the issue is more one of intrasubject factors rather than intersubject factors.) Infrahuman studies indicate the important influence of atypical early rearing patterns and sensory deficits for the development of stereotyped behavior. The sensory-stimulation model encompasses several subcomponents: the frustration hypothesis, the arousal-reduction hypothesis, and the arousal-induction hypothesis. Unfortunately, much of the research is flawed because of circularity of definition with respect to arousal, in that it is not measured directly. However, there remains substantial research support. The specificity of the arousal mechanism yields specific treatment implications, but not directionality. The sensory stimulation received by the individual must be altered, but it may require either increase or decrease. Further, specific topographies within individuals may differentially respond to increased or decreased stimulation (Romanczyk, Kistner, & Plienis, 1982).

However, sensory stimulation can serve as a powerful model to develop effective intervention strategies. Meyerson, Kerr, and Michael (1967) found that vibration, and to a lesser extent back-scratching, significantly reduced self-injurious behavior in a young boy with autism. Using a more indirect form of stimulation, Favell, McGimsey, and Schell (1982) provided toys to six individuals with profound mental retardation and found reduction in self-injurious behavior for each individual. It is important to note that the toys were specifically chosen to provide competing stimulation rather than simply a random selection of toys. The data are mixed, however, as Hollis (1965a, 1965b) found no effect of stimulation on self-injurious behavior using a detailed analysis of behavior topography. As there is no apparent relationship between diagnostic category and response of self-injurious behavior to sensory stimulation manipulation, this underscores the importance of comprehensive and individualized assessment.

## Behavioral Model

The fourth model, the behavioral, or operant model, has had the greatest impact in the treatment of self-injurious behavior. It is a deceptively simple model that suffers from oversimplifications in application and description (Romanczyk, in press). Both basic and applied research provides substantial validation. Carr (1977) provided an excellent statement of the behavioral model, and his review stands as a critical conceptual and historical contribution.

There are three specific components to the behavior model. The first is an approach component whereby self-injurious behavior is positively reinforced by attention from caregivers or other adults. Self-injurious behavior is thus an *approach behavior*, in that by engaging in this behavior, the result is positive attention from the environment. The second component is the opposite process and is termed *escape behavior*. Self-injurious behavior emitted in response to demands or unpleasant interaction or stimuli in the environment has an impact upon those making such demands, and thus serves to remove these demands or unpleasant situations. Self-injurious behavior is therefore negatively reinforced. The third component is similar and is a temporal shift of the escape response. That is, avoidance occurs when the stimuli or events associated with impending demands or unpleasant situations serves as a cue to engage in self-injurious behavior, which, because of its effect upon others in the environment, precludes the occurrence of the offending situation or stimulus.

These three mechanisms may function in isolation or in combination for a given individual. When in combination, this produces an extremely complex behavior pattern that is not necessarily readily deduced from observation (Romanczyk, in press). The implication of the behavioral model is that self-injurious behavior may be ameliorated by procedures that focus upon antecedent and consequent events. The literature documents a great variety of treatment procedures that include, but are not limited to, the following:

Extinction
Differential reinforcement of behavior
Building and strengthening repertoires of appropriate behavior
Relaxation training/desensitization
Removal or attenuation of eliciting factors
Teaching/permitting appropriate escape/avoidance behavior
Stimulus control
Restraint application or removal
Response interruption
Time-out
Response-cost
Contingent effort
Overcorrection
Contingent presentation of unpleasant stimuli
Contingent electric shock

All of these treatment procedures have been demonstrated to be effective for some individuals, and this illustrates the extreme diversity and complexity of self-injurious behavior. Because so many forms of intervention have proven effective, it may be deduced that etiological processes are likewise extremely complex and that individual differences must be of paramount focus (Romanczyk, 1989).

## Complex Behavioral Model

The complex behavioral, or operant–respondent model (Romanczyk, 1986; Romanczyk, in press; Romanczyk, Kistner, & Plienis, 1982) incorporates several etiological and maintaining factors. The behavioral model does not adequately account for the initial occurrence of self-injurious behavior and has not incorporated physiological variables. The operant–respondent model does emphasize respondent aspects of self-injurious behavior and, in particular, emphasizes the role of arousal as an important maintaining factor. Previous research has described the possible relationship between arousal and self-injurious behavior (Davenport & Menzel, 1963; Frankel & Simmons, 1976; Gluck & Sackett, 1974; Levinson, 1970; Newsom, Carr, & Lovaas, 1977; Romanczyk & Goren, 1975; Tinklepaugh, 1928), but difficulty in conducting specific research investigation has limited the impact of this hypothesis.

By acknowledging the contribution of both operant and respondent components, self-injurious behavior may be initially elicited by arousal, which in turn is elicited by stressors in the environment. As self-injurious behavior is emitted, environmental events shape and maintain the behavior through operant conditioning. Physiological variables serve to mediate arousal, as described in the sensory stimulation model.

This is perhaps best illustrated in the case of individuals who have undergone a period of severe restraint as a protective mechanism for their self-injurious behavior. Such individuals are often seen to behave in a frenzied fashion when restraints are removed. Their self-injurious behavior appears quite uncontrollable, and the individuals display severe distress and what may be termed *panic*. Given the operant–respondent model, the hypothesis is that experience with restraint has led to a conditioning history wherein restraint is associated with the removal of demands and aversive environmental events, as well as the cessation of self-injurious behavior. Because self-injurious behavior produces pain, which in turn produces arousal, it is therefore the case, in a respondent fashion, that restraint is associated with the reduction of arousal and thus becomes a powerful positive conditioned stimulus. In the diagram shown in Figure 4.1, the process is illustrated wherein self-injurious behavior, quite paradoxically, can be seen as its own eliciting event and serves to illustrate the frenzied self-injurious behavior characteristic of some individuals when removed from restraint. As indicated in the schematic shown in Figure 4.1, self-injurious behavior results in an unconditioned stimulus, that of pain. This is immediately followed by the unconditioned response of arousal, which in turn serves to motivate escape behavior.

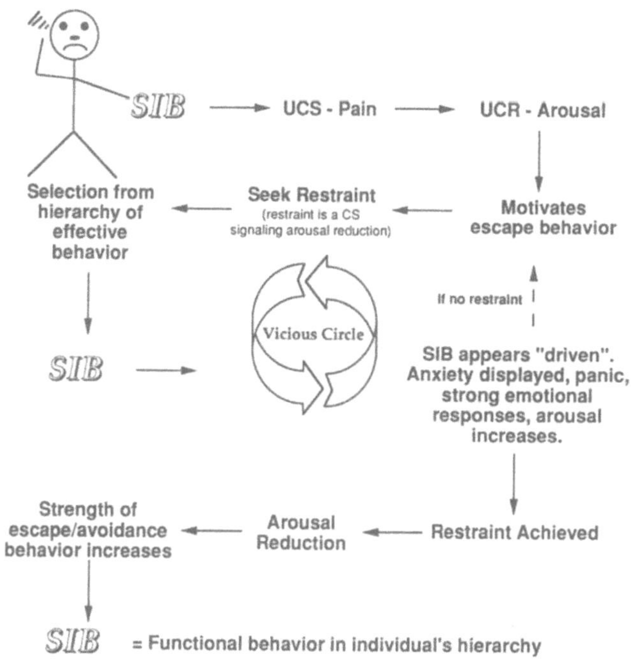


FIGURE 4.1. Diagram of the possible vicious circle that maintains SIB.

Escape behavior is selected from a hierarchy of behavior that has been effective in the past in producing escape from the aversive state or stimuli. For an individual with a history of restraint, seeking restraint is an effective method of arousal reduction. Once achieved, the negative reinforcement value of arousal reduction serves to increase the probability that this form of escape behavior will be utilized in the future. Of course, because the behavior that results in restraint is self-injurious behavior, this completes the vicious circle.

## Basic Psychophysiology

Human psychophysiological measurement and interpretation is a highly complex topic area. Because of this, there has been perhaps too cautious an atmosphere with respect to research and clinical utilization in the area of self-injurious behavior, and no doubt, there has been influence by the relative lack of sensitivity to issues of arousal/anxiety in the developmentally disabled population (Romanczyk, in press). Advances in measurement devices have occurred at an astounding rate, and it is no longer a prohibitive process to employ psychophysiological measurement on a routine basis, as required.

The following is a very brief overview of two often-used indices of arousal and attention that are relevant to our discussion.

## Heart Rate

Although the heart's primary function is one of a closed-system circulating pump, measurements of cardiac activity have been broadly utilized by psychophysiologists in a variety of areas, such as the study of fear and anxiety and in biofeedback. The widespread usage of heart rate in psychophysiological research and treatment reflects the commonly held belief that cardiac activity parallels level of arousal. However, researchers have found that the association between heart rate and arousal is not a simple linear relationship (Siddle & Turpin, 1980). There is a long history of research indicating that response patterns differ as a function of type of stimuli, as well as individual differences. Malmo and Shagass (1949) found that individuals who had somatic complaints had greater cardiac responsiveness to stress than those who did not have somatic complaints. For example, heart rate was found to decrease in response to simple stimuli (Davis, Buchwald, & Frankmann, 1955), and to increase in response to threatening or "startling" stimuli (e.g., a gun shot, Sternbach, 1960), or to stimuli that require some type of cognitive processing, such as mental arithmetic (Blair, Glover, Greenfield, & Roddie, 1959).

Heart rate is a very basic measure of cardiac functioning. A more comprehensive measure of the cardiovascular system would include heart rate as an index of blood volume supplied to the tissues and stroke volume, an index of volume of blood ejected by the heart at each beat (Siddle & Turpin, 1980). Heart rate is simply a measure of frequency of contractions of the heart initiated by spontaneous depolarization in the sinoatrial node per unit of time. Increases in heart rate are related to activation of the sympathetic division of the autonomic nervous system. Decreases in heart rate are related to activation of the parasympathetic division, specifically from the vagus nerve (Siddle & Turpin, 1980). For example, during exercise, heart rate increases due to increase in sympathetic activity and overall decrease in activity of the vagus nerve (Wolf, 1979). Heart rate can be influenced by stress, arousal, or emotion as well (Wolf, 1979).

Because heart rate measurements typically use electrodes, which result in a physical connection to the subject, many potential artifact problems exist. Generally, an active electrode is placed on a person's right wrist while a second electrode used as ground is located on the left leg. It is important to obtain adequate contact with the skin, and use of electrode cream is recommended. Extreme care must be taken to prevent ground fault, which would allow a current to flow across the heart. Thus while electrodes placed at various sites permits very accurate measurement, for the purposes of measuring heart rate rather than obtaining cardiac diagnostic profiles, the use of electrodes on a highly localized basis is desirable, rather than on opposing limbs. Another area of concern is movement. Any movement of the electrode or the cable connecting the electrode to the output device can cause artifact in the measure and can significantly affect estimates of heart rate.

An alternative method to measure heart rate is photoelectric plethysmography. *Plethysmography* operates on the basic observation that with every heartbeat there also occurs a change in blood flow to various parts of the body. This change in blood flow can be measured by the change in volume of a particular body part. Typically, a plethysmograph monitors the change in optical density through the skin region (Cromwell, Weibell, Pfeiffer, & Usselman, 1973). Photoelectric plethysmography is a very basic type of plethysmography, which can only measure the arrival time of the blood flow "pulse" that is used as an indicator of heartrate. A photoelectric plethysmograph is typically placed on the subject's fingertip or earlobe. A photocell picks up the light that is reflected by some medium such as bone or deep tissue. As the blood volume increases, less light is able to reach the photocell as it is transmitted through the capillaries. This produces changes in the resistance of the photocell, which can then be recorded. This device is not designed to measure absolute or relative volume, as other types of plethysmographs do.

The photoelectric plethysmograph also has some difficulties. For example, movement of the finger can cause a shift of the photocell or the light source and can thereby add artifact to the measurement (Cromwell et al., 1973). A second source of error results from the light source. Heat can be produced by the light source, and some increase in circulation beneath the light is evident, which will change the resistance of the photocell, producing artifact (Cromwell et al., 1973). However, current devices utilizing light-emitting diode technology effectively address this problem.

## *Electrodermal Activity*

Skin conductance is an indirect measurement of physiological arousal. Because arousal is highly correlated with sweat gland activity, and skin conductance is directly related to sweat gland activity, this chain permits a simple but very useful procedure. In the context of psychophysiology, sweat gland activity is often referred to as the galvanic skin reflex (GSR), or electrodermal activity (EDA) (Fowles, 1986), or as a function of measurement procedures, galvanic skin conductance (GSC). EDA is composed of both slow changes in baseline levels (tonic) and fast changes (phasic responses). Both types of responses are related to sympathetic nervous system activity. Sweat gland secretions are mediated by the sympathetic nervous system in response to acetylcholine (Venables &

Christie, 1980). The secretions contain large amounts of salt, which makes the skin electrically conductive. The more sweat on the skin, the more conductive the skin is to electricity.

The skin is a highly complex organ that serves a variety of functions. These include protecting the internal body from the outside environment, such as acting as a barrier against external chemical substances or preventing physical injury. Further, the skin is important in the regulation of body heat and maintenance of bodily fluids. However, the most important structure in the skin with respect to measurement of EDA is the eccrine sweat glands (Fowles, 1986). These glands are basically tubes of epithelial cells that open onto the skin. The eccrine sweat glands are widely distributed across the body in a nonuniform fashion. Therefore, skin resistance varies at different body sites (Fowles, 1986).

The greatest density of sweat glands is on the soles of the feet and the palms of the hands, and therefore most measurements of electrodermal activity are taken from these regions (Fowles, 1986). Furthermore, these areas do not contain hair follicles or sebaceous glands, which may affect the EDA measurement. While the center of the palm shows greater responsivity than the fingers, placement of electrodes on the palm is more difficult, and movement artifacts are likely as the hand flexes (Venables & Christie, 1980). These can be diminished by firmly fixing the electrodes on the fingers, but the finger site also has problems. Placement on the finger decreases the potential total area with which the electrode can be in contact with the skin, as opposed to the broad areas of the palm or feet (Venables & Christie, 1980). This leads to fewer sweat glands in the current loop, thereby decreasing the absolute skin conductance level (Venables & Christie, 1980). It is therefore important to standardize the placement and the size of the electrode to ensure equally sized areas in contact with the electrode (Lykken & Venables, 1971) and to maximize the comparability of measurements across sessions.

Sweat glands can be schematized as resistors in parallel (Venables & Christie, 1980). Each resistor is analogous to the conductive path of a sweat gland. Each sweat gland can be activated, thus forming a low resistance pathway from the skin to the inner layers; or it can be inactivated, forming a high resistance path to the deeper layers of skin (Venables & Christie, 1980). When electrodes are placed on the skin and a voltage is applied, an electrical circuit is formed. The amplitude of the electric current that flows through this circuit is directly related to the number of sweat glands activated, which is the resistance of the skin (Venables & Christie, 1980).

Two forms of electrical activity of the skin are typically studied. These are endosomatic and the more commonly recorded exosomatic EDA. Physiologists measure exosomatic EDA by passing an external electrical current through the skin to obtain skin conductance (SC) or skin resistance (SR) readings (Venables & Christie, 1980). These indicate the amount of electrical current that the skin will allow to pass. The type of method employed determines whether SC or SR is the outcome measure. SR is linearly related to the voltage change across the skin when a constant current is utilized (Fowles, 1986). Resistance is measured in units of ohms. However, with a constant voltage, the current through the skin is linearly related to SC (Fowles, 1986). Because SC is the reciprocal of SR, the unit of measurement is the mho (unit of skin conductance). With endosomatic EDA, skin potential (SP) is recorded by measuring voltage differences at two points on the skin (Venables & Christie, 1980). A committee report in 1981 recommended the use of SC over SP for a number of reasons (Fowles, Christie, Edelberg, Grings, Lykken, & Venables, 1981). First, SC measures are easier to interpret than the biphasic response of SP. Also, SP responses are more sensitive to minor fluctuations in the hydration of the skin than SC responses. This leads to more artifact in the SP recordings. Further, the simple linear relationship between SC and sweat gland secretion found by Darrow (1964) makes this measure conceptually appealing.

EDA measurement is laden with difficulties, many of which are not readily controlled. Room temperature, humidity, and movement on the part of the subject can alter the skin conductance measurements, making comparisons within a session or across sessions difficult. Increases in room temperature or humidity can activate the thermal regulatory function of the skin (Venables & Christie, 1980). This would stimulate secretion of larger amounts of the sweat and subsequently produce higher skin-conductance-level readings (Venables & Christie, 1980). Another potential problem is movement of the surface on which an electrode is attached, which changes the total area that is in contact with the electrode (Venables & Christie, 1980). This is more pronounced with dry electrodes than with electrodes used in combination with electrode gel. As mentioned earlier, firm attachment reduces this artifact.

Further complications arise from changes in skin condition, such as hydration and electrolyte concentration. For example, skin that is callused tends to be thick and dry, which leads to higher resistance readings and therefore lower skin conductance measures. Also, washing the hands with soap and water removes the salt from the skin, causing decreases in skin conductance readings (Venables & Martin, 1967). This problem can be alleviated by standardizing the procedures such that all participants wash and dry their hands immediately before the electrodes are affixed to the surface (Venables & Christie, 1980).

Further difficulty involves the choice of electrode materials. For example, when DC current loops are used, polarization may occur, thus affecting the skin conductance readings. This problem can be minimized by using Ag/Ag chloride electrodes. These are reversible electrodes, which are considered to have the lowest values of bias and polarization potentials (Venables & Christie, 1980). Reversible electrodes are composed of metal in contact with a solution of the same ions. Therefore, when a current is passed through the electrodes, there is very little chemical reaction (Venables & Christie, 1980), but it is nevertheless wise to routinely check electrodes for bias.

## Assessment and Intervention Examples

### *Relaxation*

While there has been much speculation, as well as intriguing data, concerning the relationship between arousal and anxiety and self-injurious behavior, there has been little formalized in the literature concerning treatment of self-injurious behavior based upon this type of conceptual approach. Therefore, it is all the more interesting to note that the use of relaxation as treatment or as a treatment component for self-injurious behavior has been used for quite some time but without the explicit conceptual underpinning. Thus, because relaxation or counterconditioning procedures would appear to be one very reasonable approach to take with respect to intervention, a number of studies are reviewed briefly that utilized relaxation as a component for intervention. Unfortunately, however, none of these published studies have utilized psychophysiological measurement in conjunction with their intervention programs to assess arousal directly.

Cautela and Baron (1973) report the case of a 20-year-old male college student who engaged in intense self-injurious behavior for a period of 6 months. The subject's eye-rubbing and self-biting had been previously treated by a variety of interventions, including electroshock (electroconvulsive shock treatment—ECT) protective equipment, and medication. At the time of the present intervention, the patient was completely blind, and he had bitten off a portion of his lips. Initially, the investigators examined the eliciting stimuli and the consequences that maintained the behavior. The treatment was designed to decrease the effectiveness of the controlling stimuli and to remove the observable maintaining consequences. The package included a variety of components, such as relaxation, thought stopping, covert sensitization, reinforcement of incompatible behaviors and systematic desensitization. While the success of no one procedure could be assessed in this case, the overall package was highly successful, and maintenance was excellent. The authors conclude that in some situations, several approaches may be necessary to achieve the desired effects and that both the antecedent and consequent events should be targeted.

LeBoeuf (1974) also describes a 23-year-old normal male who exhibited head-banging. The behavior started as rocking when he was an infant but changed to head-banging around the age of 10 years. At the time of the study, the client estimated that he indulged in the self-injurious behavior approximately 4–5 times a day for an average of 15 minutes. The client reported that he engaged in the behavior to relieve tension as well as to overcome boredom. The intensity had increased prior to referral, causing headaches and calluses.

Because the client reported that he engaged in the behavior to relieve tension, the relaxation treatment was implemented first. This included taped relaxation instructions to be used when the subject felt the urge to bang his head. The treatment proved to be ineffective after 2 weeks. Next, an aversive contingency arrangement was tried. Because the client often would bang his head to the rhythm of music while he was lying on the floor, he was required to wear a headband with a pressure sensitive switch linked to an amplifier of a record player. This device would detect a hit to the head and would terminate the music. This approach did extinguish the head-banging associated with being on the floor. However, head-banging was also associated with going to sleep. Again the headband was utilized, but now it was attached to an alarm that sounded when the subject activated it. This method proved highly successful. Extinction of head-banging in both settings was maintained at a 1-year follow-up.

Azrin and Wesolowski (1975) report the case of a 36-year-old woman with profound retardation who exhibited chronic vomiting. This study did not include a specific analysis of possible anxiety-related factors. However, after a 6-week baseline phase, a required relaxation procedure was implemented for 7 days. This method consisted of having the subject remain in her bed for 2 hours after each vomiting episode. It was followed by a time-out intervention phase where the individual was removed to a special room without any furniture where she was required to remain for 30 minutes. Finally, a self-correction procedure was implemented that required the subject was to clean herself and her clothing or bed sheets after every episode. This was followed by positive practice trials of the correct procedure to be followed when the subject felt as if she would vomit.

While the first two phases produced no change in the frequency of the vomiting episodes, the positive practice and self-correction procedures virtually eliminated the behaviors. Because no formal analysis of the maintaining variables was carried out prior to the intervention, an assumption must be made post hoc. Because the self-correction procedure was so effective, the maintaining variables for the vomiting behavior might have been some form of social reinforcement.

Azrin, Gottlieb, Hughart, Wesolowski, and Rahn (1975) studied 11 subjects who all had severe or profound mental retardation with the exception of one client, who was diagnosed as schizophrenic with autistic symptoms. All clients displayed head or face hitting with their hand or fist. Furthermore, visible marks or swelling were evident on all subjects. Some of the clients displayed other forms of self-injurious behavior as well, such as eye gouging, biting, and scratching. Clients ranged in age from 10 to 46 years. The chronicity of self-injurious behavior varied across subjects. Previous interventions included medications, electroconvulsive shock, time-out, and protective equipment. The researchers utilized what they termed "educative procedures," which included four components: (1) positive reinforcement for non-self-injurious behavior, (2) required relaxation, (3) overcorrection including arm and hand exercises, and (4) hand awareness training, designed to help control the self-injurious behavior by teaching incompatible behaviors.

The treatment package greatly decreased self-injurious behavior of the 11 patients in a short amount of time. However, it is not possible to evaluate the effectiveness of the relaxation component because all treatments were implemented. The authors note that relaxation was most effective with clients who displayed "outward-directed" behavior, while the patients who emitted "inward-directed" behavior actually increased self-injurious behavior under these procedures. The authors suggest that the relaxation procedure served as a reinforcer for self-injurious behavior for these inward-directed subjects and actually increased their responding.

A relaxation procedure also was applied by Cox and Klinge (1976), who treated a 20-year-old college female who exhibited severe self-burning and cutting of her arms and her legs. She was previously treated using antidepressant medications, ECT, bioenergetic techniques (diet and excercise) and traditional talk therapy. Analysis of the antecedent and consequent events failed to reveal consistent maintaining variables. The subject did report that the burning behavior was preceded by an "urge to punish" herself and that she felt relieved only when she had inflicted enough pain and physical damage. Therefore, the treatment package included thought-stopping and relaxation training, which were designed to weaken the association between the urge and the actual burning. Another component of the treatment was covert sensitization to pair the behavior with a feeling of nausea. Because the authors believed there was a strong social component, they included assertiveness training and a procedure to decrease negative self-evaluative statements. The package produced a slow decrease in the frequency of the burning episodes, and the subject was able to return to college after a 2-year absence.

Relaxation training was utilized by Steen and Zuriff (1977) with a 21-year-old woman who had profound retardation. The woman exhibited severe biting and scratching and had been placed in full restraint for the 3 years prior to treatment. When the restraints were removed for a brief baseline phase, the subject engaged in high rates of self-injurious behavior. The treatment consisted of gradually training the woman to relax her hand and arm while continually reinforcing her with food, verbal praise, and physical contact. As she was able to learn to relax, more and more restraints were removed. Scratching, a less frequent behavior, was eliminated early on in the training; while the more intense behavior, biting, took much longer to eliminate. The training procedure took a total of 115 sessions to be completed. The procedure was highly effective, and the frequency of self-injurious behavior remained low even at a 1-year follow-up. Furthermore, the staff was able to teach the woman self-help skills now that she was out of restraints. While no specific hypothesis as to the maintaining variables was made, the success of the relaxation training suggests an anxiety component.

Bull and LaVecchio (1978) reported the case of a 10-year-old boy with Lesch–Nyhan syndrome. The boy engaged in such severe self-injury that he was restrained in a wheelchair with his arms in splints. The authors described the treatment as systematic desensitization for the patient's phobic reaction to a lack of restraint. The authors sought to analyze the anxiety-provoking effects of objects associated with the restraint. A traditional desensitization program was then used, as well as exercises in relaxation, which was induced intermittently by nitrous oxide.

Furthermore, the authors suggested an attentional component to both the self-injurious behavior and the wounds that were inflicted. A time-out procedure, where the therapist would leave the room whenever the subject engaged in self-injury, was followed. Also, treatment of any wound was carried out while the boy was anesthetized, so that he did not receive attention that may have been reinforcing. This treatment was quite successful. They authors reported not only a decrease in the frequency of self-injurious behavior but also a decrease in the subject's anxiety level. However, the authors note infrequent continued episodes of self-injurious behavior during what they termed "high-anxiety situations."

Schloss, Smith, Smaldino, Field, Tiffin, and Ramsey (1983) described a teenage boy with a severe hearing impairment who engaged in intense self-injurious behavior. The boy previously was treated using time-out procedures, pharmacotherapy, and insight therapy. The authors suggested several possible hypotheses for the boy's behavior. First, negative comments often elicited the self-injurious behavior. Also, it was proposed that the teenager was unable to predict when positive consequences would occur and therefore he was unable to maintain a "positive attitude." Another possible problem was the boy's inability to relax under stress. Finally, the self-injurious behaviors appeared satisfying to the boy.

Because there were many possible maintaining variables, a multifaceted approach was designed. The program included increasing the positive components in the child's environment, including such things as praise and affection. Also, to increase his ability to predict positive consequences, a more structured schedule was implemented, where aversive and positive events were alternated. The child also underwent specific relaxation training. Finally, a token economy system was implemented, where he could earn specific activities by not engaging in self-injurious behavior for a given amount of time. Over a 1-year period, the package was quite effective. Because this was a multifaceted program, each component cannot be assessed separately. However, within this package of treatment, the relaxation component was utilized to induce a response incompatible with self-injurious behavior.

Kaminer and Shahar (1987) described an unusual case of a 32-year-old woman with severe self-injurious behavior. Initially, she began to cut her hair in a symmetrical fashion every day for long time periods, in response to internal "impulses." This behavior changed to cutting her daughter's hair in this fashion. She was referred for treatment when she injured her daughter during one of these episodes. She was treated in psychodynamic therapy for approximately 4 years, and during this time, she began engaging in severe scratching of the left side of her face.

The authors hypothesized that the behavior was anxiety reducing because it was triggered by looking in the mirror, thinking about her scarred face, and having anxiety-provoking thoughts about her husband. Therefore, the treatment package included several procedures to reduce tension, including relaxation and coping self-verbalizations. The authors also taught her to think of aversive images that could result from the behavior, and she was taught to say the word "stop" and hit her hand down from her face whenever she attempted to scratch. The treatment package was quite successful, and excellent maintenance was obtained. Again, however, with the multifaceted approach, it is not possible to determine the effects of the relaxation component.

## *Cyclicity and Self-injurious Behavior*

Although they are often not taken seriously by scientific investigators, due to distortions in the popular press with often fantastic and exaggerated claims, circadian rhythms are naturally occurring biological oscillations that have a period of approximately 24 hours. Developmentally, adult rhythmicity patterns are seen for most oscillations by 1 year of age, with some displayed much earlier: galvanic skin resistance (GSR) at 1 week, the rest–activity cycle at 16–20 weeks, and internal body temperature cycle at 5–9 months (Hellebrugge, Ehrengut, Rutenfranz, Stehr, 1964). For adults, some complex behavior patterns have also been found to demonstrate a circadian rhythm, such as physiological arousal, as measured by GSR (Doctor & Friedman, 1966), and emotional lability (McFarland, 1975). Several authors have reported on cyclicity and self-injurious behavior, such as Francezon, Visier, and Mennesson (1981) and Lewis, MacLean, Johnson, and Baumeister (1981). Romanczyk, Gordon, Crimmins, Wenzel, and Kistner (1980) observed altered circadian rhythms for a small sample of children with autism and schizophrenia. For the present topic, their data for one of the subjects are particularly intriguing. While the focus of the study was to compare deep body temperature circadian rhythmicity between children labeled "psychotic" versus "normal," the data concerning self-injurious behavior and arousal/attention is our current focus.

The subject was a 5-year-old girl with a diagnosis of psychosis with neurological impairment, receiving a score of 7 out of 9 on the Creak Scale. She was nonverbal, untestable on standard psychometric tests of intellect, and had virtually no self-help skills. There was little play and social behavior, but she seemed to enjoy social and physical contact that was initiated by an adult.

The data for self-injurious behavior and self-stimulatory behavior were quite interesting. The pattern of self-stimulatory behavior appeared consistent in that there was little daily variability in the high rates of this behavior. Only self-injurious behavior showed indication of cyclicity, but with poor day-to-day replication. While self-stimulatory behavior can have an operant component, it did not demonstrate an extinction curve. Such data lend support to researchers such as Berkson (1967), who state that, "most stereotyped acts are organized without important reference to the environment," (p. 2) and it is reasonable to conclude that certain subtypes of self-stimulation may not react to environmental influences. Given the relationship that can exist between self-stimulatory behavior and self-injurious behavior (Romanczyk, in press), it is interesting that, for this subject, the pattern of self-injurious behavior also did not demonstrate an extinction pattern. While previous research has clearly indicated an operant component for self-injurious behavior (Bachman, 1972; Bucher & Lovaas, 1968; Carr, 1977), these data should be seen as complementary rather than contradictory. As with self-stimulatory behavior, certain typographies and/or frequencies of self-injurious behavior do not exhibit functional relationships with environmental events (Romanczyk, in press).

Along with self-injurious behavior, a measure of general activity demonstrated a cyclic pattern with poor day-to-day replication. Sleep periods did demonstrate a consistent pattern, with a short sleep period usually occurring between 16:00 (4:00 P.M.) and 18:00 and a longer sleep period between 3:00 A.M. and 11:00. Thus, this child demonstrated a mixed pattern of rhythmicity with respect to various behaviors, but a stable pattern of body temperature, which can be seen as the anchor variable.

A second study was conducted with the same 5-year-old girl who was the subject in the first study. Axillary temperature was monitored hourly, using a validated thermistor procedure (Romanczyk, Crimmins, Gordon, & Kashinsky, 1977). Concurrently, the subject's psychophysiological reactivity (heart rate and skin conductance) to repeated auditory stimulus presentation was assessed. A computer controlled stimulus delivery and processed and analyzed heart rate and skin conductance data during each trial (for a period of 15 seconds prior to stimulus onset and 15 seconds poststimulus).

Two separate paradigms were used in this investigation, the first a standard habituation–dishabituation paradigm. Fifteen tone presentations were made during each 20-minute session, with tone presentations of 87 dB, 2900 Hz, and 1-second duration made on Trials 1–9 and 11–15. A dishabituation stimulus of 105 dB, broad-band noise, and 1-second duration was presented on the Trial 10. Eight sessions were scheduled over the course of 36 hours, and times were selected to represent different points in the temperature rhythm. The subject was on an ad libitum sleep schedule. A temperature rhythm was evident during the subject's 72-hour stay, with a peak at 20:00 (8:00 P.M.) and a trough at 4:00 A.M.

Psychophysiological measures were taken at 1:00 (1:00 A.M.), 2:10, 11:50, and 16:00 (4:00 P.M.). There was a dramatic difference in cardiac response to the auditory stimulus at different times of day. At 1:00, there was no heart rate change in response to the stimulus. At 2:10, only 70 minutes later, there was clear cardiac acceleration. At 11:50, cardiac deceleration, followed by acceleration in response to the stimulus, was observed.

GSC was recorded concurrently with heart rate during each 30-second sampling period. Mean SC level in micromhos (1 micromho = 1 millionth of a mho) was measured, and the number of skin conductance responses (SCRs) during the pre- and poststimulus intervals for each trial was calculated.

There were no SCRs observed in any of the prestimulus periods. There were also no SCRs noted in the poststimulus periods at 1:00 and 11:50, but SCRs were observed in the poststimulus periods at 2:10 and 16:00, the two sessions where both higher mean SC levels and cardiac acceleration occurred.

Although only mentioned briefly in the Romanczyk et al. (1980) study, Romanczyk (in press) reports additional data indicating that specific intervention for self-stimulation had effectiveness and side effects as a function of the time of day during which it was implemented. Utilizing a multiple stimulus design, where intervention and free operant sessions were conducted in an alternating sequence for both morning and afternoon sessions, specifically for the morning sessions it was found that when self-stimulation was punished, self-stimulation was substantially reduced, while self-injurious behavior remained at the levels comparable to the morning free operant rates. However, with identical procedures implemented in the afternoon hours, punishment of self-stimulatory behavior not only resulted in substantial reduction of self-stimulatory behavior, but also resulted in virtually complete suppression of self-injurious behavior. Further, simultaneous measurement of GSC activity also demonstrated dramatic changes, with a mean level of 10.9 micromhos observed in the morning sessions, and a mean level of 1.4 micromhos observed in the afternoon hours. Thus, concurrence was seen for both the behavioral and the physiological measures in terms of interaction with time of day. While such correlational results present difficulty of interpretation, in context, such findings raise intriguing questions as to relationships of physiological factors and interaction with treatment modality, timing, and outcome.

## *Case Illustrations*

Kohlenberg, Levin, and Belcher, (1973) studied the relationship between self-injurious behavior and GSC for a 7-year-old girl who had severe mental retardation, was nonverbal, and had been in restraint for several years because of the severity of her self-injurious behavior. This was an experimental investigation, as opposed to a clinical intervention. Consistent with the model presented earlier concerning arousal, they found consistent increase in GSC level when restraints were removed. However, they state that based on their data, "The lack of relationship, however, between rates of self-destructive behavior or amount of increase in skin conductance level to the initial arousal levels measured immediately before removal of restraints, does not support the arousal hypothesis. That is, if an optimal arousal level is responsible for self-destructive behavior, then higher initial values of arousal should result in lower rates of self-destruction. The data do not support such a contention" (p. 13).

The authors appeared to have conceptualized self-injurious behavior as the mechanism to produce arousal within an arousal modulation hypothesis, as opposed to viewing arousal as a contributing factor in the elicitation and maintenance of self-injurious behavior. When viewed in the context of the complex behavioral model presented earlier, their data are quite consistent.

Also of importance with respect to the Kohlenberg et al. (1973) study was that contingent electric shock was used during the experimental intervention phase to decrease the frequency of self-injurious behavior. During their experimental sessions, self-injurious behavior rapidly decreased to zero frequency, and the authors were interested in whether arousal levels as measured by GSC would rise proportionately, thus indicating that contingent electric shock was serving an arousal-increasing function and therefore substituting for the self-injurious behavior. This, in fact, did not take place and as the authors state that "the punishment and subsequent reduction in rates of self-destructive behavior did not produce effects on arousal similar to those observed for self-destructive behavior itself. Therefore, it does not appear that punishment is simply a substitute arousal producing stimulus for self-destructive behavior" (p. 13).

In an extensive, long-term treatment program for extremely severe self-injurious behavior (Romanczyk, in press) presents a case study for which physiological measurement was utilized during both the assessment and the intervention procedure. Given that the young woman displaying self-injurious behavior was, at the time of initial intervention, in 24-hour complete restraint and that the intensity of her self-injurious behavior was such that severe tissue damage resulted immediately when restraints were removed, the approach to functional analysis and assessment had to be undertaken that was different from the norm. In this context, psychophysiological measurement was utilized as an indicator of arousal given that there appeared to be concern that the limited overt behavior on the part of the individual was adequately representative of actual arousal state. During the assessment period, heart rate and skin conductance were measured during periods of offering various food items that apparently the individual preferred, as well as engaging in limited activities and stimulation exercises. In this manner, it was possible to gauge both by the individual's verbal behavior, as well as physiological monitoring, a crude hierarchy of preferred items and also activities that appeared to elicit high levels of arousal that could be counterproductive to intervention. It was hypothesized that high arousal levels could interfere with conditioning trials and, therefore, should be avoided. An assessment was also performed regarding reaction to the various restraints utilized and to the various sites on her body. Thus, it became quickly apparent that manipulation of ankle and leg restraints produced far less arousal than manipulation of torso restraints, which, in turn, were less arousing than arm and hand restraints, and chin and head restraint produced a maximum level of arousal.

Initial intervention procedures utilized the psychophysiological monitoring in an on-line biofeedback type of paradigm where the feedback was not directed primarily at the individual, but rather at the therapist. This was done in order to attempt to modulate arousal levels and to proceed at a pace that would minimize displays of self-injury and maximize the learning taking place in conditioning trials. Contingent electric shock was used to suppress self-injurious behavior and as Kohlenberg et al. (1973) found, the application of contingent electric shock per se did not either produce the highest arousal levels or even increase general arousal levels. Rather, the consistent pairing of contingent electric shock with self-injurious behavior resulted in clear patterns of arousal reduction. However, through the use of this feedback mechanism, the absolute number of applications of contingent electric shock were kept at a very low level, and the author hypothesized that by utilizing observation of both the individual's behavior as well as arousal level, that it provided the clinician with sufficient information to maximize learning while minimizing the number of trials required. This, of course, is speculative, as it is not possible within a single-subject design to ascertain whether, in fact, the outcome could have been significantly different in the absence of physiological monitoring. However, given the gravity of the individual's self-injurious behavior, the extreme history of restraint, as well as the concerns within an arousal–anxiety model for a stimulus such as contingent electric shock to "energize" and to thus provide higher levels of arousal, all these factors made the use of psychophysiological monitoring appropriate and desirable. Certainly, continued research will be necessary in order to ascertain the precise functional valuc of such procedures.

For two individuals having less severe, non-life-threatening self-injurious behavior, a similar paradigm has been used, for both a 3-year-old girl classified as autistic and a 10-year-old girl with a dual classification of mental retardation and schizophrenia. In both instances, GSC was used as the measure of choice, as heart rate was much more difficult to obtain and was fraught with artifact and difficulty of interpretation. GSC, however, proved to be very stable and relatively easy to obtain, although the problem nevertheless persists with individuals who are displaying severe behavior problems, to fashion a procedure in which they will comply with wearing electrodes and not disturb them.

In the instance of the 3-year-old girl, her self-injurious behavior was quite intense with respect to biting fingers and self-slapping, as well as occasional head-banging, and the self-injurious behavior appeared quite episodic and not easily tied to environmental events, other than that it occurred more in social/teaching contexts rather than isolate activities. Initially, psychophysiological monitoring was attempted in the context of a teacher engaging in habilitative activities. Some overall patterns emerged such that high arousal levels tended to precede bouts of self-injurious behavior. However, the pattern was more of interest rather than clinically significant. Subjectively, there still appeared to be some variation and cyclicity to her behavior, although not a stable pattern. The child had a sporadic history of ear infections, and given the occasional relationship between ear infections and self-injurious behavior, consultation was obtained with the child's physician to ensure that it was not a current problem, but testing was negative. However, given that the child was reasonably compliant with the assessment procedures, tympanograms were obtained on a daily basis. A *tympanogram* simply records the pressure on the eardrum, which, in turn, is reflective of various medical conditions, most important of which in the present context was inner-ear infections. The tympanogram is a very sensitive measure but is typically used only for routine screening and not on such a frequent daily basis. Interestingly, over the course of several weeks, it was found that, in fact, there were extremely wide variations in the tympanogram and it appeared that the child was experiencing strong inner ear pressure in the absence of easily diagnosed external signs of ear infection. Consultation with the physician resulted in a more aggressive medication regimen, and subsequent levels of intensity of self-injurious behavior began to attenuate.

This type of assessment indicates the complexity of variables associated with self-injury, and it should be underscored that, in this case in particular, this process did not result in the elimination of self-injurious behavior but rather produced greater insight into some of the cyclical aspects of the behavior and allowed attenuation of its frequency. Other aspects of the self-injurious behavior were found to be clearly under the control of demand and frustration situations, and thus a multifaceted treatment program was necessary.

For the second child, self-injurious behavior was very intense and often resulted in bleeding wounds and disfigurement. In addition to the more severe self-injurious behavior, she also would frequently pull out her hair such that it was routinely kept quite short, but still had numerous bald spots. In addition to the lacerations she produced, she would also engage in extremely intense head-banging that was cause for grave concern for her physical safety. She would often engage in self-restraint by wrapping her arms within her shirt and sitting with legs folded. This child would often avoid interaction with other individuals, but at other times, she would approach them and quite violently begin to engage in aggressive behavior. Many of these events were characterized as "unpredictable," and she presented an extreme treatment problem for her parents and the staff at the residential facility she attended. She also was quite verbal and could engage in limited conversations but would lapse into very bizarre psychotic speech and would appear to have hallucinations. She had participated in an extreme range of polypharmacy for both self-injurious and aggressive behaviors, with little apparent result.

The assessment process was similar to the previously reported cases in which GSC was utilized, and assessment took place in a structured teaching situation. Here, the results tended to confirm the initial clinical impression, in that arousal levels rose precipitously in response to physical contact and close physical proximity. Somewhat paradoxically, however, rises in arousal could also be seen after periods of quiescence or noninteraction with an individual. However, this turned out to be simply complementary aspects of the same factor: She had extreme difficulty modulating any form of arousal and at one and the same time was both attention seeking as well as contact avoiding.

The initial intervention procedure was simply to establish a very low demand situation in a small treatment intervention room where only the child and a therapist were present, and efforts were made to keep gross stimulation levels at a minimum but also not to retreat from aggressive and self-injurious behavior episodes. These responses were simply blocked, and the person neither intruded further nor withdrew. A reduction in such outbursts was seen and given this reduction, it was possible to observe reliable behavioral patterns. A program of in vivo systematic desensitization occurred, in which she was taught to tolerate closer and closer physical proximity, task demand, social interaction, and general "commotion." By permitting her a very clearly designated physical space in which she could literally retreat, she was taught to modulate her arousal by changing the physical distance between her and the other children and staff. Slowly, over time, self-control was encouraged through the use of a symbolic system in which she could earn time to be by herself for greater and greater tolerance of social interaction and physical contact. During this period, a telemetric device was utilized to transmit GSC measurement to a computer in the classroom that monitored arousal level on-line and could display a continuous visual display for staff in order to assist in choreographing the classroom situation, not to minimize arousal, but rather to ensure that it was kept at a moderate level for which she could exert control and achieve success.

## Summary

It is important to point out that as with most instances of severe self-injurious behavior, the intervention programs described were complex and multifaceted. Also, problems arose with the use of psychophysiological measurement, as oftentimes the individual's boredom, curiosity, or displeasure with wearing the monitoring electrodes could serve in itself to precipitate an inappropriate interaction, and thus, such procedures could only be used sporadically. Nevertheless, such information served to both enhance and confirm more typical observational and performance information and thus served as an important adjunct in the treatment of difficult and intense self-injurious behavior and particularly where the maintaining factors were multifaceted.

Sensitivity to possible physiological variables that influence both etiology and maintenance of self-injurious behavior is advocated. Investigation of such variables need not automatically lead to use of medication as opposed to behavioral, educative procedures as illustrated in the examples. However, the more selective and accurate use of appropriate pharmacology could also result as the determination of causative factors is expanded. Further, factors related to pain perception and drug effects may also assist in understanding important interaction of behavioral and pharmacological intervention (e.g., Durand, 1982).

Focus upon the individual's characteristics that sets the person apart with respect to unique abilities, learning history, biological status, physiological response patterns, reaction to stimuli and events, and speed and capacity for change must take precedence over focus upon specific treatment approaches, techniques, or ideologies. Emphasis must be placed upon assessment to determine the specific etiological and maintaining factors for self-injurious behavior rather than simply evaluating treatment effects in a trial-and-error fashion). From this assessment and analysis, treatment procedures are then derived that address, in the most expedient manner possible, the *individual's* treatment needs, while weighing and balancing the important factors of the individual's reaction, possible side effects of intervention, speed of effect, social acceptability, potential for success, resources available for treatment, and distress. In this process, appropriate investigation of physiological variables may add significant clinical incremental information.

## *References*


Azrin, N. H., Gottlieb, L., Hughart, L., Wesolowski, M. D., & Rahn, T. (1975). Eliminating self-injurious behavior by educative procedures. *Behaviour Research and Therapy*, *13*, 101–111.

Azrin, N. H., & Wesolowski, M. D.(1975). Eliminating habitual vomiting in a retarded adult by positive practice and self-correction. *Journal of Behavior Therapy and Experimental Psychiatry*, *6*, 145–148.

Bachman, J. A. (1972). Self-injurious behavior: A behavioral analysis. *Journal of Abnormal Psychology*, *80*, 211–224.

Baumeister, A. A., & Rollings, J. P. (1976). Self-injurious behavior. In N. R Ellis (Ed.), International review of research in mental retardation, Vol. 8. NY: Academia Press.

Berkson, G. (1967). Development of abnormal stereotyped behaviors. *Developmental Psychology*, *1*, 118–132.

Blair, D. A., Glover, W. F., Greenfield, A. D. M., & Roddie, I. C. (1959). Excitation of cholinergic vasodilator nerves to human skeletal muscles during emotional stress. *Journal of Physiology*, *148*, 633–47.

Bucher, B., & Lovaas, O. I. (1968). Use of aversive stimulation in behavior modification. In M. Jones (Ed.), *Miami Symposium on the Prediction of Behavior, 1967: Aversive stimulation* (pp. 77–145). Coral Gables, FL: University of Miami Press.

Bull, M., & LaVecchio, F. (1978). Behavior therapy for a child with Lesch–Nyhan syndrome. *Developmental Medicine & Child Neurology*, *20*(3), 368–375.

Cain, A. C. (1961). The presuperego turning inward of aggression. *Psychoanalytic Quarterly*, *30*, 171–208.

Carr, E. G. (1977). The motivation of self-injurious behavior: A review of some hypotheses. *Psychological Bulletin*, *84*, 800–816.

Carr, E. G., & McDowell, J. J. (1980). Social control of self-injurious behavior of organic etiology. *Behavior Therapy*, *11*, 402–409.

Cataldo, M. F., & Harris, J. (1982). The biological basis for self-injury in the mentally retarded. *Analysis and Intervention in Developmental Disabilities*, *2*(1), 21–39.

Cautela, J. P., & Baron, M. G. (1973). Multifaceted behavior therapy of self-injurious behavior. *Journal of Behavior Therapy and Experimental Psychiatry*, *4*, 125–131.

Cox, M. D., & Klinge, V. (1976). Treatment and management of a case of self-burning. *Behaviour Research and Therapy*, *4*, 201–213.

Cromwell, L., Weikell, F. J., Pfeiffer, E. A., & Usselman, L. B. (1973). *Biomedical instrumentation and measurements*. Englewood Cliffs, NJ: Prentice-Hall.

Darrow, C. W. (1964). The rationale for treating the change in galvanic skin response as a change in conductance. *Psychophysiology*, *1*, 31–38.

Davenport, R. K., & Menzel, E. W. (1963). Stereotyped behavior in the infant chimpanzee. *Archives of General Psychiatry*, *8*, 99–104.

Davis, R. C., Buchwarld, A. M., & Frankmann, R. W. (1955). Autonomic and muscular responses and their relation to simple stimuli. *Psychological Monographs*, *69*, 1–71.

DeLissovoy, V. (1963). Head banging in early childhood: A suggested cause. *Journal of Genetic Psychology*, *102*, 109–114.

Doctor, R. F., & Friedman, L. F. (1966). Thirty-day stability of spontaneous galvanic skin responses in man. *Psychophysiology*, *2*, 311–315.

Durand, V. M. (1982). Analysis and intervention of self-injurious behavior. *Journal of the Association for the Severely Handicapped*, *7*, 44–53.

Farber, J. (1987). Psychopharmacology of self-injurious behavior in the mentally retarded. *Journal of American Academy of Child and Adolescent Psychiatry*, *26*(3), 296–302.

Favell, J. E., McGimsey, J. F., & Schell, R. M. (1982). Treatment of self-injury by providing alternate sensory activities. *Analysis and Intervention in Developmental Disabilities*, *2*(1), 83–104.

Fowles, D. C. (1986). The accrine system and electrodermal activity. In M. G. H. Coles, E. Donchin, & S. W. Porges, (Eds.), *Psychophysiology systems, processes, and applications*. New York: Guilford Press.

Fowles, D. C., Christie, M. J., Edelberg, R., Grings, W. W., Lykken, D. T., & Venables, P. H. (1981). Committee report: Publication recommendations for electrodermal measurements. *Psychophysiology*, *18*, 232–239.

Francezon, J., Visier, J. P., & Mennesson, J. F. (1981). Circannual fluctuation of a sterotype behaviour with possible self-mutilation in a mentally deficient adolescent. *International Journal of Chronobiology*, *7*(3), 129–140.

Frankel, F., & Simmons, J. Q. (1976). Self-injurious behavior in schizophrenic and retarded children. *American Journal of Mental Deficiency*, *80*, 512–522.

Gluck, J. P., & Sackett, G. P. (1974). Frustration and self-aggression in social isolate rhesus monkeys. *Journal of Abnormal Psychology*, *83*, 331–334.

Harkness, J. E., & Wagner, J. E. (1975). Self-mutilation in mice associated with otitis media. *Laboratory Animal Science*, *25*, 315–318.

Hellebrugge, R., Ehrengut, L. J., Rutenfranz, J., & Stehr, K. (1964). Circadian periodicity of physiological functions in different stages of infancy and childhood. *Ann. N. Y. Academy Science*, *117*, 361–373.

Hollis, J. H. (1965a). The effects of social and nonsocial stimuli on the behavior of profoundly retarded children: I. *American Journal of Mental Deficiency*, *69*, 755–771.

Hollis, J. H. (1965b). The effects of social and nonsocial stimuli on the behavior of profoundly retarded children: II. *American Journal of Mental Deficiency*, *69*, 772–789.

Kaminer, Y., & Shahar, A. (1987). The stress inoculation training management of self-mutilating behavior. *Journal Behavior Therapy & Experimental Psychiatry*, *18*(3), 289–292.

Kohlenberg, R. J., Levin, M., & Belcher, S. (1973). Skin conductance changes and the punishment of self-destructive behavior: A case study. *Mental Retardation*, *11*, 11–13.

Lapierre, Y. D., & Reesal, R. (1986). Pharmacologic management of aggressivity and self-mutilation in the mentally retarded. *Psychiatric Clinics in North America*, *9*(4), 745–754.

LeBoeuf, A. (1974). Aversive treatment of headbanging in a normal adult. *Journal of Behavior Therapy and Experimental Psychiatry*, *5*, 197–199.
Levinson, C. A. (1970). The development of headbanging in a young rhesus monkey. *American Journal of Mental Deficiency*, *75*, 323–328.
Lewis, M. A., MacLean, W. E., Johnson, W. L., & Baumeister, A. A. (1981). Ultradian rhythmns in stereotyped and self-injurious behavior. *American Journal of Mental Deficiency*, *85*, 601–610.
Lykken, D. T., & Venables, P. H. (1971). Direct measurement of skin conductance: A proposal for standardization. *Psychophysiology*, *8*, 656–672.
Malmo, R. B., & Shagass, C. (1949). Physiologic study of symptom mechanisms in psychiatric patients under stress. *Psychophysiology*, *Med.*, *11*, 25–9.
McFarland, R. A. (1975). Air travel across time zones. *American Scientist*, *63*, 23–30.
Menninger, K. (1935). A psychoanalytic study of the significance of self-mutilations. *Psychoanalytic Quarterly*, *4*, 408–466.
Meyerson, L., Kerr, N., & Michael, J. L. (1967). Behavior modification in rehabilitation. In S. W. Bijou & D. M. Baer (Eds.), *Child development: Readings in experimental analysis* (pp. 214–239). New York: Appleton–Century–Crofts.
Newsom, C. D., Carr, E. G., & Lovaas, O. I. (1977). The experimental analysis and modification of autistic behavior. In R. S. Davidson (Ed.), *Modification of Pathological behavior* (pp. 109–187). New York: Gardner Press.
Romanczyk, R. G. (1986). Self-injurious behavior: Conceptualization, assessment and treatment. In K. D. Gadow (Ed.), *Advances in learning and behavioral disabilities*. Greenwich, CT: JAI Press.
Romanczyk, R. G. (1989). A review of the literature on self-injurious behavior: Factors that should influence clinical decision making. *In Proceedings of the NIH Consensus Development Conference on Treatment of Destructive Behaviors in Persons with Developmental Disabilities*. Rockville, MD: National Institutes of Health.
Romanczyk, R. G. (in press). *Self-injurious behavior: Etiology and treatment*. New York: Plenum Press.
Romanczyk, R. B., Crimmins, D. B., Gordon, W. C., & Kashinsky, W. M. (1977). Measuring circadian cycles: A simple temperature recording preparation. *Behavior Research Methods & Instrumentation*, *9*, 393–394.
Romanczyk, R. G., Gordon, W. C., Crimmins, D. B., Wenzel, A. M., & Kistner, J. A. (1980). Childhood psychosis and 24-hour rhythms: A behavioral and psychophysiological analysis. *Chronobiologia*, *7*, 1–14.
Romanczyk, R. G., & Goren, E. R. (1975). Severe self-injurious behavior: The problem of clinical control. *Journal of Consulting and Clinical Psychology*, *43*, 730–739.
Romanczyk, R. G., Kistner, J. A., & Plienis, A. (1982). Self-stimulatory and self-injurious behavior: Etiology and treatment. In J. Steffen & J. J. Karoly (Eds.), *Advances in child behavior analysis and therapy* (pp. 189–254). Lexington, MA: Lexington Books.
Schloss, P. J., Smith, M., Smaldino, S., Field, M., Tiffin, R., & Ramsey, D. (1983). Social learning treatment of self-injurious and aggressive behaviors of a hearing impaired youth. *Journal of Rehabilitation of the Deaf*, *17*(2), 16–22.

Siddle, D. A., & Turpin, G. (1980). Measurement, quantification, and analysis of cardiac activity. In I. Martin & P. H. Venables, (Eds.), *Techniques in psychophysiology*. New York: Wiley.

Singh, N. N., & Millichamp, C. J. (1984). Effects of medication on the self-injurious behavior of mentally retarded persons. *Psychiatric Aspects of Mental Retardation Reviews*, *3*(4), 13–16.

Steen, P. L., & Zuriff, G. E. (1977). The use of relaxation in the treatment of self-injurious behavior. *Journal of Behavior Therapy and Experimental Psychiatry*, *8*, 447–448.

Sternbach, R. A. (1960). A comparative analysis of autonomic responses in startle. *Psychosomatic Medicine*, *22*, 204–10.

Tinklepaugh, O. L. (1928). The self-mutilation of a male macacus monkey. *Journal of Mammalogy*, *9*, 293–300.

Venables, P. H., & Christie, M. J. (1980). Electrodermal activity. In I. Martin & P. H. Venables (Eds.), *Techniques in psychophysiology*. New York: Wiley.

Venables, P. H., & Martin, I. (1967). The relation of palmar sweat gland activity to level of skin potential and conductance. *Psychophysiology*, *3*, 302–311.

Wolf, S. (1979). Anatomical and physiological basis for biofeedback. In J. V. Basmajian (Ed.), *Biofeedback—Principles and practices for clinicians*. Baltimore, MD Williams and Wilkins.

# 5
# Functional Analysis and Treatment of Self-injury

F. CHARLES MACE, JOSEPH S. LALLI, and MICHAEL C. SHEA

Self-injurious behavior (SIB) is perhaps the most severe behavior problem encountered by mental health professionals. The debilitating and often life-threatening nature of SIB has attracted considerable research and discussion regarding the etiology and treatment of the disorder (see Carr, 1977; Favell et al., 1982a; Frankel & Simmons, 1976; Matson & Taras, 1989; Picker, Poling, & Parker, 1979; Schroeder, Schroeder, Rojahn, & Mulick, 1981). Yet, despite this attention, there are few behavior problems that have moved researchers and practitioners to adopt interventions that are as highly controversial as those used to treat SIB. Among the treatments used to suppress self-injury are overcorrection (Harris & Romanczyk, 1976), physical and mechanical restraint (Favell, McGimsey, & Jones, 1978; Luiselli, 1986; Pace, Iwata, Edwards, & McCosh, 1986) aversive electrical stimulation (Iwata, 1988), applications of various noxious stimuli (Tanner & Zeiler, 1975), and highly sedative medications (Altmeyer, Locke, Griffen, Ricketts, Williams, Mason, & Stark, 1987; Ferguson & Breuning, 1982). The restrictive and intrusive nature of many SIB treatments reflects both the immediate extraordinary needs of the population, as well as our limited understanding of the behavioral etiology of self-injury (Iwata, 1988).

Many believe that advances in nonaversive treatment will follow from increased knowledge of how the environment influences self-injury (Axelrod, 1987; Durand & Carr, 1985). Behavior analysis has led this field with testable conceptualizations of the etiology of self-injury that focus on the role that reinforcement contingencies play in the development and maintenance of SIB (Bachman, 1972; Carr, 1977; Skinner, 1953). During the past 10 years, the methods of the experimental analysis of behavior have been used to investigate theoretical accounts of the operant basis of self-injury. This approach of analyzing behavior–environment interactions has become known as the *functional analysis of behavior*. Functional analysis methods have been used to analyze a wide range of aberrant behaviors, including SIB, often leading to the design of treatment procedures that are linked to a behavior analysis of the problem

(Axelrod, 1987; Carr, 1977; Durand & Carr, 1985; Favell et al., 1982a; Mace, Lalli, & Pinter, 1991; Newsom, in press).

A functional analysis approach to the study and treatment of self-injury offers several unique benefits to the field of severe behavior disorders. First, in many respects, functional analysis research is basic research in applied settings. Because a principal goal of this approach is to empirically identify functional relations between specific environmental events and SIB, functional analysis research creates a data base that describes the nature of self-injury. Unlike treatment evaluation studies and basic research with animals, functional analysis research can shed light on the fundamental operant processes that support aberrant behavior in non-laboratory settings. Second, by linking treatment development to an understanding of how a particular environment maintains SIB, intervention procedures tend to be parsimonious and tailored to the individual case. This contrasts with treatment selection based on evaluation studies in which the goal is to use the least restrictive intervention that has proven to be effective with a given population and target behavior. Finally, analysis-derived interventions tend to be less intrusive than many other treatments for self-injury (Axelrod, 1987; Demchak & Halle, 1985). Strategies aimed at interrupting the maintaining contingencies and at teaching adaptive responses with the same function as self-injury can rely less on aversive contingencies to suppress maladaptive behavior.

Our goal in this chapter is to provide an overview of functional analysis methods, with particular attention to applications with self-injurious behavior. We review the classes of variables shown or believed to control self-injury and describe a comprehensive functional analysis methodology. We begin, however, with a discussion of the characteristics of SIB that merit special consideration when embarking on a functional analysis.

## Important Characteristics of Self-injury

SIB has several features that combine to pose unique and formidable challenges to behavior analysts. In general, we believe that functional analysis and treatment of self-injury is more likely to meet with success when these features of SIB are considered during both the analysis and the treatment phases. Most of the challenges posed by SIB arise either directly or indirectly from the topographies of behavior that constitute self-injury. Although numerous forms of SIB have been reported, their common denominator is responses that result in self-inflicted damage to tissue or physiological function. This includes (a) self-striking, (b) biting, pinching, scratching, poking, or pulling various body parts, (c) repeated vomiting or vomiting and re-ingesting food, and (d) consuming inedible substances (Favell et al., 1982a).

These topographical features of self-injury make it a highly effective response. Environments that are unresponsive to milder forms of aberrant behavior are often compelled to react to self-injury in a manner that may reinforce the behavior. For example, several studies have noted that clients' self-injury was preceded either developmentally or contiguously by tantrums (e.g., Edelson, 1984). Whereas caregivers may have been able to ignore or maintain task-related demands in the face of tantrumous behavior, the change in response topography to self-injury can elicit visceral reactions from observers as few other aberrant behaviors can. Moreover, the reactions of caregivers may be motivated by powerful escape contingencies. For many, observing a person engage in SIB is a highly aversive event. Any action on the part of the caregiver which terminates the self-injury, albeit temporarily, is likely to be negatively reinforced. Moreover, this can occur despite the caregiver's knowledge that his or her response to self-injury may maintain the behavior (Anderson, Dancis, & Alpert, 1978; Carr & McDowell, 1980).

The capacity of SIB to evoke responses from others has important implications for analysis and treatment of the disorder. First, self-injury that has evolved through a shaping process of differential reinforcement of increasingly extreme forms of aberrant behavior may eventually be maintained by a thin schedule of reinforcement. Many caregivers may be able to resist responding to SIB temporarily but not indefinitely. In such cases, the consequences maintaining the behavior may occur too intermittently to be detected by a functional analysis.

Second, the capacity of SIB to compel reactions from others suggests that interventions include treatment components, in addition to extinction, that prescribe specific actions on the part of the caregiver. Placing self-injury on extinction without other interventions to discourage SIB or to increase alternative behavior would probably result in initial higher rates of harmful behavior that may not be justified. Caregivers should receive specific training on how to respond to SIB to minimize possible reinforcement effects when the severity of the behavior necessitates a response. For these reasons, a physician should closely monitor each client's medical condition throughout the analysis and treatment process (Iwata, Dorsey, Slifer, Bauman, & Richman, 1982).

Third, there are many cases in which a client's self-injurious behavior is of such severity that it is unethical to allow the behavior to occur freely. However, conducting a functional analysis of self-injury requires that the response be observed under various environmental conditions until a pattern of differential responding emerges. Necessary abbreviation of this process due to ethical considerations may unfortunately result in an incomplete analysis and inadequate information upon which to design an intervention.

A final characteristic of self-injury that may affect a functional analysis is that, for some cases, there is a clear association between SIB and specific medical conditions. Most behavior problems may be considered primarily operant in nature. Because the aberrant behavior was probably shaped and maintained by its consequences, a functional analysis of reinforcement contingencies may permit good prediction and control of the problem behavior. However, some cases of SIB occur with predictable topographies coincident with specific medical conditions, such as Lesch–Nyhan syndrome (Lesch & Nyhan, 1964) and, to a lesser extent, Cornelia de Lange syndrome (Bryson, Sakati, Nyhan, & Fish, 1971), and it can be a cofactor of other conditions, such as otitis media (De Lissovoy, 1963), contact dermatitis, and impaired pain mechanisms (Cataldo & Harris, 1982). For these individuals, an operant analysis alone may not account for the occurrence of self-injury.

This is not to say that the environment does not influence the behavior of a client whose biological condition may precipitate self-injury, in ways that can be predicted by an operant analysis. For example, individuals with Lesch–Nyhan syndrome, a sex-linked genetic disorder, engage generally in lip-, tongue-, and finger-biting. Yet, despite the clear relationship between this medical condition and SIB, the frequency of self-injury has been shown to vary considerably and predictably with environmental changes (Anderson et al., 1978; Duker, 1975).

The obstacle to effective analysis and treatment of self-injury with a correlated biological factor is that at least a portion of the processes maintaining SIB may be either unknown, unobservable, and/or difficult to interrupt. Accordingly, a functional analysis may yield inconclusive findings, such as undifferentiated responding across environmental conditions (Iwata et al., 1982), or may prove difficult to reduce to acceptable levels. Advances in medical treatments may at some point neutralize biological factors and permit a more conclusive analysis of the social contingencies that may have developed to maintain SIB. However, medical intervention alone may be insufficient to eliminate a response with a history of influencing the environment in a predictable manner (Carr & McDowell, 1980; Favell et al., 1982a).

## Variables Controlling Self-injury

Carr (1977) reviewed available experimental research, case studies, and anecdotal reports concerning possible motivational hypotheses for self-injury. In his comprehensive critique of existing evidence, he found support for three major propositions: (1) Self-injury is an operant behavior maintained by positive social reinforcement (positive reinforcement hypothesis); (2) self-injury is an operant behavior maintained by the termination of an aversive stimulus (negative reinforcement hypothesis); and (3) self-injury is maintained by the production of sensory stimulation (sensory reinforcement hypothesis). These hypotheses provided a conceptual framework that stimulated considerable research aimed primarily at identifying variables that were functionally related to self-injury. Many studies further evaluated the effectiveness of treatments derived from the functional analysis findings. As the research evolved, the methodology used to study functional relations was refined and extended to the analysis and treatment of a wide range of maladaptive behaviors (Axelrod, 1987; Mace et al., 1991).

In this section, we review recent developments in functional analysis research, most of which followed Carr's (1977) seminal review. We summarize the major research findings in support of each of the preceding hypotheses, as well as a recent hypothesis concerning the communicative function of aberrant behavior, including self-injury.

## Attention

*Attention* refers to a broad class of social responses others have to a individual's behavior. The topography of these social responses can vary greatly from a mild disapproving look or comment to a loud admonishing reprimand, from a look of sympathetic concern to a physical embrace and expression of sorrowful consolation, and from an inconspicuous prompt to engage in constructive activity to the programmatic redirection of a misbehaving client. Although varied in form, such responses may have a common functional relationship to aberrant behaviors such as self-injury. Attention in this case is a reaction to aberrant behavior, or stated alternatively, it is the consequence of aberrant behavior.

When the contingent relationship between SIB and attention results in a maintenance or increase in the class of self-injurious responses that produce attention, self-injury is maintained, at least in part, by positive reinforcement (Skinner, 1938). The potential for aberrant behavior to be positively reinforced by attention is especially acute for persons with developmental disabilities (Picker et al., 1979). Frequently, these individuals have limited adaptive repertoires and are subjected to environments with sparse social interaction. When inconspicuous or innocuous behaviors go unnoticed by caregivers, conditions are conducive for response topographies to vary until a response occurs that produces reinforcement. Environments that are particularly unresponsive to adaptive behavior and generally, but not consistently, ignore maladaptive behavior, can foster extreme topographies, which may culminate in self-injury.

For ethical reasons, laboratory studies with animals have provided the only experimental evidence that the onset and maintenance of self-injurious behavior can be attributed exclusively to environmental contingencies. For example, Shaefer (1970) used a shaping process to initiate the occurrence of head-hitting in an adult rhesus monkey in 12–20 minutes by differentially reinforcing approximations of self-injury with food pellets. Initially, reinforcement was delivered for raising a paw, then positioning the paw above the head, and finally, bringing the paw down on the head. In a subsequent experiment, sympathetic comments were provided to the monkey only during sessions in which self-injury was reinforced with food. Sessions of nonreinforcement were paired with ignoring the monkey. This procedure resulted in social responses to self-injury becoming discriminative for the delivery of reinforcement.

Indirect evidence for the hypothesis that human aberrant behavior may be positively reinforced by attention comes from several studies in which withholding social responses to aberrant behavior resulted in a decrease in maladaptive behavior. Ayllon and Michael (1959) conducted one of the first empirical studies that extinguished clinically aberrant behavior by withholding attention. When nursing staff stopped replying to the bizarre speech of a woman in a psychiatric hospital, the rate of her bizarre comments dropped sharply. This general strategy of withholding attention was extended to self-injury by either removing sources of social consequences for SIB (e.g., Budd, Green, & Baer, 1976; Ferster, 1961; Lovaas & Simmons, 1969; Tate & Baroff, 1966) or removing the client from the source of social reinforcement via time-out contingent on the occurrence of SIB (e.g., Carr & McDowell, 1980; Hamilton, Stephens, & Allen, 1967; Romanczyk & Goren, 1975; White, Nielsen, & Johnson, 1972; Wolf, Risley, & Mees, 1964). The majority of studies employing these strategies reported marked reductions in self-injurious responses (see Carr, 1977 for a discussion of studies with negative results).

Another source of support for the attention hypothesis is gleaned from research manipulating noncontingent presentation or withdrawal of attention. A number of studies have reported that some subjects engage in self-injury relatively less often when noncontingent social interaction is readily available. For example, Burke, Burke, and Forehand (1985) observed eight institutionalized youth with severe developmental disabilities under natural conditions and found that SIB was least likely to occur following positive social interactions. Similar results have been reported when the level of noncontingent social interaction has been manipulated directly by the experimenters (e.g., Carr & Durand, 1985a; Iwata et al., 1982, Mace & Knight, 1986). These findings are bolstered by other studies in which periods of isolation arranged noncontingently resulted in gradual reductions of SIB to near-zero levels (e.g., Jones, Simmons, & Frankel, 1974). Presumably, the absence of relevant social stimuli removes the function of self-injury maintained by social consequences.

The most compelling evidence in support of the positive reinforcement via attention hypothesis comes from experimental studies in which attention is arranged as a consequence of self-injury. In order to attain sufficient experimental control, most researchers have created analogue conditions in which relevant antecedent and consequent stimuli are under the control of the experimenter. Attentive responses to self-injury in these studies have generally been of two qualities. The most commonly arranged form of attention is termed social disapproval and includes comments such as "Don't do that, you're going to hurt yourself," "Look at your hand, don't hit yourself" (Iwata et al., 1982, p. 10; see also Carr & McDowell, 1980; Parrish, Iwata, Dorsey, Bunck, & Slifer, 1985). Other researchers have supplied sympathetic and reassuring comments contingent on SIB to analyze its influence on the behavior (e.g., Anderson et al., 1978; Lovaas, Freitag, Gold, & Kassorla, 1965). Examples of this type of attention include "You're hurting yourself" (Parrish et al., 1985) and "I don't think you're bad" (Lovaas et al., 1965).

The results of many experimental analogue studies have shown that only some subjects presented with these experimental arrangements engaged in self-injury primarily when the behavior produced attention. For example, Iwata et al. (1982) found the self-injury of only one of nine subjects to be controlled mainly by social disapproval. We can speculate as to why a greater proportion of self-injury is not controlled by attention. The most obvious and plausible reason is that the varied environments, learning histories, and organic conditions of different subjects results in self-injury with different functions. Thus, although similarities in topography of self-injury may be evident, individual environments and organisms can be expected to result in different classes of controlling variables across subjects. Another contributing factor may be that, for some self-injurious clients, attention may not have been established as a positive reinforcer. While the austere social environments of many persons with severe developmental disabilities who present SIB may foster extraordinary acts to access attention, for others, these environments may simply fail to cultivate and reinforce any social interaction.

Finally, methodological refinements in the manner and schedule in which attention is arranged may result in the identification of more subjects whose SIB is controlled by attention. For instance, the quality or topography of attention supplied contingent on SIB is often determined a priori and then standardized across subjects (e.g., Iwata et al., 1982). To the extent that social responses to self-injury in the subject's natural environment differ substantially from those arranged in analogue conditions, the true effects of attention may not be identified. In addition, the ratio of self-injurious responses to instances of contingent attention often approaches 1.0 in many studies (e.g., Carr & McDowell, 1980). As it seems unlikely that reinforcement occurs naturally in such rich ratios, the motivating influence of attention may only be exposed when subjects are deprived of interaction for longer intervals (e.g., a VI-5 minute schedule of reinforcement). As functional analysis methodologies are refined to identify the controlling variables unique to each subject, attention may prove to be a more prevalent reinforcer of SIB.

## *Access to Materials or Activities*

A second class of variables found to positively reinforce self-injurious behavior is contingent access to materials or activities (Durand & Carr,

1985). For some individuals, the effect of their self-destructive behavior on the environment is to gain access to tangible reinforcers, such as food, toys, or the opportunity to engage in preferred activities. The evolution of such an extreme form of behavior, in lieu of countless benign alternatives, seems perplexing. In the absence of experimental evidence documenting the genesis of human self-injury, we can hypothesize, as with attention, that the unresponsive environments of many persons with severe disabilities may encourage topographical variations that may become increasingly aberrant. That is, in some environments, ordinary behavior may become a discriminative stimulus for nonreinforcement, whereas extraordinary behavior may occasion reinforcing reactions from the same environment. This seems especially likely when the environment fails to actively teach (i.e., reinforce) socially acceptable means of obtaining tangible reinforcers.

Some indirect empirical support for this hypothesis may be found in studies showing an inverse relationship between the degree of environmental enrichment and the degree of aberrant behavior observed, including self-injury. For example, Madden, Russo, and Cataldo (1980) exposed three children hospitalized for lead poisoning due to pica to three different settings: a group play environment, an impoverished individual play environment, and an enriched individual play environment. The group play and enriched individual play environments contained numerous and varied toys and educational activities plus opportunities for social interaction. By contrast, the impoverished environment contained no toys, five common household items, and an observer who did not interact with the child. Pica rates were consistently three to five times greater in the impoverished environment than in either of the enriched settings (for similar results with pica and other aberrant behaviors, see Favell, McGimsey, & Schell, 1982b; Horner, 1980; and Mosely, Faust, & Reardon, 1970). Such findings suggest that nonreinforcement conditions alone may be a potent setting event for maladaptive behavior (Wahler & Fox, 1981).

More direct evidence that self-injury may be maintained by tangible reinforcers is available from studies that manipulated access to recreational and edible items. For example, Day, Rea, Schussler, Larsen, and Johnson (1988) conducted sessions in which preferred items were offered to a self-injurious student's peers. Contingent on the occurrence of self-injury, the teacher permitted the student access to the items for 20–30 seconds. Two of the three subjects in the experiment engaged in high rates of SIB when exposed to this condition, in alternation with a negative reinforcement and a sensory input condition. Similar results were reported by Durand and Crimmins (1988) for two of eight subjects studied. However, in this study, high rates of SIB were observed when tangible reinforcers were continually visible to subjects and delivered on a fixed ratio schedule of one reinforcer for nine correct task responses (FR-9).

In sum, substantial evidence has accumulated during the past 10 years to support the hypothesis that, for some individuals, self-injury is maintained by positive reinforcement via attention or tangible items (Carr, 1977). For others, however, self-injury may be an effective response to escape or avoid aversive situations.

## *Escape–Avoidance of Aversive Demand Conditions*

Of the three hypotheses identified by Carr (1977), the one that has attracted the most research and support is the view that self-injury may be an operant behavior maintained by negative reinforcement. Negative reinforcement is an operant process by which a response or class of responses becomes more probable when the behavior results in (a) complete avoidance of some (aversive) stimulus condition, (b) a delay in the presentation of aversive stimuli, (c) attenuation of the strength of the aversive stimuli, or (d) alleviation of aversive stimuli. As with positive reinforcement, environmental conditions that are correlated with the onset of aversive stimuli may set the occasion for escape–avoidance behavior, even though reinforcement of the response (i.e., removal or postponement of the stimulus) may be on an intermittent schedule.

The incipient etiology of escape-motivated self-injury is not well-documented, although some plausible scenarios have been suggested (e.g., Bachman, 1972; Carr, 1977; Skinner, 1953). As noted previously, some individuals with impaired physiological functions may also reside in impoverished teaching environments (Altmeyer et al., 1987). Without effective instruction and sufficient reinforcement for performing tasks such as dressing, self-feeding, academic activities, and even social interaction, the effort involved in performing particular tasks may outweigh the reinforcement derived from it. When such conditions prevail, the introduction of task-related demands may evoke protestant responses (e.g., tantrums, aggression), some of which may be strengthened because they alleviate demands. In extreme cases, the topographies of aggressive tantrums may be shaped into self-injurious responses.

Task-related demands may not be the only aversive stimuli that can motivate self-injury (Carr, 1977). For example, when a standard assessment protocol (Iwata et al., 1982) failed to identify maintaining conditions for a client with chronic medical problems, Pace and colleagues devised a novel condition to test the hypothesis that this subject's SIB was maintained by escape from intrusive medical procedures (Pace, February, 1989, personal communication). These researchers found that when medical personnel conducted routine medical examinations, the individual engaged in very high rates of head-hitting and hand-biting until the examination was interrupted. In another study, Ross, Meichenbaum, and Humphrey (1971) reported anecdotal information to suggest that an adolescent girl awoke herself at night by head-banging, the effect of which was believed to be escape from nightmares.

Two general strategies have been used to experimentally analyze the effects of demand conditions on self-injury. The first and most common strategy has been to compare rates of self-injury during gradients of instructional demands. For example, Carr, Newsom, and Binkoff (1976) alternately exposed a child with mild mental retardation to various demand and no-demand conditions. During demand periods, the instructional procedures remained in effect regardless of the occurrence of SIB. Onset of demand conditions reliably evoked high rates of self-injury, which gradually decreased in a manner consistent with an extinction curve. By contrast, two types of conditions were correlated with little or no SIB: the no-demand conditions, and conditions in which a stimulus that signaled the end of demand sessions was presented.

Several other studies have tested the negative reinforcement hypothesis by presenting different task conditions graded according to difficulty. For example, Weeks and Gaylord-Ross (1981) had self-injurious children perform easy and difficult two-choice discrimination problems. In the easy condition, for example, students were required to distinguish between open and closed figures, while the difficult condition called for discriminations between reversed form figures. Durand (1982) assessed self-injury during easy and difficult form-box tasks in which difficulty level was based on the subject's prebaseline accuracy. Finally, Mace, Browder, and Lin (1987) compared SIB during low (snack preparation) and high (table games) response activities, and during familiar versus novel snack activities. All of these studies arranged positive reinforcement for appropriate responses in all conditions. A consistent finding across this research is that self-injury occurred at higher rates during tasks in which the response requirements were greatest. However, in some cases, these effects were found to be dependent on a combination of task type and experimenter requests during the task (Gaylord-Ross, Weeks, & Lipner, 1980). Viewed collectively, these studies suggest that, for some clients, difficult tasks may constitute aversive stimuli, which may occasion SIB maintained by negative reinforcement.

The second strategy used to test the negative reinforcement hypothesis has been to directly manipulate the consequences for self-injurious responses during task conditions. That is, if the function of self-injury is to alter the presence or presentation of task-related demands, SIB can be expected to occur at a relatively high rate when an arranged consequence of self-injury is to temporarily escape the demand. A recent study by Steege, Wacker, Berg, Cigrand, and Cooper (1989) illustrates a tactic used commonly in this line of research. The self-injurious hair-pulling (trichotillomania) of a 4-year-old boy with moderate mental retardation was assessed under various analogue conditions. In the demand condition, a trainer presented academic tasks to the subject using a prescriptive prompt procedure (Steege, Wacker, & McMahon, 1987). Contingent on each occurrence of hair-pulling, the prompting procedure was discontinued for a 20-second time-out period, after which the task was resumed at the point it had been interrupted. For this subject, the demand condition was associated with the highest rate of self-injury, suggesting this individual's SIB was maintained by negative reinforcement. Using similar procedures, several other studies have reported findings that support the hypothesis that self-injury may be escape motivated for many persons with this disorder (e.g., Day et al., 1988; Iwata et al., 1982; Mace et al., 1987; Repp, Felce, & Barton, 1988).

## *Sensory Reinforcement*

There remains a segment of this population whose SIB is not clearly correlated with observable reinforcement contingencies. The pattern of self-injurious behavior for these individuals is either undifferentiated under varying reinforcement conditions or, alternatively, is most likely to occur when environmental stimulation is low. Self-injury of this type has led some researchers to speculate that SIB may be maintained by sensory reinforcement (Carr, 1977; Baumeister & Forehand, 1973; Favell et al., 1982a, 1982b; Iwata et al., 1982; Kulka, Fry, & Goldstein, 1960; Lovaas, Newsom, & Hickman, 1987).

According to the self-reinforcement hypothesis, organisms require some minimum level of sensory stimulation from the tactile, vestibular, and kinesthetic modalities (Carr, 1977; Edelson, 1984). When this input is restricted due to physical anomalies or an impoverished environment, individuals may behave in a manner that augments available sensory input. Such behavior may consist of stereotyped acts such as body rocking, hand or finger waving, posturing, or repetitive manipulation of objects. The topography of sensory-producing behaviors may include self-injurious responses when sensory deprivation is acute. Sensory reinforcement is said to occur because the stimulation that results from performing the behavior reinforces or maintains the occurrence of stereotypy or self-injury. An alternative view is that some individuals may be in a state of overstimulation, which stereotypy or self-injury may attenuate (Murphy, 1982). Because stereotypy and SIB that is maintained by sensory reinforcement may be viewed as topographical variants along a response-class continuum, research related to stereotypy is also discussed in this section (Cataldo & Harris, 1982; Edelson, 1984).

Sensory reinforcement differs in two important respects from the contingencies of positive and negative reinforcement in operant psychology (Skinner, 1969). First, operant behavior, as usually conceived, is a function of the environmental response to the behavior. Often, the ratio of behaviors to reinforcing consequences is less than 1.0. Further, operant behavior generally occurs in the context of antecedent environmental (discriminative) stimuli, which are correlated with reinforcement for that behavior. These features give operant behavior a probabilistic nature: Not all presentations of discriminative stimuli occasion the response, and not all occurrences of the response yield reinforcement (Skinner, 1938, 1953, 1969). The behavior analyst's task is to discover which antecedent stimuli evoke behavior and which consequences maintain it. However, sensory reinforcement presumably does not work quite like this. We must assume that each cycle of the behavior results in sensory stimulation that is sufficient to reinforce the behavior. In other words, the schedule maintaining the behavior is roughly equivalent to a continuous reinforcement schedule (CRF). However, because there is a one-to-one relationship between behavior and reinforcement, there is no reason to believe that antecedent environmental events will acquire discriminative control because the availability of reinforcement for the target response is constant across all environmental conditions.

A second difference between operant behavior maintained by external consequences and behavior controlled by internal (sensory) consequences is that the latter are not amenable to direct measurement or direct manipulation. By necessity, we rely on our common experience of sensory stimulation to infer presence, contingency, and schedule.

These two features of reinforcement by sensory stimulation pose formidable obstacles to experimental analysis. Clearly, the usual method of introducing and withdrawing antecedent or consequent variables believed to exert operant control of the behavior is not possible when these variables cannot be manipulated by the experimenter. Instead, researchers have used indirect methods to test the viability of the sensory-reinforcement hypothesis. One strategy has been to place a self-injurious client in an environment with sparse environmental stimulation (e.g., Favell et al., 1982b; Iwata et al., 1982; Madden et al., 1980; Parrish et al., 1985). This arrangement may be viewed as altering the available concurrent schedules of reinforcement in a manner that will induce self-injury maintained by sensory consequences. For instance, if sensory stimulation is a potent reinforcer for an individual at a given time, responses that produce this stimulation are likely to occur. In an austere environment that provides few external sources of sensory reinforcement, the alternative that is most likely to be reinforced may be stereotypy or SIB. When these behaviors occur most often in environments with low sensory stimulation, a plausible explanation is that they are reinforced by sensory stimulation.

A second strategy used to investigate the sensory-reinforcement hypothesis is to alter the environment in a manner that reduces or masks the sensory consequences produced by self-injury or stereotypy (Lovaas et al., 1987). By interfering with the sensory consequences that maintain these behaviors, their frequency can be reduced via sensory extinction. Rincover and his colleagues decreased stereotypic movements by masking auditory, proprioceptive, or visual stimulation that accompanied stereotypy (Rincover, Cook, Peoples, & Packard, 1979; Rincover, Newsom, & Carr, 1979). For example, stereotypic behavior was reduced for one subject by attaching a small vibrator to the back of the hand in an attempt to mask the proprioceptive stimulation resulting from finger and arm waving. By carpeting a table top, another subject's repetitive plate spinning decreased, presumably because the auditory consequences for this behavior were minimized. Similar approaches have also been applied to self-injury. For instance, Rincover and Devany (1982) evaluated the effects of different sensory extinction procedures for three children whose SIB occurred across various environmental conditions. Head-banging was eliminated for one subject by placing foam pads on the floor and walls and for another subject by having the child wear a padded helmet. A third subject's face scratching discontinued after thin rubber gloves were placed on her hands. These kinds of treatments were thought to be effective by masking or attenuating the stimulus consequences that presumably had maintained the behaviors.

A third indirect test of the sensory reinforcement hypothesis is to provide frequent opportunities for a client to engage in adaptive behavior that produces sensory consequences that are similar to those generated by self-injury. This approach involves a concept known as *functional equivalence* (Carr, 1988). When topographically different behaviors are maintained by the same reinforcer class, the responses are said to be functionally equivalent. Favell et al. (1982b) demonstrated that it may be possible to reduce sensory-motivated self-injury by encouraging alternative behaviors with sensory consequences that are as reinforcing as or more reinforcing than stimulation from SIB. Simply providing a client access to a bowl of popcorn resulted in a sharp reduction in pica, a response that was believed to be maintained by tactile or gustatory reinforcement.

Viewed collectively, this research provides ample support for the idea that the self-injury of some individuals is maintained to some degree by the sensory stimulation produced by the behavior itself. Future research may identify the environmental conditions that interact with sensory reinforcement to heighten and suppress the occurrence of self-injury.

## *Communication Hypothesis*

Carr and Durand have suggested another hypothesis for the behavioral etiology of severe behavior problems, including self-injury (Carr, 1982, 1988; Carr & Durand, 1985a, 1985b; Durand, 1982; Durand & Carr, 1985). They argue for conceptualizing behavior problems as functional communication. According to this view, problematic forms of behavior such as aggression, tantrums, and self-injury may have functions similar to socially acceptable forms of verbal and nonverbal communication. The former topographies may develop in individuals whose physical limitations and impoverished environments interfere with shaping and maintenance of appropriate means of producing attention or assistance. Thus, a child's head-banging that reliably attracts adult attention may be functionally equivalent to palatable forms of behavior that access attention (e.g., requests or task completion).

Viewing behavior problems as having a communicative function may have heuristic value for the development of treatments and treatment philosophy. This view considers problem behaviors to be adaptive inasmuch as the responses function to produce access to important social and material reinforcers (Carr & Durand, 1985b). This contrasts with traditional philosophies, which conceptualize behaviors such as self-injury as aberrant or maladaptive. Instead, SIB would be seen as a form of behavior that may impede developmental progress, but that has a legitimate function. The goal of treatment then becomes to teach a socially appropriate form of communication that is functionally equivalent to self-injury. Such a framework may alter the philosophical approach to intervention in ways that may benefit individuals with self-injury by emphasizing the acquisition of substitute adaptive behaviors in lieu of the traditional focus on suppressing the problem behavior.

Carr, Durand, and others have demonstrated the potential value of the communication hypothesis for treatment development. In the first of two studies, Carr and Durand (1985a) assessed disruptive behavior during easy and difficult task conditions. Both task conditions also varied in the amount of adult attention that was provided to the students. The results of this assessment showed that three students were most disruptive during difficult tasks, one student was disruptive during easy tasks with low levels of adult attention, and one child misbehaved during difficult tasks and during low adult attention. During the treatment phase, all students were taught to request assistance ("I don't understand") and attention ("Am I doing good work?"). Disruptive behavior was reduced for all students when verbal requests were reinforced, which, based on the pretreatment assessment, were functionally equivalent to the individual's disruptive behavior. As expected, reinforcement of the irrelevant communication failed to reduce disruption below baseline levels. A similar application to escape-motivated stereotypic behavior proved successful when students were taught to use the phrase "Help me" during task-related demands (Durand & Carr, 1987). Finally, Day et al. (1988) found this treatment approach to be effective with self-injury subsequent to conducting an analogue functional analysis. Large reductions in SIB were observed after training clients to request tangible reinforcers.

In our view, the value of the communication hypothesis is dependent on conducting a valid pretreatment analysis of the operant function of self-injury (as in Carr & Durand, 1985a; Durand & Carr, 1987). In a sense, any behavior that produces a response from others may be conceptualized as communicative (Skinner, 1957). It is this aspect of the term *communicative* (i.e., the functional relation between problem behavior and the responses of others) that leads to training a verbal response that is functionally equivalent to SIB. However, there is another meaning of the term *communicative* that leads to speculation regarding the *intent* or the *message value* of the behavior problem (Donnellan, Mirenda, Mesaros, & Fassbender, 1984). This intent or message-value connotation of the term takes the focus off an analysis of behavior–environment interactions and places it instead on the interpretation of private motivations of persons with behavior problems. For example, Donnellan et al. (1984) suggest assessing the communicative functions of problem behavior by having the practitioner record ongoing *impressions* regarding the possible communicative function(s) of the target behavior (p. 205). When this occurs, behavior becomes a sign of an underlying motivational condition rather than a function of its environmental consequences. In our view, the best way to discover the communicative function of an individual's self-injury is to observe its effect on the environment. As Carr and Durand (1985a) illustrated, the effectiveness of intervention will depend on training a verbal response that has a function equivalent to the problem behavior.

### *Summary*

This section reviewed research supporting five major hypotheses regarding the function of self-injurious behavior. According to two of these hypotheses, self-injury is positively reinforced by the consequential attention provided by others, or, alternatively, by the access to tangible reinforcers SIB provides. A third hypothesis states that the function of self-injury is to escape or avoid certain situations, especially those calling for performance of tasks. There is growing evidence to support a fourth hypothesis that self-injury may be maintained by the sensory consequences the behavior produces. Finally, we reviewed research that views behavior problems as having a communicative function (i.e., to command or demand attention or assistance). The communication hypothesis has stimulated approaches to intervention that supplant the function of self-injury with appropriate verbal responses. It is important to note that these variables can operate singularly or in combinations to maintain the self-injury of a particular individual.

Methodologies used to identify the functions of self-injury have varied considerably. In the following section, we propose a comprehensive functional analysis methodology, which combines methods reported across studies.

## A Comprehensive Functional Analysis Methodology

The methodologies used in the functional analysis of self-injury range from interviews and casual observations to well-controlled analogue experimentation. We believe that a comprehensive approach to the functional analysis and treatment of self-injury involves a multistage process, which includes (a) descriptive analysis under natural conditions, (b) hypothesis formation, (c) experimental analysis under analogue conditions, (d) intervention development, implementation, and evaluation, and (e) maintenance and generalization of intervention effects.

## *Descriptive Analysis Under Natural Conditions*

A step included rarely in functional analysis studies is a descriptive analysis of the aberrant behavior under natural conditions. Descriptive analysis entails assessment of the individual's behavior in the context of the home, school, or occupational environment. The goal is to identify covariations between self-injurious responses and specific environmental events that occur antecedent or subsequent to the behavior. This is usually achieved by conducting systematic observations of the client in various naturally occurring situations (e.g., Bijou, Peterson, & Ault, 1968; Bijou, Peterson, Harris, Allen, & Johnson, 1969; Touchette, MacDonald, & Langer, 1985). These data provide an empirical basis for the formulation of hypotheses concerning possible functions of the problem behavior that may be tested experimentally or that may suggest potentially effective interventions.

The descriptive phase of a functional analysis can contribute significantly to the long-range success of analysis-derived interventions, as well as to the development of a general theory of human behavior in natural environments. Most functional analysis studies identify functional relations during controlled analogue conditions in which the variable(s) suspected to control SIB are systematically applied and withdrawn in order to observe their effect on the behavior. For example, to test the escape–avoidance hypothesis, the experimenter may prompt a client through an academic task, permitting temporary escape from the task contingent on occurrences of self-injury (e.g., Day et al., 1988; Iwata et al., 1982; Mace et al., 1987; Parrish et al., 1985; Steege et al., 1989). Yet, for many self-injurious individuals, SIB is a high-probability response that is likely to occur at some level across environmental situations. Although an escape contingency applied to self-injury may result in relatively high rates of SIB, there is some risk in concluding that a similar contingency maintains the behavior under natural conditions. Carr, Newsom, and Binkoff (1980) illustrated this point by alternately applying an escape contingency to aggression and to finger-tapping. Both responses occurred at high rates when they resulted in escape from demands. However, the unlikelihood that finger tapping is maintained naturally by escape from demands also casts doubt as to whether this is the contingency that reinforces aggression in the natural environment.

The problem may be exacerbated when interventions are designed on the basis of an invalid analysis. Suppose an analogue analysis shows that

SIB is maintained by attention. A reasonable intervention in this case may be to ignore self-injury and to teach the client appropriate means of evoking attention. Although this intervention may reduce self-injury under analogue conditions, its effectiveness in the client's natural environment depends on whether attention maintains SIB at home and at school. It may be that the client's SIB is escape-motivated at school, but because of differences in tasks, teachers, and competing schedules of reinforcement, the analogue analysis may not reveal this finding.

We are suggesting that the validity of a functional analysis may depend on the extent to which conditions in the analogue analysis are representative of those that operate naturally on self-injury. There may be some cases in which SIB is highly responsive to an escape contingency, for example, such that self-injury will occur at high rates regardless of the task materials used, the schedule in which escape is arranged, the learning history with the instructor, and the contingencies that exist for other behaviors. However, other cases may be sensitive to these variables, resulting in different response patterns in natural and analogue conditions.

A variety of methodologies have been used to conduct a descriptive analysis of natural conditions. Common to most methodologies are repeated direct observations of the target behavior and specific environmental events that occur contiguous to the target response. Because observations are taken in the absence of experimental arrangements, the resulting data must be considered correlational rather than confirmatory. For example, Patterson (1969), Saudargas and Lentz (1986), Strain and Ezzell (1978), and Wahler (1975) employed complex observational codes to identify behavior–environment relations or behavioral sequences that were suggestive of reinforcement contingencies that may maintain child, parent, or teacher behaviors. Others have used traditional interval recording procedures. For example, Vyse, Mulick, and Thayer (1984) recorded multiple classroom behaviors using partial-interval and momentary time-sampling procedures. Correlational analyses on these data showed that some problem behaviors tended to co-vary in clusters such that the occurrence of one response was predictive of others in that cluster.

We have adopted a descriptive analysis methodology, which is based largely on early studies by Bijou and his colleagues (Bijou et al., 1968, 1969). The first step is to obtain several unstructured narrative accounts of the subject's behavior and the environmental events that surround its occurrence. This information is used to formulate operational definitions of the target response class and to identify 3–5 categories each of antecedent and subsequents events that cooccur naturally with the problem behavior. For a self-injurious client, response topographies may include hand-biting and head-banging. Antecedent events may be task demands, others present—no interaction, social interaction, and alone. Possible subsequent events may be discontinuation of task performance, reprimands, prompts to engage in an activity, and consoling comments.

Data on self-injury and the antecedent and subsequent event categories are collected concurrently, using a continuous 10-second partial-interval recording procedure. Events in the antecedent categories are recorded throughout the observation session. When a target response occurs, it is recorded, along with events in the subsequent categories for the next two 10-second intervals, or up to 30 seconds following the target behavior. Subsequent events with this temporal relation to self-injury may function to reinforce the behavior. Observation sessions should be of sufficient length to observe several occurrences of self-injury per session in a variety of environmental situations.

We have found it useful to express descriptive analysis data as conditional probabilities (cf. Bijou et al., 1968, 1969) that relate to the viability of different reinforcement contingencies that may maintain self-injury. One class of questions asked is, "Given the occurrence of a particular antecedent event, what is the probability of observing a contiguous self-injurious response?" This question is related to the power each antecedent event has to evoke SIB and may be suggestive of conditions that are discriminative for self-injury. For example, data for one subject might show that 50% of the intervals that are scored as task demands are followed by self-injury, while for another subject, this value may be only 10%. When SIB is more probable following task demands, an escape–avoidance hypothesis seems plausible. Another relevant question may be "Given the occurrence of self-injury, what is the probability of observing a particular subsequent event?" This question assesses the natural covariation between SIB and subsequent events that may reinforce the behavior. Here, the relationship need not be strong in order to suspect a reinforcement relation because the reinforcement schedule may be intermittent. However, this analysis may suggest that some hypotheses are unlikely to be valid because the response–reinforcer relation is never observed to occur naturally.

## *Hypothesis Formation*

The results of a descriptive analysis are by nature suggestive. Their primary value is to provide an empirical basis for formulating hypotheses concerning the contingencies that may maintain self-injury in the client's natural environment (Bijou et al., 1968; Kohler & Greenwood, 1986; Wahler, 1975). Such natural observations may also identify unique instructions, task materials, or qualitative reactions of others that are more or less likely to be associated with SIB. A descriptive analysis is considered successful when careful examination of the data reveals the environmental circumstances in which self-injury is most likely to occur, thus providing a basis for postulating about the function of an individual's self-injury.

Specific hypotheses usually follow directly from the data patterns observed in the descriptive analysis. In our experience, correlations are often most apparent between antecedent events and the aberrant behavior. This is consistent with the idea that, in general, discriminative stimuli reliably evoke more responses than are reinforced (Ferster & Skinner, 1957), making this relationship easier to detect with uncontrolled observations than is the response–reinforcer relation. The general practice is to consider viable any hypothesis that has a correlated antecedent event that is associated with a relatively high level of self-injury. For example, if the antecedent event *others present—no interaction* is followed an average of 30% of the time by SIB, a reasonable hypothesis would be that self-injury is maintained by attention. Additional support for the attention hypothesis would follow from observations that self-injury that occurred under these antecedent conditions was in fact followed by attention from others. Similar tactics may be used to assess the plausibility of the escape–avoidance hypothesis (e.g., high rates of SIB during task demands and occasional alleviation of demands following SIB), and the sensory reinforcement hypothesis (i.e., high rates of SIB during periods of low stimulation).

At this juncture, observed response–event and event–response covariations must be viewed tentatively. Firm conclusions regarding the function(s) of self-injury require experimental manipulation of the variable suspected to influence self-injury.

## *Experimental Analysis Under Analogue Conditions*

A successful descriptive analysis culminates in one or more *testable* hypotheses regarding the variables that control self-injury. In the experimental analysis phase, the validity of each hypothesis is assessed by performing well-controlled experiments, which attempt to isolate the variable in question and observe its relation to the subject's self-injury. A variable that is functionally related to SIB should, when introduced to the client's environment, result in comparatively higher levels of self-injury than when variables without a functional relation to SIB are in effect.

Variables suspected to influence self-injury are presented to the subject during analogue condition. An *analogue condition* is a situation that simulates environmental circumstances in the client's natural environment. The important distinction between the natural environment and an analogue condition is that, unlike natural settings, where environmental influences occur in uncontrolled combinations, the behavior analyst arranges the environment so as to observe the effect of one variable at a time. This is generally achieved by holding constant factors that, if allowed to vary, may affect self-injury, while the suspect (independent) variable is systematically introduced and withdrawn across a series of experimental sessions. The conclusions that can be drawn from an experimental analysis of analogue conditions warrant much more confidence than the functional relations suggested by the descriptive analysis. When self-injury is observed to reliably co-vary with an experimenter-controlled variable, a functional relation is established.

As noted in the previous section, the generality of a functional relation identified in an experimental analysis of analogue conditions depends on the validity of the simulation. Generality may be enhanced by using information obtained during the descriptive analysis to design the procedures for the analogue conditions (cf. Kohler & Greenwood, 1986; Stokes & Baer, 1977). For example, observations in the natural setting may reveal that SIB is more likely to occur under some task conditions than others. It may be the type of task (Mace et al., 1987), the manner in which the task is presented (Carr et al., 1976; Gaylord-Ross, Weeks, & Lipner, 1980), the instructional pace (Carrine, 1976), the availability of reinforcement for concurrent behaviors (Favell et al., 1982b), or the type and schedule of reinforcement supplied for task performance (Carr & Durand, 1985a) that are important cofactors in controlling an individual's self-injury. That is, self-injury may be maintained by negative reinforcement (escape from demands) only under certain task conditions. Most of these factors can be incorporated into the design of analogue conditions in order to make them more representative of natural circumstances. When this is done, the functional relations identified through experimental analysis are more likely to be useful to design interventions for natural settings.

Various approaches have been used to design analogue conditions. One strategy has been to design a different experimental condition for each hypothesis being tested (e.g., Carr et al., 1976; Day et al., 1988; Durand & Crimmins, 1988; Iwata et al., 1982; Mace, Page, Ivancic, & O'Brien, 1986; Parrish et al., 1985; Steege et al., 1989). For example, to test the positive-reinforcement-via-attention hypothesis, Parrish et al. (1985) placed a self-injurious child in a room with play materials, and then the therapist withdrew from him and sat in a chair across the room. Each time the child hit his head, the therapist provided a statement of social disapproval. The negative-reinforcement hypothesis was evaluated in this study with a separate condition in which academic tasks were presented by a therapist using a graduated prompt hierarchy. Each occurrence of self-injury resulted in the therapist discontinuing the task demands for 30 seconds.

Another approach to the design of analogue conditions is to design two or more separate conditions to test a single hypothesis. This strategy attempts to vary as few environmental factors as possible across analogue conditions, in order to isolate the effects of one variable. For example, Mace and Knight (1986) assessed the effects of varying levels of noncontingent attention on self-injurious pica by comparing three different attention conditions. Room location, persons present, and seating arrangements, activity, and reinforcement for appropriate behavior were held constant. The three conditions differed only in the schedule on which noncontingent attention was supplied, thus permitting the differences in pica across conditions to be attributed solely to the rate of attention provided.

In order to draw valid inferences from the analogue analysis, conditions are generally presented to the client in the context of a single-case experimental design. Many functional analysis studies expose clients individually to analogue conditions according to an alternating-treatments design (e.g., Durand & Crimmins, 1988; Favell et al., 1982b; Iwata et al., 1982; Mace & Knight, 1986). In this arrangement, sessions of each analogue condition are usually conducted in a random or counterbalanced order each day of the study. Rates of self-injury are graphed by condition as concurrent time-series to illustrate the relative effect each situation has on SIB.

An alternative design option is the withdrawal design. This approach involves conducting a series of sessions of a single analogue condition until data on SIB are stable. A second condition is then introduced, followed by a succession of replication phases to establish the control each experimental condition has on self-injury (e.g., Anderson et al., 1978; Carr et al., 1980; Durand & Carr, 1987). Both design strategies can yield experimentally valid results upon which to design interventions to reduce self-injury.

## *Intervention Development, Implementation, and Evaluation*

The clinical objective of a functional analysis is to design intervention procedures that are linked to a valid behavioral analysis of the problem behavior. When the experimental analysis of analogue conditions isolates one or more contingencies or antecedent variables that maintain SIB, the applied behavior analyst is equipped to design interventions that interrupt the maintaining contingencies and that promote alternative behaviors that have a function equivalent to the SIB (Axelrod, 1987).

Table 5.1 presents some interventions that are derived logically from the function that self-injury is shown to have in the descriptive and experimental analysis phases. Notice that, in many cases, intervention strategies appropriate for one function of self-injury would probably prove ineffective or even counterproductive when self-injury has another function. For example, the use of time-out with escape-motivated self-injury runs the risk of strengthening rather than reducing the behavior (e.g., Durand & Carr, 1987; Iwata et al., 1982). Similarly, guided com-

TABLE 5.1. Listing of potential intervention strategies based on the function of self-injury.

- Negative reinforcement via escape–avoidance of task demands
  - Extinction
    - Guided compliance (Repp et al., 1988)
    - Continued instruction (Mace et al., 1987; Repp et al., 1988)
  - Teach an appropriate escape response
    - Request assistance (Carr & Durand, 1985a)
    - Request breaks (Day et al., 1988; Durand & Kishi, 1987)
  - Reduce task difficulty (Weeks & Gaylord-Ross, 1981)
  - Schedule frequent breaks (Gaylord-Ross et al., 1980)
  - Increase reinforcement for task engagement (Gaylord-Ross et al., 1980; Steege et al., 1989)
- Positive reinforcement via attention
  - Extinction
    - Provide minimal attention for self-injury (Lovaas & Simmons, 1969; Carr & McDowell, 1980; Repp et al., 1988)
    - Nonexclusionary time-out contingent on SIB (Anderson et al., 1978; Steege et al., 1989)
  - Teach an appropriate request for attention
    - Conversation initiation and expansion training (Carr & Durand, 1985a)
    - Prompt noninteractional attention (for persons with sèvere handicaps) (Tarpley & Schroeder, 1979)
  - Increase the rate of noncontingent attention (Anderson et al., 1978; Lovaas et al., 1965)
  - Increase opportunities for social interaction (Favell et al., 1982b; Horner, 1980)
  - Seating arrangements, interactive activities
- Positive reinforcement via tangible rewards
  - Extinction
    - Withhold tangible rewards following SIB (Allen & Harris, 1966; Repp et al., 1988)
  - Teach appropriate request for tangible rewards (Day et al., 1988; Durand & Kishi, 1987)
  - Use tangible rewards to reinforce appropriate behavior
    - Varied reinforcer menus (Allen & Harris, 1966; Durand & Kishi, 1987; Repp & Deitz, 1974)
  - Increase rate of noncontingent access to tangible rewards (Horner, 1980)
- Sensory reinforcement
  - Sensory extinction (where possible and practical)
    - Mask sensory stimulation (Rincover & Devany, 1982)
    - Response blocking (Favell et al, 1982b; Pace et al., 1986)
  - Environmental enrichment
    - Increased social interaction (Mace & Knight, 1986; Parrish et al., 1985)
    - Increased access and training with interesting materials (Favell et al., 1982b; Parrish et al., 1985; Steege et al., 1989)
  - Teach appropriate requests
    - Access to social interaction and materials (Day et al., 1988)

pliance, which supplies a degree of attention in its execution, would be contraindicated for individuals whose SIB is maintained by attention. This approach of linking treatment to preintervention assessment data casts a new light on the effectiveness of behavioral interventions. This view suggests that many treatment procedures are effective under specific conditions, which are linked to the function of the problem behavior.

In our view, severe behavior problems such as self-injury are best treated by incorporating as many potentially effective intervention components as possible. However, the general strategy is to minimize the reinforcement derived from self-injury to the greatest extent possible. This extinction strategy will be most effective when applied in conjunction with procedures to prompt and reinforce alternative responses that produce the same class of reinforcers found to maintain SIB (Carr, 1988; Carr & Durand, 1985b). Another general strategy to weaken the response–reinforcer relation maintaining self-injury is to schedule response-independent reinforcement whenever it is practical and appropriate. Interventions such as scheduling breaks and increasing the rate of social interaction illustrate this strategy.

The effectiveness of analysis-derived interventions is evaluated in the usual manner, using single-case experimental designs. However, the health-threatening nature of self-injury raises ethical questions about using designs that involve the withdrawal of effective interventions (e.g., reversal or withdrawal designs). In most cases, the experimental control offered by multiple baseline designs should be sufficient to draw valid conclusions about treatment effectiveness.

## *Maintenance and Generalization of Intervention Effects*

It has been hypothesized that generalization and maintenance of treatment gains can be facilitated by implementing interventions utilizing a functional-equivalence approach for the treatment of aberrant behavior (Durand & Kishi, 1987). The basis for teaching a functionally equivalent adaptive response is to provide the individual with an alternative behavior that has a function equivalent to the maladaptive response. Carr (1988) proposed that functional equivalence occurs when two or more response classes are maintained by the same reinforcer class. The responses can be topographically similar or distinct, yet serve the same function. The goal of the therapist is to determine the function of the aberrant response and then to empirically demonstrate and equivalence between the maladaptive the and appropriate behaviors. From this information, interventions can be developed that emphasize the training of the functionally equivalent response that provides the individual a method of actively obtaining the preferred reinforcer in an appropriate manner.

Recently, a number of studies have been presented that have applied the knowledge of the function of an aberrant response to select and train a functionally equivalent adaptive behavior. In addition to the initial decelerative effect on the frequency of self-injury, the interventions also produced generalization and maintenance of the treatment gains. Durand and Kishi (1987) determined that the self-injury of five students with severe mental retardation and dual sensory impairments functioned to escape from work or to obtain either tangible reinforcers or adult attention. The authors used the pretreatment assessment data to teach each student how to communicate basic requests by presenting tokens to their teachers. Results indicated that the procedures were effective in reducing the levels of the behavior problems for four of the five students through a 9-month follow-up. Similar findings were presented by Day and colleagues (1988). In this investigation, the authors used a series of analogue assessments to determine that the self-injury emitted by three students enabled them to obtain preferred reinforcers. Interventions based on teaching the students to request the preferred item resulted in substantial decreases in self-injury during the treatment conditions, as well as across conditions (i.e., generalization), which lasted through the 5 months of the study.

Carr (1988) presented an interesting view in regard to the effectiveness of a functional-equivalence approach for facilitating response generalization and maintenance. Based on the concept of functional equivalence, when the adaptive response is strengthened, problem behavior should decrease. What is the mechanism responsible for this covariation? Given that both behaviors were effective in producing the preferred reinforcer, why would an individual not retain both types of behavior? Carr (1988) proposed that we must take the analysis one step further and examine the relative efficiency of the two behaviors in producing the environmental consequence. Reinforcement consistency and reinforcement delay can be used as starting points in an analysis of an aberrant response's efficiency (Carr, 1988). *Reinforcement consistency* refers to the schedule of reinforcement produced by a given response. If the aberrant response produces the preferred reinforcer 50% of the time, and the appropriate response does so 90% of the time, we can then state that the latter was more efficient in producing the preferred reinforcer. *Reinforcement delay* refers to the amount of time between the aberrant response and the presentation of the environmental consequent event. An individual's adaptive response may produce an environmental stimulus event in one half the time of that required for the aberrant response to produce the same reinforcer class. In this case, the appropriate response is more efficient than the self-injury in terms of the reinforcement delay. An experimental analysis along these dimensions may help explain the natural covariation between the functionally equivalent responses.

## Summary and Conclusion

In this chapter, we reviewed literature in which a behavior-analytic approach was utilized to treat individuals' self-injury. Functional analysis research has identified several contributing factors to self-injury. An individual's self-injury may be positively reinforced by some form of social attention (Iwata et al., 1982), access to materials or activities (Durand & Carr, 1985), or sensory and perceptual consequences produced by the self-injury (Favell et al., 1982b). A negative-reinforcement paradigm may also maintain self-injury by resulting in escape or avoidance of aversive conditions (Carr et al., 1976).

An analytic approach to the treatment of self-injury has provided a number of benefits to the field of behavior analysis. By conducting pre-treatment functional analyses, therapists have provided a link between basic and applied research by contributing to the existing data base with respect to the operant processes that support aberrant behavior in natural settings. Knowledge of the contributing factors of an individual's self-injury has enabled therapists to develop parsimonious and effective interventions and, in many cases, without resorting to the use of intrusive procedures. In addition, the identification of the possible motivational sources of an individual's aberrant behavior can assist the therapist in the selection of alternative adaptive behaviors to teach in the treatment package.

We have also detailed the characteristics of self-injurious behavior that may hinder the implementation of comprehensive functional analysis procedures. These include (a) the schedule of reinforcement produced by the aberrant response (i.e., maintained by a thin schedule of reinforcement); (b) the severity of the behavior, which may necessitate a response from the caregiver, and which may preclude observations of naturally occurring conditions for a sufficient length of time; and (c) the association of self-injury with medical conditions that may be unknown and difficult to observe.

In the second half of the chapter, we described a comprehensive procedure for conducting functional analyses of aberrant behavior. The procedures described included (a) a descriptive analysis of natural conditions (Bijou et al., 1968), (b) hypothesis formation of functional relationships, (c) experimental analysis of analogue conditions (Iwata et al., 1982), (d) intervention development, implementation, and evaluation, and (e) maintenance and generalization of intervention effects.

It is our hope that by utilizing a comprehensive functional analysis, therapists can develop interventions that avoid the use of aversive procedures and that are based on teaching alternative adaptive behaviors. In addition to providing initial benefits, these interventions may also facilitate the generalization and maintenance of treatment gains.

## References

Allen, K. E., & Harris, F. R. (1966). Elimination of a child's excessive scratching by training the mother in reinforcement procedures. *Behaviour Research and Therapy*, *4*, 79–84.

Altmeyer, B. K., Locke, B. J., Griffen, J. C., Ricketts, R. W., Williams, D. E., Mason, M., & Stark, M. T. (1987). Treatment strategies for self-injurious behavior in a large service-delivery network. *American Journal of Mental Deficiency*, *91*, 333–340.

Anderson, L., Dancis, J., & Alpert, M. (1978). Behavioral contingencies and self-mutilation in Lesch–Nyhan disease. *Journal of Consulting and Clinical Psychology*, *46*, 529–536.

Axelrod, S. (1987). Functional and structural analyses of behavior: Approaches leading to reduced use of punishment procedures? *Research in Developmental Disabilities*, *8*, 165–178.

Ayllon, T., & Michael, J. (1959). The psychiatric nurse as a behavioral engineer. *Journal of the Experimental Analysis of Behavior*, *2*, 323–334.

Bachman, J. A., (1972). Self-injurious behavior: A behavioral analysis. *Journal of Abnormal Psychology*, *80*, 211–224.

Baumeister, A. A., & Forehand, R. (1973). Stereotyped acts. In N. R. Ellis (Ed.), *International review of research in mental retardation* (Vol. 6, pp. 55–96). New York: Academic Press.

Bijou, S. W., Peterson, R. F., & Ault, M. H. (1968). A method to integrate descriptive and experimental field studies at the level of data and empirical concepts. *Journal of Applied Behavior Analysis*, *1*, 175–191.

Bijou, S. W., Peterson, R. F., Harris, F. R., Allen, K. E., & Johnson, M. S. (1969). Methodology for experimental studies of young children in natural settings. *Psychological Record*, *19*, 177–210.

Bryson, Y., Sakati, N., Nyhan, W., & Fish, C. (1971). Self-mutilative behavior in the Cornelia de Lange syndrome. *American Journal of Mental Deficiency*, *76*, 319–324.

Budd, K. S., Green, D. R., & Baer, D. M. (1976). An analysis of multiple misplaced parental social contingencies. *Journal of Applied Behavior Analysis*, *9*, 459–470.

Burke, M. M., Burke, D., & Forehand, R. (1985). Interpersonal antecedents of self-injurious behavior in retarded children. *Education and Training of the Mentally Retarded*, *20*, 204–208.

Carnine, D. W. (1976). Effects of two teacher-presentation rates on off-task behavior, answering correctly, and participation. *Journal of Applied Behavior Analysis*, *9*, 199–206.

Carr, E. G. (1977). The motivation of self-injurious behavior: A review of some hypotheses. *Psychological Bulletin*, *84*, 800–816.

Carr, E. G. (1982). *How to teach sign language to developmentally disabled children*. Lawrence, KS: H & H Enterprises.

Carr, E. G. (1988). Functional equivalence as a mechanism of response generalization. In R. H. Horner, R. L. Koegel, & G. Dunlap (Eds.), *Generalization and maintenance: Life-style changes in applied settings* (pp. 221–241). Baltimore: Paul H. Brookes.

Carr, E. G., & Durand, V. M. (1985a). Reducing behavior problems through functional communication training. *Journal of Applied Behavior Analysis*, *18*, 111–126.

Carr, E. G., & Durand, V. M. (1985b). The social communicative basis of severe behavior problems in children. In S. Reiss & R. Bootzin (Eds.), *Theoretical issues in behavior therapy* (pp. 219–254). New York: Academic Press.

Carr, E. G., & McDowell, J. J. (1980). Social control of self-injurious behavior of organic etiology. *Behavior Therapy*, *11*, 402–409.

Carr, E. G., Newsom, C. D., & Binkoff, J. A. (1976). Stimulus control of self-destructive behavior in a psychotic child. *Journal of Abnormal Child Psychology*, *4*, 139–153.

Carr, E. G., Newsom, C. D., & Binkoff, J. A. (1980). Escape as a factor in the aggressive behavior of two retarded children. *Journal of Applied Behavior Analysis*, *13*, 101–117.

Cataldo, M. F., & Harris, J. (1982). The biological basis for self-injury in the mentally retarded. *Analysis and Intervention in Developmental Disabilities*, *2*, 21–39.

Day, R. M., Rea, J. A., Schussler, N. G., Larsen, S. E., & Johnson, W. L. (1988). A functionally based approach to the treatment of self-injurious behavior. *Behavior Modification*, *12*, 565–589.

De Lissovoy, V., (1963). Head banging in early childhood: A suggested cause. *Journal of Genetic Psychology*, *102*, 109–114.

Demchak, M. A., & Halle, J. W. (1985). Motivational assessment: A potential means of enhancing treatment success of self-injurious individuals. *Education and Training of the Mentally Retarded*, *20*, 25–38.

Donnellan, A. M., Mirenda, P. L., Mesaros, R. A., & Fassbender, L. L. (1984). Analyzing the communicative functions of aberrant behavior. *Journal of the Association for the Severely Handicapped*, *9*, 201–212.

Duker, P. (1975). Behavior control of self-biting in a Lesch–Nyhan patient. *Journal of Mental Deficiency Research*, *19*, 11–19.

Durand, V. M. (1982). Analysis and intervention of self-injurious behavior. *Journal of the Association for the Severely Handicapped*, *7*, 44–53.

Durand, V. M., & Carr E. G., (1985). Self-injurious behavior: Motivating conditions and guidelines for treatment. *School Psychology Review*, *14*, 171–176.

Durand, V. M., & Carr, E. G. (1987). Social influences on "self-stimulatory" behavior: Analysis and treatment application. *Journal of Applied Behavior Analysis*, *20*, 119–132.

Durand, V. M., & Crimmins, D. B. (1988). Identifying variables maintaining self-injurious behavior. *Journal of Autism and Developmental Disorders*, *18*, 99–117.

Durand, V. M., & Kishi, G. (1987). Reducing severe behavior problems among persons with dual sensory impairments: An evaluation of a technical assistance model. *Journal of the Association for Persons with Severe Handicaps*, *12*, 2–10.

Edelson, S. M. (1984). Implications of sensory stimulation in self-destructive behavior. *American Journal of Mental Deficiency*, *89*, 140–145.

Favell, J. E., Azrin, N. H., Baumeister, A. A., Carr, E. G., Dorsey, M. F., Forehand, R., Foxx, R. M., Lovaas, O. I., Rincover, A., Risley, T. R., Romanczyk, R. G., Russo, D. C., Schroeder, S. R., & Solnick, J. V. (1982a). The treatment of self-injurious behavior. *Behavior Therapy*, *13*, 529–554.

Favell, J. E., McGimsey, J. F., & Jones, M. L. (1978). The use of physical restraint in the treatment of self-injury and as positive reinforcement. *Journal of Applied Behavior Analysis*, *11*, 225–242.

Favell, J. E., McGimsey, J. F., & Schell, R. M. (1982b). Treatment of self-injury by providing alternate sensory activities. *Analysis and Intervention in Developmental Disabilities*, *2*, 83–104.

Ferguson, D. G., & Breuning, S. E. (1982). Antipsychotic and antianxiety. In S. E. Breuning & A. D. Poling (Eds.), *Drugs and mental retardation* (pp. 168–214). Springfield, IL: Charles C. Thomas.

Ferster, C. B. (1961). Positive reinforcement and behavioral deficits in autistic children. *Child Development*, *32*, 437–456.

Ferster, C. B., & Skinner, B. F. (1957). *Schedules of reinforcement*. Englewood Cliffs, NJ: Prentice-Hall.

Frankel, F., & Simmons, J. Q. (1976). Self-injurious behavior in schizophrenic and retarded children. *American Journal of Mental Deficiency*, *80*, 512–522.

Gaylord-Ross, R., Weeks, M., & Lipner, C. (1980). An analysis of antecedent, response, and consequence events in the treatment of self-injurious behavior. *Education and Training of the Mentally Retarded*, *15*, 35–42.

Hamilton, J., Stephens, L, & Allen, P. (1967). Controlling aggressive and destructive behavior in severely retarded institutionalized residents. *American Journal of Mental Deficiency*, *71*, 852–856.

Harris, S. L., & Romanczyk, R. G. (1976). Treating self-injurious behavior of a retarded child by overcorrection. *Behavior Therapy*, *7*, 235–239.

Horner, R. D. (1980). The effects of an environmental "enrichment" program on the behavior of institutionalized profoundly retarded children. *Journal of Applied Behavior Analysis*, *13*, 473–491.

Iwata, B. A. (1988). The development and adoption of controversial default technologies. *The Behavior Analyst*, *11*, 149–157.

Iwata, B. A, Dorsey, M. F., Slifer, K. J., Bauman, K. E., & Richman, G. S. (1982). Toward a functional analysis of self-injury. *Analysis and Intervention in Developmental Disabilities*, *2*, 3–20.

Jones, F. H., Simmons, J. Q., & Frankel, F. (1974). An extinction procedure for eliminating self-destructive behavior in a nine-year-old autistic girl. *Journal of Autism and Childhood Schizophrenia*, *4*, 241–250.

Kohler, F. W., & Greenwood, C. R. (1986). Toward a technology of generalization: The identification of natural contingencies of reinforcement. *The Behavior Analyst*, *9*, 19–26.

Kuulka, A., Fry, C., & Goldstein, F. J. (1960). Kinesthetic needs in infancy. *American Journal of Orthopsychiatry*, *30*, 562–571.

Lesch, M., & Nyhan, W. L. (1964). A familial disorder of uric acid metabolism and central nervous system function. *American Journal of Medicine*, *36*, 561–570.

Lovaas, O. I., Freitag, G., Gold, V. J., & Kassorla, I. C. (1965). Experimental studies in childhood schizophrenia: Analysis of self-destructive behavior. *Journal of Experimental Child Psychology*, *2*, 67–84.

Lovaas, O. I., Newsom, C., & Hickman, C. (1987). Self-stimulatory behavior and perceptual reinforcement. *Journal of Applied Behavior Analysis*, *20*, 45–68.

Lovaas, O. I., & Simmons, J. Q. (1969). Manipulation of self-destruction in three retarded children. *Journal of Applied Behavior Analysis*, *2*, 143–157.

Luiselli, J. K. (1986). Modification of self-injurious behavior: An analysis of the use of contingently applied protective equipment. *Behavior Modification*, *10*, 191–204.

Mace, F. C., Browder, D. M., & Lin, Y. (1987). Analysis of demand conditions associated with stereotypy. *Journal of Behavior Therapy and Experimental Psychiatry*, *18*, 25–31.

Mace, F. C., & Knight, D. (1986). Functional analysis and treatment of severe pica. *Journal of Applied Behavior Analysis*, *19*, 411–416.

Mace, F. C., Lalli, J. S., & Pinter, E. (1991). Functional analysis and treatment of aberrant behavior. *Research in Developmental Disabilities*, *12*, 155–180.

Mace, F. C., Page, T. J., Ivancic, M. T., & O'Brien, S. (1986). Analysis of environmental determinants of aggression and disruption in mentally retarded children. *Applied Research in Mental Retardation*, *7*, 203–221.

Madden, N. A., Russo, D. C., & Cataldo, M. F. (1980). Environmental influences on mouthing in children with lead intoxication. *Journal of Pediatric Psychology*, *5*, 207–216.

Matson, J. L. & Taras, M. E. (1989). A 20 year review of punishment and alternate methods to treat problem behaviors in developmentally delayed persons. *Research in Developmental Disabilities*, *10*, 85–104.

Mosely, A., Faust, M., & Reardon, D. M. (1970). Effects of social and nonsocial stimuli on the stereotyped behaviors of retarded children. *American Journal of Mental Deficiency*, *74*, 809–811.

Murphy, G. (1982). Sensory reinforcement in the mentally handicapped and autistic child: A review. *Journal of Autism and Developmental Disorders*, *12*, 265–278.

Newsom, C. (in press). Self-stimulatory behavior. In O. I. Lovaas, L. Schreibman, E. G. Carr, C. Newsom, & D. C. Russo (Eds.), *Experimental analysis of autistic behaviors*. New York: Irvington.

Pace, G. M., Iwata, B. A., Edwards, G. L., & McCosh, K. C. (1986). Stimulus fading and transfer in the treatment of self-restraint and self-injurious behavior. *Journal of Applied Behavior Analysis*, *19*, 381–389.

Parrish, J. M., Iwata, B. A., Dorsey, M. F., Bunck, T. J., & Slifer, K. J. (1985). Behavior analysis, program development, and transfer of control in the treatment of self-injury. *Journal of Behavior Therapy and Experimental Psychiatry*, *16*, 159–168.

Patterson, G. R. (1969). Behavioral intervention procedures in the classroom and in the home. In A. E. Bergin & S. L. Garfield (Eds.), *Handbook of psychotherapy and behavior change*. New York: Wiley.

Picker, M., Poling, A., & Parker, A. (1979). A review of children's self-injurious behavior. *The Psychological Record*, *29*, 435–452.

Repp, A. C., & Deitz, S. M. (1974). Reducing aggressive and self-injurious behavior of institutionalized retarded children through reinforcement of other behaviors. *Journal of Applied Behavior Analysis*, *7*, 313–325.

Repp, A. C., Felce, D., & Barton, L. E. (1988). Basing the treatment of stereotypic and self-injurious behaviors on hypotheses of their causes. *Journal of Applied Behavior Analysis*, *21*, 281–289.

Rincover, A., Cook, R., Peoples, A., & Packard, D. (1979). Sensory extinction and sensory reinforcement principles for programming multiple adaptive behavior change. *Journal of Applied Behavior Analysis*, *12*, 221–233.

Rincover, A., & Devany, J. (1982). The application of sensory extinction procedures to self-injury. *Analysis and Intervention in Developmental Disabilities*, *2*, 67–81.

Rincover, A., Newsom, C. D., & Carr, E. G. (1979). Use of sensory extinction procedures in the treatment of compulsive-like behavior of developmentally disabled children. *Journal of Consulting and Clinical Psychology*, *47*, 695–701.

Romanczyk, R. G., & Goren, E. R. (1975). Severe self-injurious behavior: The problem of clinical control. *Journal of Consulting and Clinical Psychology*, *43*, 730–739.

Ross, R. R., Meichenbaum, D. H., & Humphrey, C. (1971). Treatment of nocturnal headbanging by behavior modification techniques: A case report. *Behavior Research and Therapy*, *9*, 151–154.
Saudargas, R. A. & Lentz, F. E. (1986). Estimating percent of time and rate via direct observation: A suggested observational procedure and format. *School Psychology Review*, *15*, 36–48.
Schroeder, S. R., Schroeder, C. S., Rojahn, J., & Mulick, J. A. (1981). Self-injurious behavior: An analysis of behavior management techniques. In J. L. Matson & J. R. McCartney (Eds.), *Handbook of behavior modification with the mentally retarded* (pp. 61–115). New York: Plenum Press.
Shaefer, H. H. (1970). Self-injurious behavior: Shaping "head-banging" in monkeys. *Journal of Applied Behavior Analysis*, *3*, 111–116.
Skinner, B. F. (1938). *The behavior of organisms*. New York: Appleton-Century-Crofts.
Skinner, B. F. (1953). *Science and human behavior*. New York: Macmillan.
Skinner, B. F. (1957). *Verbal behavior*. Englewood Cliffs, NJ: Prentice-Hall.
Skinner, B. F. (1969). *Contingencies of reinforcement: A theoretical analysis*. Englewood Cliffs, NJ: Prentice-Hall.
Steege, M. W., Wacker, D. P., Berg, W. K., Cigrand, K. K., & Cooper, L. J. (1989). The use of behavioral assessment to prescribe and evaluate treatments for severely handicapped children. *Journal of Applied Behavior Analysis*, *22*, 23–33.
Steege, M. W., Wacker, D., & McMahon, C. (1987). Evaluation of the effectiveness and efficiency of two stimulus prompt strategies with severely handicapped students. *Journal of Applied Behavior Analysis*, *20*, 293–299.
Stockes, T. F., & Baer, D. M. (1977). An implicit technology of generalization. *Journal of Applied Behavior Analysis*, *10*, 349–367.
Strain, P. S., & Ezzell, D. (1978). The sequence and distribution of behaviorally disordered adolescents' disruptive/inappropriate behaviors. *Behavior Modification*, *2*, 403–425.
Tanner, B., & Zeiler, M. (1975). Punishment of self-injurious behavior using aromatic ammonia as the aversive stimulus. *Journal of Applied Behavior Analysis*, *8*, 53–57.
Tarpley, H., & Schroeder, S. (1979). Comparison of DRO and DRI on rate of suppression of self-injurious behavior. *American Journal of Mental Deficiency*, *84*, 188–194.
Tate, B. G., & Baroff, G. S. (1966). Aversive control of self-injurious behavior in a psychotic boy. *Behaviour Research and Therapy*, *4*, 281–287.
Touchette, P. E., MacDonald, R. F., & Langer, S. N. (1985). A scatter plot for identifying stimulus control of problem behavior. *Journal of Applied Behavior Analysis*, *18*, 343–351.
Vyse, S., Mulick, J. A., & Thayer, B. M. (1984). An ecobehavioral assessment of a special education classroom. *Applied Research in Mental Retardation*, *5*, 395–408.
Wahler, R. G. (1975). Some structural aspects of deviant child behavior. *Journal of Applied Behavior Analysis*, *8*, 27–42.
Wahler, R. G., & Fox, J. J. (1981). Setting events in applied behavior analysis: Towards a conceptual and methodological expansion. *Journal of Applied Behavior Analysis*, *14*, 327–338.

Weeks, M., & Gaylord-Ross, R. (1981). Task difficulty and aberrant behavior in severely handicapped students. *Journal of Applied Behavior Analysis*, *14*, 449–463.
White, G. D., Nielsen, G., & Johnson, S. M. (1972). Time-out duration and the suppression of deviant behavior in children. *Journal of Applied Behavior Analysis*, *5*, 111–120.
Wolf, M., Risley, T., & Mees, H. (1964). Application of operant conditioning procedures to the behavior problems of an autistic child. *Behaviour Research and Therapy*, *1*, 305–312.

# Part 3
## Treatment

# 6
# Behavioral Diagnostic Interventions

DAVID A. M. PYLES and JON S. BAILEY

Over the past 20 years, great strides have been made in the analysis and treatment of self-injurious behavior (SIB). Although a few of the early studies (Lovaas, Freitag, Gold, & Kassorla, 1965) investigated controlling conditions, most of the research literature focused on the manipulation of consequences to reduce the frequency and/or severity of SIB. Little attention was paid to causes (i.e., the *function* the behavior served).

That tradition began to change with the publication of Iwata, Dorsey, Slifer, Bauman, and Richman (1982). This research showed that SIBs of similar topography could be caused by different operant variables. The logical extension of this investigation is that for ethical and effective treatment, interventions should be based on the *function* of the behavior, not topography alone. Bailey and Pyles (1989) illustrated the importance of basing treatment of maladaptive behavior on its causes with the example of a client who engaged in SIB when demands were made. Placing the client in time-out contingent upon SIB would be contraindicated, as that intervention would positively reinforce escape behavior—clearly an unacceptable treatment.

Recently, other innovations have been made in the analysis of maladaptive behaviors. Bailey and Pyles (1989) describe a new approach to analyzing and treating maladaptive behaviors: behavioral diagnostics. This method involves collecting all possible information about a client and the events surrounding the behavior, both antecedent and consequent. Behavioral diagnostics places much more emphasis on antecedent conditions than historically has been the case. Examples of the data collected include nutrition variables, such as caloric intake or food allergies; physiological variables, such as menstrual cycles or constipation; medication variables, such as drug dosage and side effects; and operant variables, such as demands made, or attention received for maladaptive behavior.

When designing interventions using the behavior diagnostics method, two different approaches are used. The first, *active behavior management*, utilizes the manipulation of consequence variables to affect the rates of the targeted maladaptive behaviors. This approach is exemplified by the

$S \rightarrow R \rightarrow S^{R+}$ model (stimulus–response–reinforcing stimulus) and is the method most commonly taught for addressing maladaptive behaviors. The second, *passive behavior management*, involves manipulating antecedent variables so that maladaptive behaviors are not occasioned, either by reducing an aversive condition the client attempts to escape, or by removing the stimulus cues indicating that reinforcement for a given behavior is forthcoming. This method is diagrammed $S -//\rightarrow R \rightarrow S^{R+}$, showing that the discriminative or eliciting stimuli for the response has been removed, thus reducing the probabilities the behavior will occur.

## Active Behavior Management

Active behavior management represents the vast majority of methods in the research literature for reducing SIB. The positive reinforcement approaches involve reinforcement for *not* engaging in self injury (DRO), for engaging in alternative or incompatible behaviors (DRA/DRI), or teaching the client to comply with requests.

The punishment procedures involve presentation of an aversive stimulus contingent upon the client's engaging in SIB. The active behavior management approaches for reducing SIB will be described briefly here; for more detail, the reader is referred to the other chapters of this volume. These procedures are briefly described, with a description of the advantages, disadvantages and limiting conditions of the approaches. The same analysis is done later in the chapter with the aversive and the Passive Behavior Management approaches to reducing self-injurious behavior.

### *Positive Reinforcement Interventions*

Positive reinforcement has been used to reduce SIB in the research literature. The typical approach is to reinforce the subject for *not* engaging in the targeted responses, also known as **d**ifferential **r**einforcement of **o**ther behavior(s) (DRO). Variations on this theme include **d**ifferential **r**einforcement of **a**lternative behaviors (DRA) and **d**ifferential **r**einforcement of **i**ncompatible (DRI) behaviors. Compliance training has also been used to reduce self-injurious and other disruptive behaviors caused by demands made on the subjects. Figure 6.1 summarizes the major features of positive-reinforcement interventions.

#### Differential Reinforcement

The differences between differential reinforcement methods are slight and vary with regard to the behavior to be reinforced. DRO approaches usually reinforce the client for *not* engaging in SIB, whereas DRA and

Active behavior management

| Positive Reinforcement Interventions | | | |
|---|---|---|---|
| Procedure | Advantages | Disadvantages | Limiting conditions |
| DRO | • Positive<br>• No escape–avoidance emotional behaviors<br>• Little/No outside review necessary | • Ineffective by itself as an intervention<br>• Slow to obtain behavior change<br>• Does not address function | • Must have identified reinforcer<br>• Can client respond to schedule of reinforcement for nonoccurrence of behavior?<br>• Must have adequate staff ratio |
| DRA/DRI | • Positive<br>• No escape–avoidance emotional behaviors<br>• Addresses skill deficit<br>• Little/No outside review necessary | • Little research to document effectiveness<br>• Slow to obtain behavior change | • Must have identified reinforcer<br>• Can client respond to schedule of reinforcement for nonoccurrence of behavior?<br>• Must have adequate staff ratio |
| Compliance training (DRC) | • Positive<br>• Addresses function<br>• Little/No outside review necessary | • Can be slow to obtain behavior change | • Must have identified reinforcer<br>• Must have adequate staff ratio<br>• Not recommended for strong/resistive clients<br>• Little research with SIB applications to document effectiveness |

FIGURE 6.1. Advantages, disadvantages, and limiting conditions of positive-reinforcement interventions.

DRI target specific behaviors to be reinforced, which are anything other than SIB. The difference between DRA and DRI is that the behavior reinforced under a DRA schedule can physically occur at the same time as the SIB, but the behavior reinforced under a DRI schedule precludes the possibility of SIB occurring. For example, suppose a client engages in the SIB of hitting his head with his hand. Under a DRA, the client may be reinforced for listening to music. Using a DRI, however, the client may be reinforced for assembling puzzles—a use of the hands being incompatible with SIB. There is, however, little if any, literature documenting the use of DRA/DRI to reduce self-injury (cf. Tarpley & Schroeder, 1979).

Corte, Wolf, and Locke (1971) used a DRO to reduce the SIB of two profoundly retarded children. Initially, they attempted to reinforce the subjects for not engaging in SIB for 15 seconds. If they did become self-injurious, there was a 45-second delay before being eligible for receiving reinforcement in a subsequent trial. With one subject, the DRO did not work until the researchers deprived the subject of food (the subject was not given lunch; the sessions were not run until 3:00 P.M.) and changed the edible reinforcer to one that was more salient under the same 15-second schedule of reinforcement. The other subject did not respond under either the nondeprived or the food-deprived DRO.

Rolider and Van Houten (1985) analyzed the effects of a DRO alone versus DRO plus movement-suppression time-out for SIB with two subjects. For both subjects, the DRO was ineffective in reducing the maladaptive behaviors by itself; however, the DRO plus movement-suppression time-out was effective in eliminating the SIB (see also, Luiselli, Myles, Evans, & Boyce, 1985).

## Compliance Training

Iwata et al. (1982) found, when demands were made on subjects in analogue settings, some of the subjects increased their rates of SIB, indicating that the subjects engaged in the behavior to escape the demand situation. The SIB was maintained by negative reinforcement—an escape–avoidance paradigm.

Carr and Durand (1985) found that as task difficulty increased, two subjects engaged in increased rates of aggressive, disruptive, and self-injurious behaviors (data were not presented by individual behavior); thus lending additional support for demands maintaining maladaptive behaviors with some clients.

The treatment of choice for maladaptive behaviors maintained by escape from demands is typically compliance training. In such a paradigm, the behavior analyst teaches the client to comply with requests by providing reinforcement contingent upon compliance to a request (e.g., Carr & Durand, 1985). Graduated guidance is used to teach clients to perform tasks using a least-to-most intrusive instructional prompt sequence (Cuvo & Davis, 1983). With this procedure, a client is given the opportunity to perform a skill on her or his own. If unsuccessful, verbal prompts, demonstration prompts, then physical guidance are provided until the client performs the task.

Steege, Wacker, and McMahon (1987) described a procedure called "prescriptive training," whereby a baseline was taken of prompting required to perform the steps of a task. Training then involved using a level of prompt one step less restrictive than required previously to perform the step. If that level of prompt was unsuccessful, the trainer then escalated to the next level of prompt, which had been successful to get the client to perform the step previously. Prescriptive training has not been used as a means of compliance training in the research literature, but it may provide an alternative means of obtaining compliance.

Behavioral momentum is another technique for obtaining compliance to requests (Mace, Hock, Lalli, West, Belfiore, Pinter, & Brown,

1988). This procedure entails giving several simple, high-probability-of-compliance requests before making other, lower-probability-of-compliance requests.

In our work in applied settings, we have also used a procedure we call "differential reinforcement for compliance" (DRC). With this procedure, staff members approach a client and make requests on a schedule. If she complies, she is reinforced heavily; if she does not, staff members walk away. This procedure is a slow but useful one for clients whose strength and/or extreme resistance make physical guidance difficult or impossible.

Little, if any, research has been done examining the effects of compliance training per se on SIB. However, data from other studies indicate that rates of maladaptive behaviors can be decreased by teaching clients to comply with requests.

## Advantages of Positive-Reinforcement Interventions

There are several advantages of using positive-reinforcement interventions to reduce SIB. The focus on reinforcing appropriate behaviors rather than using aversive procedures to reduce inappropriate behaviors has widespread appeal. The approach is positive, and few can argue with trying less intrusive measures before more intrusive ones (if necessary), so long as they are effective.

Another advantage in using positive-reinforcement approaches is that they do not result in escape or avoidance behaviors by the client. There are no emotional or countercontrol (Skinner, 1969) measures taken to avoid the aversive interventions.

## Disadvantages of Positive-Reinforcement Interventions

Despite the positive press (LaVigna & Donellan, 1986), the major disadvantage to using positive-reinforcement interventions for reducing SIB is that they are largely ineffective. All studies reviewed showed little or no effect in reducing SIB, unless the researchers increased deprivation or combined differential reinforcement with other procedures. The positive-reinforcement intervention holding the most promise is compliance training, but this procedure would only be effective with escape-motivated SIB.

Another disadvantage to using positive-reinforcement interventions is that even if changes do occur, dramatic decreases in SIB take a long time. If rapid behavior change is desired, others procedures are indicated.

Not all clients engaging in SIB have identifiable reinforcers, a third disadvantage to using positive-reinforcement procedures. Unless a client has an identified, relatively powerful reinforcer, providing preferred stimuli contingent upon compliance or the nonoccurrence of a behavior is unlikely to affect rates of SIB.

### Limiting Conditions for Positive-Reinforcement Interventions

One major limiting condition for using positive-reinforcement interventions is the relative lack of effectiveness compared to other procedures. The behavioral literature does not support the efficacy of DRO/DRA/DRI without other contingencies as well—it is the rare case where these interventions have been effective in reducing SIB by themselves (Corte, Wolf, & Locke, 1971; Dorsey, Iwata, Ong, & McSween, 1980).

A further concern is that many clients have no identified reinforcers, or do not respond when the *occurrence* of a behavior is reinforced. We have found even slower progress providing reinforcement for the *nonoccurrence* of a behavior. Typically, the durations used in a DRO with profoundly mentally retarded persons are so short that the trainer must continuously reinforce (more accurately, *feed*) the client on a 5–30-second schedule.

It is physically impossible for direct-care staff to reinforce even one, let alone several clients simultaneously on such schedules of reinforcement. Even if it were possible, one should have reservations about attempting to reinforce (especially with edibles) every 30 seconds throughout the day for nonoccurrence of SIB. The clients would most likely quickly satiate, making food (or any other stimulus) even *less* of a reinforcer. Such food intake would interfere with the client's dietary regimen, most likely resulting in weight gain, possibly putting the client at health risk.

## *Aversive Interventions*

Aversive procedures have been successful in reducing SIB. Procedures range from annoying stimuli such as water mist to painful stimuli such as electric shock (Corte, Wolf, & Locke, 1971; Foxx & Azrin, 1973; Lovaas & Simmons, 1969; Rolider & Van Houten, 1985; Tanner & Zeiler, 1975). The fact that they work is the reason systematic oversight and peer review is necessary—to reduce their potential for abuse. Figure 6.2 outlines the major features of aversive procedures.

Aversive procedures are discussed in greater detail in Chapter 10 of this volume, and thus are only briefly reviewed here, to illustrate the types of methods employed using an active behavior management approach to reduce SIB.

### Water Mist

Dorsey et al. (1980) used a "fine mist of water directed toward the participant's face contingent upon the occurrence of a target SIB" to reduce the rates of self-abuse with eight profoundly retarded clients. The sprayer was held about 0.3 meters form the subjects' faces and dispensed approximately 0.6 cc (cubic centimeters) of water each spray. The mist was described as "annoying," rather than painful by the experimenters.

Active behavior management

| Procedure | Aversive Interventions<br>Advantages | Disadvantages | Limiting conditions |
|---|---|---|---|
| Water mist | • Quick to obtain behavior change<br>• Not painful | • May not be strong enough stimulus to cause behavior change<br>• Does not address function | • Moderately restricted procedure—must obtain consent<br>• Must have adequate staff ratio<br>• Little published research |
| Aversive taste (Lemon juice, Tabasco Sauce) | • Not painful<br>• Quick results in literature | • May function as reinforcer for some clients<br>• May not be strong enough stimulus to cause behavior change<br>• Does not address function | • Moderately restricted procedure—must obtain consent<br>• Must have adequate staff ratio<br>• Little published research |
| Overcorrection | • Quick results in literature<br>• May address function (positive practice) | • May result in escape-avoidance behaviors<br>• Time consuming to implement | • Moderately restricted procedure<br>• May not be appropriate for strong/combative clients |
| Protective equipment | • Prevents tissue damage<br>• Quick results in literature | • Does not address function | • Moderately to very restricted procedure—must obtain consent<br>• Little published research<br>• Requires adequate staff ratio and supervision |
| Restraint | • Prevents tissue damage<br>• Quick results in literature | • Does not address function<br>• May function as a positive reinforcer for some clients | • Moderately to very restricted procedure—must obtain consent<br>• Requires adequate staff ratio and supervision |
| Aromatic ammonia | • Quick results in literature | • Subjects may struggle<br>• Smell lingers on person implementing procedure<br>• Does not address function | • Moderately to very restricted procedure; may not be permited in some states/agencies.<br>• May not be appropriate for strong/agile clients<br>• Little published research |
| Electric shock | • Very quick results in literature | • Subjects resist/ attempt to escape<br>• Very aversive to subjects<br>• Does not address function<br>• Results do not maintain or generalize to new situations—very high stimulus specificity | • Very restricted or prohibited procedure<br>• Requires intensive supervision and oversight |

FIGURE 6.2. Advantages, disadvantages, and limiting conditions of positive aversive interventions.

With each subject, providing water mist contingent upon SIB resulted in rapid and substantial decreases of the targeted behaviors for each subject. Two of the subjects were exposed to DRO conditions, which had no effect until paired with water mist. Combining water mist with a DRO plus verbal reprimand ("No") allowed the experimenters to withdraw the water mist while maintaining treatment effects.

### Lemon Juice

Sajwaj, Libet, and Agras (1974) used lemon juice as a punisher to reduce life-threatening rumination with a 6-month-old infant. They squirted 5 to 10 cc of lemon juice (unsweetened Realemon brand) into her mouth, contingent upon rumination, with a 30-cc medical syringe. This intervention resulted in rapid reductions of her rumination to near-zero rates. The subject also gained nearly 3 pounds from the initiation of treatment to her discharge from the medical center.

Favell, McGimsey, and Jones (1978) used lemon juice to reduce eye-poking with a profoundly retarded girl, reducing the rates of the behavior. Further treatment gains were achieved using a treatment package of lemon juice contingent on occurrences of SIB, restraint (as a reinforcer) for not engaging in SIB, and "distraction" (providing alternative activities).

### Overcorrection

Foxx and Azrin (1973) used an overcorrection procedure to reduce hand-mouthing (described as self-stimulation in this study) with two severely retarded girls. The method described by Foxx and Azrin involved brushing the child's teeth and gums with an antiseptic solution and wiping her outer lips with a washcloth dampened with the antiseptic. The overcorrection procedure reduced hand-mouthing to rates below those obtained using reinforcement for not hand-mouthing, noncontingent reinforcement, physical punishment, or distasteful solution on the hands.

Overcorrection procedures have been successful in reducing a number of maladaptive behaviors in the research literature. Overcorrection, however, is *not* appropriate for clients whose size, strength, and/or resistance allows them to escape implementation of the procedure (see Chapter 8, this volume).

### Restraint

Use of restraints, including protective equipment, is probably the most commonly used treatment for severe SIB. Implemented either alone or as part of an intervention package, restraint is primarily utilized to prevent tissue damage or to terminate the ongoing maladaptive behavior quickly. Rapoff, Altman, and Christophersen (1980) used brief periods of restraint (30 seconds) to reduce head hitting.

Protective equipment has also been used to decrease SIB (Dorsey, Iwata, Reid, & Davis, 1982), although some behavior management guidelines consider this procedure to be a form of restraint. Advantages of protective equipment include its not being as likely to function as a reinforcer with some clients, its preventing of tissue damage, and its decreasing of possible sensory stimulation reinforcement received by engaging in SIB. (Protective equipment interventions are reviewed extensively in Chapter 9.)

There have been abuses of restraint in the past, with some clients remaining in restraints 24 hours or longer at a time. Federal and state ICF/MR guidelines (Intermediate Care Facilities for the Mentally Retarded) provide strict instructions for oversight and implementation of restraints to consequate maladaptive behaviors. However, these guidelines do not cover *all* facilities treating developmentally disabled persons. Any use of restraint should be implemented only with stringent human rights, behavioral, and medical staff oversight.

A further caveat about using restraint to reduce SIB is that with some clients, restraint can function as a positive reinforcer (Favell, McGimsey, & Jones, 1978). When using restraint for SIB, data must be monitored carefully to make sure the restraint itself does not *increase* the rates of the behavior.

### Aromatic Ammonia

Tanner and Zeiler (1975) investigated the use of aromatic ammonia contingent upon face-slapping. They crushed capsules of aromatic ammonia and held them under the subject's nose upon occurrence of the target behavior. This intervention produced very rapid and substantial reductions in her SIB; an effect replicated using an A-B-A-B design.

Tanner and Zeiler (1975) reported that the smell of the ammonia pellets was mildly annoying up to about 2 feet from the source but was aversive only when the capsules were brought close to the nose. They also noted that bringing the pellets into direct contact with the skin could result in tissue damage. During one intervention phase (when she had a cold), scabs appeared on the subject's nose. It was unknown whether the cold or ammonia pellets were responsible.

### Electric Shock

Electric shock contingent upon occurrences of SIB has been shown to produce rapid decreases in SIB responding in the literature (Corte, Wolf, & Locke, 1971; Lovaas & Simmons, 1969; Risley, 1968; Tate & Baroff, 1966). The voltages were described as painful but did not cause tissue damage. Lovaas and Simmons (1969) raise the question of how shock even works, in view of the more intense pain associated with some forms of SIB (giving the example of one client who pulled his own nails out with his teeth). The procedures have uniformly been associated with rapid and substantial decreases in SIB.

There are a number of drawbacks to using electric shock in the studies cited. For example, Corte, Wolf, and locke (1971) reported that the subjects often tried to escape or resist the shock. They also noted that the effects were not durable. Lovaas and Simmons (1969) also reported that reductions in SIB were highly specific both to physical locales and to the attending adults.

The use of electric shock is also very controversial and highly regulated (e.g., 1989 Federal ICF/MR regulations) or prohibited (Florida's Health and Rehabilitative Services 160–4 Behavior Management Guidelines). Furthermore, there are groups actively lobbying legislatures to ban the use of aversive procedures, especially electric shock.

As such, electric shock should only be used after other attempts to reduce SIB have failed, and with the interdisciplinary team approval, following all state and federal standards. Only trained professionals should implement these procedures.

## Advantages of Aversive Procedures

One reason aversive procedures may have had such widespread exposure in the literature is that researchers have been reinforced for using them. In this case, the reinforcer is rapid behavior change: an effective treatment showing (nearly) immediate results. Practitioners, likewise, have been reinforced for using such procedures.

Nearly all the research articles reviewed here demonstrated rapid and substantial decreases in the targeted behaviors once aversive contingencies were applied. When differential reinforcement procedures have been compared to aversive ones, the latter uniformly resulted in quicker and greater decreases in rates than the former. Herein lies a major benefit of using aversive procedures: speed of significant reductions in SIB.

A second reason these procedures are used is that they work. As stated earlier, the published research demonstrates more substantial reductions in SIB using aversive procedures than reinforcement methods. The fact that they work is the very reason they are so controversial and restricted—it can be all too easy to use aversive contingencies to suppress behavior rather than finding functional controlling variables. As a result, aversive contingencies are often applied without regard to the cause. If the intervention does not correspond to the function, unethical and ineffective treatment may very well result.

A third advantage to using aversive contingencies is that, in many cases, the program only need be implemented a short while before rates decrease to zero or near-zero levels. As a result, programs are often implemented for only short periods of time before they become unnecessary and are discontinued. Thus, the client may come into contact with programmatic contingencies fewer times by using more-intrusive procedures than less-intrusive ones. The end result may be less total damage to the client.

### Disadvantages of Aversive Procedures

The disadvantages of using aversive procedures are well documented and discussed in both the research and theoretical literature. Most often cited are the emotional behaviors such as escape, avoidance, or aggression. For example, Corte, Wolf, and Locke (1971) modified their electric-shock procedure because the subjects resisted being shocked on the same arm the subject used for self-injury.

Another criticism of using aversive procedures is that the staff implementing the procedures become conditioned aversive stimuli. The clients may avoid the staff altogether, due to the generalized negative stimulation, and thus reduce the opportunities for positive contact between staff and client. Lovaas and Simmons (1969), however, found that the subjects did not avoid the staff implementing the procedures except when the staff had an angry expression on their faces (that facial expression having been paired with the electric shocks during the treatment conditions). The generalized avoidance effects of aversive stimulation contingent upon SIB are not well researched in the developmental disabilities literature, so definitive statements cannot be made.

The possibility of tissue damage occurring from painful stimuli is very real. Malfunction or misuse of electrical shock apparatuses could harm or burn the client. As described earlier, Tanner and Zeiler (1975) reported that scabs developed on the subject's nose during an aromatic ammonia treatment condition. It was not known whether the sores were due to accidental skin contact with the ammonia pellets, or to a cold the subject had. Any noxious or painful procedures should be closely monitored by both medical and behavioral staff to cnsurc that no tissuc damage results from application of aversive procedures.

### Limiting Conditions of Aversive Procedures

Aversive procedures, like any other in our technology, have conditions that must be satisfied before the procedures can work. For example, it is a truism that a procedure must be implemented consistently in order for it to be successful—and no treatment should be designed or implemented if it cannot be performed consistently. However, consistency is not the only limiting condition that must be met when implementing restrictive procedures; there are other conditions affecting the successful implementation of restrictive programming that require consideration before they are used.

State and federal regulations provide limiting conditions to the use of aversive procedures. These regulations primarily guide the implementation of behavioral procedures in ICF/MRs, and proscribe the use of certain aversive procedures, or place limitations on the uses of some procedures until specific conditions are met. Every practitioner should be aware of and should follow the regulations applicable in her or his given circumstance.

Ethical treatment involves, among other things, using the least restrictive intervention effective to reduce the targeted maladaptive behavior. Other ethical considerations include doing a behavioral diagnosis before conducting treatment, and designing interventions based upon the causes of the behaviors. This brief list covers but a few of the factors to be considered in providing treatment. They were included as a prompt: ethical considerations should play an important role in making treatment decisions and in program implementation as well.

Use of aversive procedures should be closely monitored by appropriately trained professionals. Supervision of staff implementing these procedures is absolutely necessary to ensure strict adherence to programmatic contingencies and to prevent abuse of clients. As such, much professional time and energy must be spent overseeing programs when aversive procedures are used. If adequate supervision cannot be provided, these procedures should not be used.

Some aversive procedures, such as overcorrection, or response effort require the client to engage in specified behaviors contingent upon targeted responses. For example, if a client becomes self-injurious, he or she may be required to wash any cuts, apply antiseptic and bandages, etc. However, some clients physically resist complying with the requests that are part of programmatic contingencies. If the client is able to escape demands or physical guidance, or resists strongly, these procedures are not recommended, as they could cause more problems than they solve (i.e., the client then develops a history of resisting that may be difficult to extinguish).

Even if staff can overpower a resistive client to gain compliance, using superior physical strength is still not recommended because (1) the client may learn to discriminate who can overpower him and who cannot, and differentially respond to each; (2) resorting to physical force to obtain compliance often leads to client aggression toward staff, further compounding the problem; and (3) if superior physical force needs to be used to obtain compliance, some aspect(s) of the training procedure need(s) to be examined to determine whether it is the best available treatment.

## *The Limiting Conditions of Behavior Technology*

Behavior analysis is often considered a technology without limits. The successes, especially those presented in leading journals, imply that the technology of behavior can be used to solve *any* problem. An examination of published studies is, in fact, quite impressive. Severe and long-standing behavior problems *have* been treated successfully (Bailey, Shook, Iwata, Reid, & Repp, 1989). However, readers and potential therapists must be cautioned to read the method section of such studies carefully, to learn the conditions under which such studies were carried out. Replication is at the heart of our science and, presumably, if an equally qualified person can replicate the conditions under which the study was carried out, they should be able to replicate the outcome as well.

In the treatment of severe self-injury, it is important to note several distinguishing features of this research. First, it is necessary to consider who carried out the treatment. A quick review of the most significant studies in this field suggests that the intervention was most often carried out by M.A.- or Ph.D.-level researchers/therapists. This situation is as it should be, of course, because they have a dual responsibility of treating clients *and* contributing to the research literature. For research purposes, the treatments are carried out by the same personnel every day (usually at a set time). In addition, the ratio of clients to staff is usually 1:1 (sometimes, it can be 1:2 or 1:3). Furthermore, the treatment, again for the sake of consistency and research consideratons, is usually carried out for relatively short sessions each day. Such sessions usually occur in a controlled lablike environment or a simulation of some aspect of a living or working environment for the client (e.g., a classroom). Finally, a close examination of the studies in the literature suggests that a high percentage of the applied research has been carried out with moderately or severely mentally retarded clients.

Behavior analysis technology has reached far beyond the laboratory. It is virtually mandated by state and federal regaultions and is seen as *the* treatment of choice by those working in the field.

Unfortunately, the conditions in the field under which the technology must be carried out rarely match those seen in the published research. In the real world, the most contact with clients comes from direct-care staff who, for the most part, are mimimum-wage employees with a high school (or GED) diploma. It is not unusual to have high turnover in such facilities, with 100% turnover per year found routinely. Furthermore, this staff consists of three shifts per day and may amount to as many a 16 different staff coming in contact with a client in one 24-hour period. Funding is such that a 5:1 (clients to staff) ratio is seen fairly regularly (it should be less, usually 3:1 is required by law, but with sick leave, lunch breaks, rest breaks, meetings, etc., 5:1 is common). These clients require treatment 24 hours per day, and the treatment must be carried out most often in open community and residential settings where there is little control over who comes into contact with the client. Finally, the population in most residential treatment settings is 85% profoundly retarded.

Proponents of the field, in an effort to rally support for applications, rarely mention the treatments that did not work, and such applications are never published. As an extenstion of the science of human behavior, the technology *is* limited, especially as it carried out in human service settings, by available resources. As we consider the treatment of SIB, these limiting conditions must be kept in mind. Having to face these conditions has forced us to reconsider the applicability of many of the standard behavioral treatment procedures. Those requiring considerable expertise, consistency of application, and control over the environment do not appear likely to succeed. These limiting conditions have forced us to search for other alternative treatments that will work in less than ideal conditions.

### Client Characteristics and Limiting Conditions

One further dimension needs to be considered when behavioral treatments appear appropriate for client treatment. Those procedures based on positive reinforcement (DRO, DRI, DRA) make one simple assumption: A known reinforcer exists for the client in question. In the population we have been working with for the past 5 years, the lack of a known reinforcer has been a primary limiting condition. These clients, all in the profound range, do not appear to respond to any enviromental stimuli (including food) on any consistent basis. Visual and auditory stimuli have been successful on a short-term basis with some clients, but many clients are blind and deaf, thus providing obvious limits. Social reinforcers appear very weak, and the lack of any extensive operant repertoire makes activity reinforcers untenable most of the time.

### The Need for Alternatives

The aforementioned practical limiting conditions have forced us to seek alternatives in the treatment of self-injurious behavior. In our facility, we do not always have adequate staff to carry out complex and demanding active behavior management programs. State law prohibits the use of many aversive procedures. As a result, we have been actively involved in finding other ways of treating client behavior problems. The behavioral diagnostic method and passive behavior management are the results of that search.

## Passive Behavior Management

The primary thrust of traditional behavior modification approaches has been the reduction or elimination of behavior problems by the use of consequences. This work is widely represented in the literature, and the techniques are now widely used wherever severe behavior problems arise. Typically, little attention is paid to the cause of the behavior problem because it is assumed to be buried somewhere in the past history of the individual and is unlikely to be uncovered. Recently, we have begun to

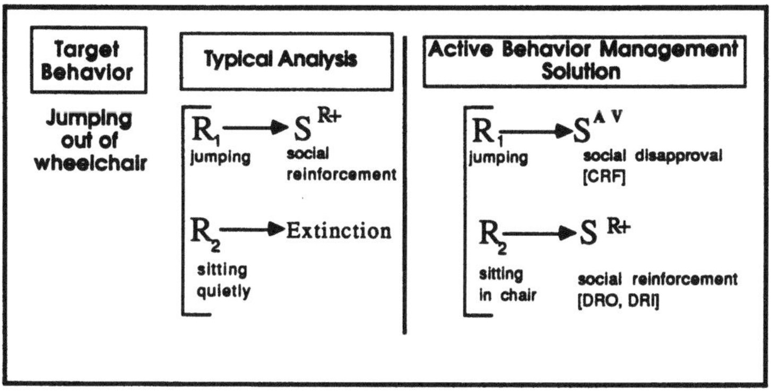


FIGURE 6.3. Standard behavior analysis and typical active behavior management solution.

discover, however, a striking number of cases where there is a fairly clear antecedent that appears to produce the maladaptive or self-injurious behavior. One case in particular serves to illustrate this point.

James was a profoundly retarded, nonverbal, nonambulatory young adult who began throwing himself out of his wheelchair onto the floor. Observations revealed staff quickly approached him when this occurred and tended to his split lip or bump on the head. When he sat quietly in his chair, he was, for the most part, ignored. A standard behavior analysis of this pattern suggests that the contingencies are simply backward: James should be reinforced when he sits appropriately and given some form of punisher (probably response interruption and social disapproval initially). Figure 4.3 illustrates this analysis and the resulting standard behavior program.

Typically, behavior programs predicated on "behavior is a function of consequences" emphasize aversive consequences for the inappropriate behavior and positive reinforcement for the incompatible behavior. In the present case, however, further investigation revealed that James may well be responding to an antecedent stimulus from which he is trying to escape. His daily schedule had him in his wheelchair almost continuously from approximately 6:30 A.M. until the time the jumping occurred (about 3–3:30 P.M. when he returned home from school). A new analysis of his behavior is shown in Figure 6.4. While still operant in nature, this anaylsis suggests the behavior is maintained by negative reinforcement (i.e. escape from the aversive stimulus).

The most appropriate treatment in this case is removal of the antecedent, which should eliminate the response. When this program was implemented (i.e., James was taken out of his wheelchair and placed on a mat or on the couch), the jumping dropped to zero. He made no other attempts to harm himself in any other way and subjectively appeared

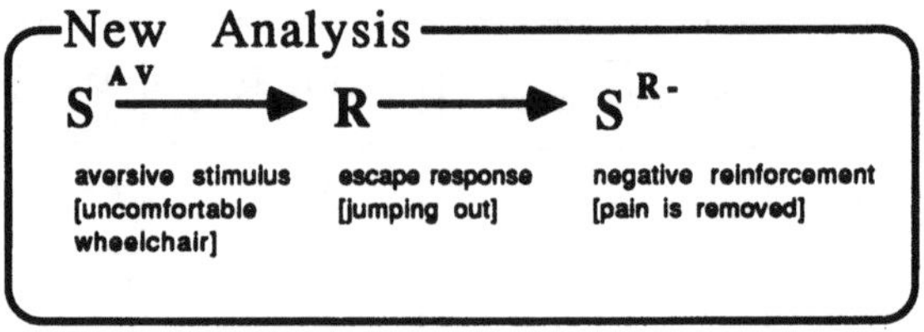


FIGURE 6.4. A new analysis of the behavior suggests that it may be a function of antecedent stimuli that are aversive and produce escape responses.

greatly relieved to be out of the chair. After a few days of this routine, he began, upon arriving back at his residence, raising his elbows in anticipation of being taken from his chair.

The success of this program reinforced our analyzing every existing client case to determine whether similar variables were operating. New cases were similarly analyzed from the outset. Over a 5-year period of using this method, we have determined a wide variety of alternative solutions to the treatment of severe behavior disorders, including SIB similar to that described previously, which are effective.

## *Categories of Passive Interventions*

### Reduce Discomfort and Pain

Pain and discomfort in particular appear to affect the nonverbal, multiply handicapped, profoundly mentally retarded person. Unable to effectively communicate their discomfort or to take action to stop it, they may engage in what appears to be maladaptive behavior. One client, who had not had previous referrals, began engaging in face slapping and face scratching and was immediately referred when the staff were unable to stop her. The SIB did not appear to occur under any consistent setting conditions (e.g., a response to demands, or at any particular time of day). About the time the behavior program had been approved and was ready for implementation, it was discovered the client had infected sinuses. Following medical treatment, the SIB ceased, and the client was treated by the nursing staff with the antihistamines for an allergy that appeared to cause the sinus infection.

Another nonverbal, nonambulatory client engaged in crying and sobbing throughout the day. A detailed analysis over several weeks revealed she was responding to being wet, constipated, and thirsty. In addition, she was bothered by menstrual cramps and was easily fatigued. When she was checked often to be sure she had not wet herself, was changed to a high-fiber diet, was offered water regularly, was given Motrin for menstrual cramps, and offered naps twice per day, she ceased the crying and sobbing.

### Improve Communications

Another client pounded his chest with sufficient force that it could be heard across the room. He was referred by the nurse for SIB. When the staff members were asked about the behavior, they readily offered an explanation. "He just does that when he wants to go to the bathroom." The treatment of choice in such cases in not a standard behavior program, which involves a DRO for non-chest-beating and social disapproval for the response but rather a training program to teach a less harmful way of getting staff attention.

### Break Up Behavior Chains

Rob's most salient behavior was his propensity to destruction. He would tear up his wheel chair, walls, bulletin boards, tile floors, or the couch. He needed a small tool to do his work, and finding paper clips, push pins, thumb tacks or any other small, hard object took up most of his time each day. When these objects were taken from him, he sometimes began engaging in severe hand-biting, head-hitting, and head-banging. As shown in Figure 6.5, frequency of SIB and attempted destructions occurred at high levels over a 3-month baseline period. In order to break up the chain of behavior, a major effort was begun in the fifth month to totally eliminate potential tools for Rob. Again, as shown in Figure 6.5, attempted destructions were reduced from an average of 300 per month to less then 100. During this same time, his SIB was reduced from 12–15 per month to 5–8 instances per month. By focusing on the antecedent rather than the target behavior, we were able to significantly reduce the SIB.

### Teach Staff More Adaptive Responses

One client repeatedly fell out of bed in the evening, causing tissue damage and requiring the nurses to apply bandages. Building an apparatus to keep her in bed was proposed, but because it was severely restrictive, it was not considered further. The night staff were aware of the problem and with some questioning explained that the client was trying to transfer to her wheelchair so she could go down to the TV room. This was not permitted as they "had too much too do" and could not be bothered watching her. However, when it was explained that young adults (she was 25 years old) often watch TV in the evenings, and that no behavior program to keep her in her bed would be approved, a new schedule for her bed time was set. Further, she was to be given some one-on-one training on wheelchair transfer. No further incidents of self-injury in the evening were reported.

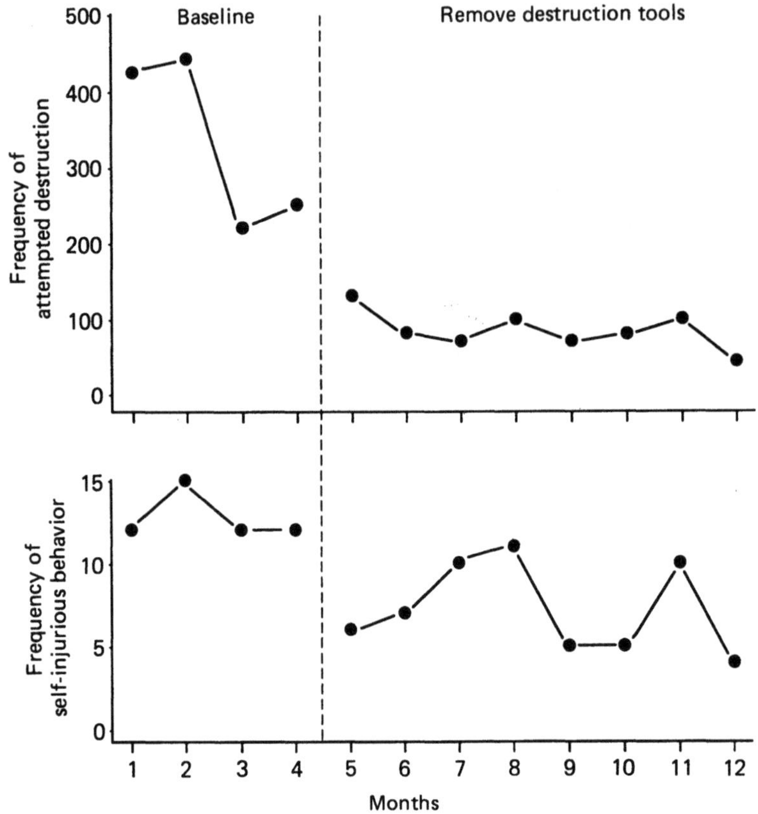


FIGURE 6.5. The effects of reducing an antecedent behavior (destruction) on frequency of SIB.

## Enrich Environment

Clients routinely engage in self-stimulatory behavior in response to boring environments. If the self-stimulation occasionally results in self-injury some staff attention may be forthcoming. It is possible, therefore, for some clients to be "shaped" into engaging in by unwitting, overworked staff. A referral to the behavior treatment team may occur, and a "program" to reduce the behavior could result. We have seen this scenario repeatedly and, thus, always closely inspect the activity schedule of any client referred for self-stimulation or self-injury. Devising activities that appeal to severely and profoundly mentally retarded clients is challenging, and designing a schedule and training supervisors to see that the activities are carried out is doubly difficult. It is, however, ethically inappropriate to do anything else. Implementing an aversive program to stop a behavior that occurs primarily because a client is bored is totally inappropriate. We have found recreation specialists to be a particularly valuable resource in evaluating clients and in designing and scheduling activities that are functional for severely and profoundly retarded clients. Outside group gross-motor activities in particular appear effective in competing with self-stimulation and SIB.

## Provide Medical/Dietary Changes

Severe screaming, yelling, and head-banging were the cause of referral for a profoundly retarded male in his mid-30s. An examination of patterns of the behavior revealed that it occurred when other clients were getting snacks or when he was requested to leave the dining area after meals. Although he received attention from staff at these times, the behavior did not appear" attention seeking" in nature (i.e., he had a variety of ways of gaining attention). After some inquiry, it became clear that food was a powerful reinforcer, and he often engaged in food begging and stealing. On a trial basis he was given larger portions at meal time and was given extra snacks. Screaming, yelling, and head-banging decreased to zero within a week.

Another client was referred for severe head-banging, which, the data showed, occurred only 2–3 times per month. The circumstances surrounding these instances varied in terms of time of day, staff present, and type of activity (he was often by himself when it happened). The second author was present one day and witnessed one of the episodes, which appeared to be a psychomotor seizure rather than head-banging. Subsequently, following extensive negotiations with the physician (EEG testing failed to reveal any seizure activity), a trial of phenobarbital was implemented. Seizures (head-banging) dropped to zero after 1 month and stayed at that level of 2 more months. Outside pressure forced the elimination of the medication, and seizures (head-banging) returned. We are presently negotiating with the new physician to attempt a second trial of phenobarbital.

Donna was profoundly mentally retarded, nonambulatory, nonverbal, blind, deaf, young woman with a seizure disorder. She would hit her head with her fists, or bang her head against objects. Behavioral and nursing data indicated that most of her head-banging occurred prior to or during her menstrual cycle and when she was constipated (Smith, Mathiasen, & Bailey, 1986). Originally, her programming consisted of a protective helmet contingent on head-banging, along with a 30-minute DRO. Subsequently, a passive behavior management approach of giving her Motrin during her menstrual cycle (see Figure 6.6) was implemented following an initial evaluation. Her cycles were irregular, so it was not possible to give her the pain reliever before it began. She also reveived a laxative if she went 3 consecutive days without having a bowel movement. The use of the helmet for protection and the 30-minute DRO continued as before.

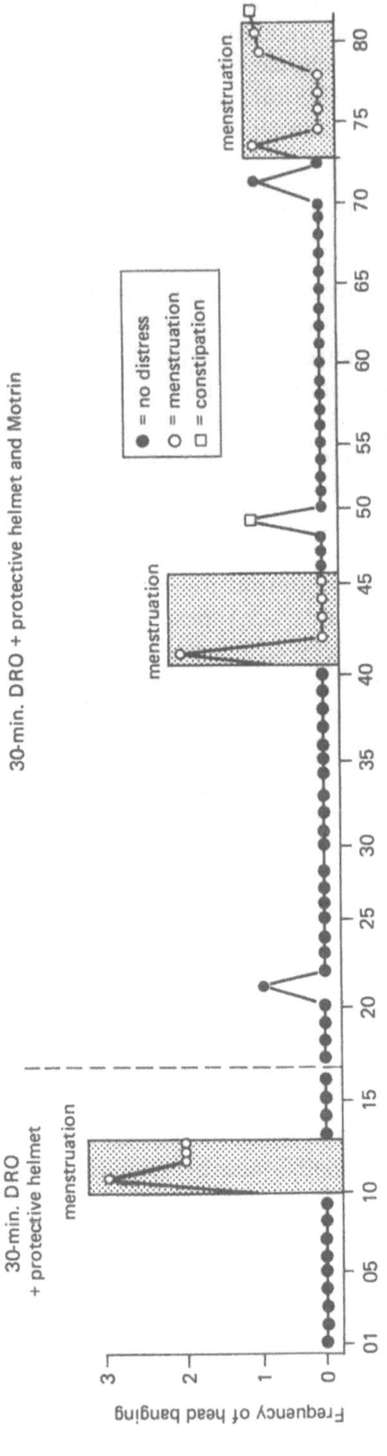


FIGURE 6.6. Adding Mortrin to a DRO + protective helmet program further reduces frequency of head-banging.

During the month prior to the implementation of this approach, Donna engaged in 12 episodes of SIB: four when constipated, seven during menstruation, and one without apparent physical distress. In the first month of treatment, she had 3 episodes of SIB: 2 during menstruation, and 1 not assoicated with apparent discomfort. In the second month of this program, Donna engaged in 6 episodes of SIB: 2 when constipated, 3 immediately prior to and during menstruation, and 1 unexplained, thus demonstrating that, for some clients, medication is an appropriate solution.

One final client illustrates a related point. Sheila pushed and poked in her ear and was causing tissue damage in the ear canal. After first being referred for behavior treatment, she was referred to the nursing staff for physical examination. No organic cause of the SIB could be found (i.e., no build-up of ear wax, no foreign object, no ear infection) and Sheila was again referred for behavior treatment. The behavior did not have any apparent function that would maintain it (i.e., it did not get Sheila any attention, did not get her out of training or allow her to escape any activity). When presented to the entire team with a recommendation that behavior modification was not indicated, Sheila's case was reviewed by the pharamacist. He immediately spotted a medication she was receiving, which, in his opinion, could cause tinnitis (ringing or whistling noise in the ear). He recommended an alternative medication, and within a week, her ear-poking SIB ceased.

### Allow Choice

Arthur was referred for severe tantrums, aggression, and SIB surrounding his refusal to cooperate with bathing in the morning. Staff were being injured because of his behavior, and no one wanted to work with him. He was referred for behavior treatment, and the staff received training in how to handle him with this daily chore. Other than this problem in the morning, Arthur was a "good citizen" and had been since his arrival at the facility a year earlier. Thus, we were puzzled and curious about the origins of such a serious problem. Upon questioning a number of staff members, it appeared that the problem had only begun in the past 2 weeks. Further inquiry revealed Arthur previously took his bath *at night* with no problems. When his bath time was rescheduled to evenings, Arthur returned to the quiet, unassuming client we knew him to be.

### Do Not Treat; Be More Tolerant

Some self-injury is topographically defined (e.g., hand-in-mouth). In some cases, the "self-injury" does not actually cause any tissue damage (although admittedly it does not enhance the client's appearance). In some cases, one option is simply not to treat the behavior (i.e., allow the client to engage in the behavior). In some cases, the "self injury" is a barometer of stimulation; observation often reveals that when activities are

Passive behavior management

| Procedure | Advantages | Disadvantages | Limiting conditions |
|---|---|---|---|
| Reduce discomfort and pain | • Humane<br>• Addresses function of behavior | • Can be difficult to eliminate variables may need months of data to determine causes | • Need high levels of cooperation within client's interdisciplinary team |
| Improve communication skills | • Client can control delivery of reinforcers; client can minimize aversive stimuli | • Can be difficult to teach to very low-functioning clients; staff must know the communication system | • Depends upon staff for maintenance |
| Teach adaptive responses | • Client controls own reinforcers<br>• Independence is fostered | • Can be difficult to teach to very low-functioning clients; client may have history of reinforcement for maladaptive behavior | • Client must be allowed to practice responses<br>• Environment must support new repertoire |
| Teach staff more adaptive responses | • Less inappropriate behavior is shaped | • May be more work for staff | • Staff must be flexible and readily adopt new patterns of response |
| Enrich environment | • Addresses client need for stimulation | • May be expensive to maintain<br>• Difficult to determine what is required for each client | • Facility must be prepared to make schedule and activity changes to meet client needs |
| Provide medical/dietery changes | • Addresses client need for medical care<br>• Addresses client need for additional food | • Some clients will need medication<br>• Clients may become overweight if special diets are modified· | • Facility must be prepared to use medication where needed<br>• Nutrition staff may have to give up control over client food consumption |
| Allow choice | • Addresses client needs | • Staff and facility must respond to client needs | • Facility and staff truly client centered |
| Do not treat; be more tolerant | • Clients are allowed to control own lives | • Some behaviors will go untreated and may appear undesirable | • Staff and administration willing to tolerate unusual behaviors without negative reaction |

FIGURE 6.7. The advantages, disadvantages, and limiting conditions of passive behavior management.

available, self-injury (actually self-stimulation or stereotypic behavior) decreases. Thus, an indirect method of treatment involving presenting the client with more stimulating activities is preferred to attempts to directly reduce the self-injury.

Figure 6.7 summarizes the advantages, disadvantages, and limiting conditions of passive behavior management.

## Balancing Advantages and Disadvantages of Treatment

Ethical, state, and federal guidelines mandate that when providing treatment for maladaptive behaviors, the least restrictive and least intrusive effective measures be used before more restrictive and intrusive ones are used. However, when working with clients engaging in severe self-injury, the first and foremost concern should be their safety. A client *must not* be allowed to cause severe and possibly irreparable damage. Initially, it may be necessary to restrain the client or to use protective equipment as emergency procedures to prevent injury.

While it is not the preferred practice to implement procedures without first taking baseline data, it may, in some cases, be necessary. At these times, the restraint/protective equipment should not be viewed as treatment in and of itself (see Luiselli, Chapter 9 this volume). Rather, it should be viewed as a client protection procedure to be used until a treatment plan is designed addressing the cause(s) of the behavior. Implementation of these procedures should always be documented according to applicable guidelines.

The baseline data taken in such situations would not be a true baseline, in the sense of the absence of any consequences provided contingent upon the behavior; rather, baseline would include implementation of the protective procedures.

The treatment procedure designed should have protection components written into it to prevent the client from injuring herself. It should also address the function of the behavior (e.g., if the client head-bangs to escape requests, evaluation of the more problematic requests and compliance training should be a component of the program). It is our experience that once the causes of the behaviors are known and addressed, implementation of restrictive procedures becomes increasingly less necessary.

## Cost–Benefit Analysis

One means of determining the appropriate treatment for clients engaging in SIB is a cost–benefit analysis. If a behavior is not a function of medical or apparent situational variables, and active behavior management is indicated, such an analysis may be useful.

For example, a decision may need to be made whether to employ a more intrusive and effective short-term treatment to reduce severe SIB quickly, or to use a less restrictive and less effective procedure that will take longer, thus allowing the client to engage in more of the self-abusive acts. (In the example of providing electric shock contingent upon severe SIB, it is very unlikely that a brief shock would be more painful than head-banging that results in a detached retina). The decision would need to be made according to what is best for the client. Would it be preferable to employ an aversive stimulus for a few sessions, with booster sessions used as needed, or would it be preferable to use a much less effective positive reinforcement intervention that would still allow the client to inflict serious damage to her-or himself?

Suggesting that a cost–benefit analysis be used to determine treatment is not likely to be popular with some people. However, the questions raised in this section are not merely rhetorical; they require answers. In some states (e.g., Florida), laws against the use of noxious or painful stimuli render many of these equestions moot. However, in other states, where these procedures are allowed, these points need to be considered. Lobbying groups are organized nationwide to legislate against the use of aversive procedures. We need to do all we can to ensure that whatever decisions are made are based on the available data with a consideration of what is best for the client.

The use of a cost–benefit analysis is not one that could (or should) be made by a given behavior analyst alone. Rather, it must be made by the client's interdisciplinary team, with consideration of the preceding issues and caveats.

## Summary

Active behavior management for the treatment of SIB has dominated the research literature for the past 20 years. However, limiting conditions imposed by the lack of resources in most facilities often prevent the proper implementation of these treatment approaches. State and federal guidelines now also limit severely the use of many well-established aversive behavioral procedures. It is just such limitations that forced us to look for alternatives, and we have, in the process, discovered a whole host of factors that appear to cause self-injurious and other maladaptive behaviors. It is now parent that the proper treatment of such cases requires a much more thorough understanding of conditions leading to the occurrence of the behavior. A variety of physiological, medical, and behavioral conditions can increase the likelihood of a SIB occurring. Using a diagnostic approach involves seeking the answers to a host of questions about the physical condition of the client and the environment in which the behavior occurs. Correcting these conditions must precede the implementation of any standard behavioral program, especially those involving aversive components.

Behavior analysis can make a positive contribution to the lives of persons with retardation if it focuses on reducing maladaptive behavior through enviromental design and elimination of those conditions that set the occasion for self-injury or other destructive behavior. We look forward to the development of a full technology of behavior change based on this passive behavior management approach and urge our colleagues to join us in this endeavor.

## References

Bailey, J. S., & Pyles, D. A. M. (1989). Behavioral diagnostics. *Monographs of the American Association on Mental Retardation. 12*, 85–106.

Bailey, J. S., Shook, G. L., Iwata, B. A., Reid, D. H., & Repp, A. C. (Eds.). (1989). *Behavior analysis in developmental disabilities 1968–1988* (2nd ed.). Lawrence, KS: Society for the Experimental Analysis of Behavior.

Carr, E. G., & Durand, V. M. (1985). Reducing behavior problems through functional communication training. *Journal of Applied Behavior Analysis, 18*, 111–126.

Corte, H. E., Wolf, M. M., & Locke, B. J. (1971). A comparison of procedures for eliminating self-injurious behavior of retarded adolescents. *Journal of Applied Behavior Analysis, 4*, 201–213.

Cuvo, A., & Davis, P. (1983). Behavior therapy and community living skills. In M. Hersen, R. Eisler, & M. Miller (Eds.), *Progress in behavior modification* (Vol. 14, pp. 125–172). New York: Academic Press.

Dorsey, M. F., Iwata, B. A., Ong, P., & McSween, T. E. (1980). Treatment of self-injurious behavior using a water mist: Initial response suppression and generalization. *Journal of Applied Behavior Analysis, 13*, 343–353.

Dorsey, M. F., Iwata, B. A., Reid, D. H., & Davis, P. (1982). Protective equipment: Continuous and contingent application in the treatment of self-injurious behavior. *Journal of Applied Behavior Analysis, 15*, 217–230.

Favell, J. E., McGimsey, J. F., & Jones, M. L. (1978). The use of physical restraint in the treatment of self-injury and as positive reinforcement. *Journal of Applied Behavior Analysis, 11*, 225 241.

Florida Department of Health and Rehabilitative Services. (1989). *Behavioral programming* (HRS Manual No. 160–4). Tallahassee, FL: Author.

Foxx, R. M., & Azrin, N. H. (1973). The elimination of autisic self-stimulatory behavior by overcorrection. *Journal of Applied Behavior Analysis, 6*, 1–14.

Iwata, B. A., Dorsey, M. F., Slifer, K. J., Bauman, K. E., & Richman, G. S. (1982). Toward a functional analysis of self-injury. *Analysis and Intervention in Developmental Disabilities, 2*, 3–20.

LaVigna, G. W., & Donnellan, A. M. (1986). *Alternatives to punishment: Solving behavior problems with non-aversive strategies*. New York: Irvington Publishers.

Lovaas, O. I., Freitag, G., Gold, V. J., & Kassorla, I. C. (1965). Experimental studies in childhood schizophrenia: Analysis of self-destructive behavior. *Journal of Experimental Child Psychology, 2*, 67–84.

Lovaas, O. I., & Simmons, J. Q. (1969). Manipulation of self-destruction in three retarded children. *Journal of Applied Behavior Analysis*, *2*, 143–157.

Luiselli, J. K., Myles, E., Evans, T. E., & Boyce, D. A. (1985). Reinforcement control of severe dysfunctional behavior of blind, multihandicapped students. *American Journal of Mental Deficiency*, *90*, 328–334.

Mace, F. C., Hock, M. L., Lalli, J. S., West, B. J., Belfiore, P., Pinter, E., & Brown, K. (1988). Behavioral momentum in the treatment of noncompliance. *Journal of Applied Behavior Analysis*, *21*, 123–141.

Rapoff, M. A., Altman, K., & Christophersen, E. R. (1980). Elimination of a blind child's self-hitting by response-contingent brief restraint. *Education and Treatment of Children*, *3*, 231–236.

Risley, T. R. (1968). The effects and side effects of punishing the autistic behaviors of a deviant child. *Journal of Applied Behavior Analysis*, *1*, 21–34.

Rolider, A., & Van Houten, R. (1985). Movement suppression time-out for undesirable behavior in psychotic and severely developmentally delayed children. *Journal of Applied Behavior Analysis*, *18*, 275–288.

Sajwaj, T., Libet, J., & Agras, S. (1974). Lemon juice therapy: The control of life-threatening rumination in a six-month-old infant. *Journal of Applied Behavior Analysis*, *7*, 557–563.

Skinner, B. F. (1969). *Contingencies of reinforcement: A theoretical analysis*. Englewood Cliffs, NJ: Prentice-Hall.

Smith, P., Mathiasen, J., & Bailey, J. S. (1986). *Passive behavior management in the reduction of aggression and tantrums*. Poster presented at the sixth annual meeting of the Florida Association for Behavior Analysis, Orlando, FL.

Steege, M. W., Wacker, D. P., & McMahon, C. M. (1987). Evaluation of the effectiveness and efficiency of two stimulus prompt strategies with severely handicapped students. *Journal of Applied Behavior Analysis*, *20*, 293–299.

Tanner, B. A., & Zeiler, M. (1975). Punishment of self-injurious behavior using aromatic ammonia as the aversive stimulus. *Journal of Applied Behavior Analysis*, *8*, 53–57.

Tarpley, H. D., & Schroeder, S. R. (1979). Comparison of DRO and DRI on rate of suppression of self-injurious behavior. *American Journal of Mental Deficiency*, *84*, 188–194.

Tate, B. G., & Baroff, G. S. (1966). Aversive control of self-injurious behavior in a psychotic boy. *Behaviour Research and Therapy*, *4*, 281–287.

# 7

# Treatments of Self-injury Based on Teaching Compliance and/or Brief Physical Restraint

RON VAN HOUTEN, AHMOS ROLIDER, and MIKE HOULIHAN

Several of the treatment approaches employed to treat self-injury involve the use of brief, contingent physical restraint. Some of these procedures have as an integral part the requirement that the person receiving treatment also comply with commands given by the therapist. All of these procedures involve the use of physical intervention because the therapist needs to physically restrain or prompt a behavior contingent upon self-injurious behavior (SIB).

Some methods that involve contingent brief restraint alone include physical immobilization, and momentary movement restraint (described in the following section). Methods that involve the use of contingent brief physical restraint plus compliance training include overcorrection, contingent exercise, and movement suppression.

## Treatments Employing Brief Restraint Alone

### *Contingent Physical Restraint*

One method of treating SIB is to apply brief physical restraint on a contingent basis (Bitgood, Crowe, Suarez, & Peters, 1980; Griffin, Locke, & Landers, 1975; Rapoff, Altman, & Christophersen, 1980; Saloviita, 1988; Singh, Dawson, & Manning, 1981). This procedure should be differentiated from blocking, which only involves interrupting the SIB (Underwood, Figueroa, Thyer, & Nzeocha, 1989). One defining characteristic of brief physical restraint is that the part of the body involved in the execution of the SIB is restrained. For example, Bitgood et al. (1980) punished hand-to-head responses in a 9-year-old autistic boy by immobilizing the seated child for 15 seconds by holding his hands at his sides. The experimenter who immobilized the child's arms was seated behind the child and only held the child's arms with the least amount of force required to keep the boy's arms at his sides. In another experiment, Rapoff et al. (1980) used a 30-second immobilization procedure to eliminate self-injury in a mentally retarded girl. Singh et al. (1981) compared a 3-minute contingent restraint condition with a 1-minute contingent restraint condition on the rate of SIB of a profoundly retarded 16-year-old girl. They found that the 1-minute restraint procedure reduced SIB to near-zero levels while the 3-minute restraint condition actually increased the level of SIB above the baseline level. The superiority of short periods of contingent restraint certainly bears further examination in future research.

Azrin, Besalel, Jammer, and Caputo (1988) examined the effects of contingent restraint procedures on the head-banging of nine mentally retarded clients. The treatment consisted of differential reinforcement of incompatible behavior (DRI) plus contingent restraint. Sessions were conducted during training activities while the client worked on a task. Each time the client attempted to engage in SIB, a trainer who was sitting or standing behind the client blocked the movement of the client's arm or fist, delivered a firm reprimand, and held the client's hands in the client's lap for 2 minutes. Head-banging was significantly reduced in all nine clients. One positive feature of this experiment was that the treatment was provided in the context of teaching appropriate skills in a highly structured setting.

A major disadvantage of the contingent-restraint procedure is that some forms of physical restraint may function as a positive reinforcer rather than a punisher for some clients. Favell, McGimsey, and Jones (1978) demonstrated that applying physical restraint whenever SIB did not occur could reduce SIB in two clients. In these subjects, making physical restraint contingent upon SIB may have increased the likelihood of SIB. It should be noted, however, that all forms of physical restraint may not prove equally reinforcing or aversive to an individual. Factors influencing whether physical restraint functions as a positive or negative reinforcer may include how uncomfortable the restraint is and the individual's prior exposure to restraint.

## *Momentary Movement Restraint*

Another form of contingent restraint is the momentary movement restraint procedure reported by Van Houten and Rolider (1989). This procedure involves placing the client's head between the client's knees with arms behind the back. Following the emission of an SIB, the therapist delivers a firm reprimand and then places a hand on the client's upper back between the shoulder blades. Next, the client is guided forward and down toward the knees so that his or her chest rests against the knees. The client's arms are placed behind his or her back with one hand on top of the other over the small of the back. In carrying out this procedure the therapist always brings the head down toward the knees by pressing on the upper back, and never by pressing on the neck or head.

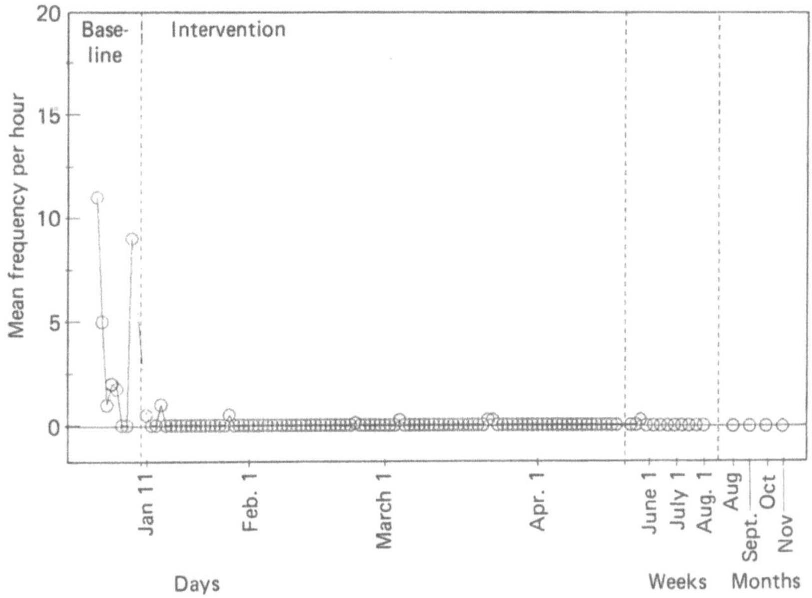


FIGURE 7.1. The number of times that a developmentally handicapped child banged his head against the windows in the home during the baseline condition and following the introduction of the momentary movement restraint condition.

Conditions that may preclude its use include conditions of the spine, Down syndrome, high blood pressure, obesity, or asthma. Therefore, a physician should be consulted prior to employing this procedure if any of these conditions are suspected.

One advantage of the momentary movement restraint procedure is that it is relatively easy to prevent injury or escape once someone is maintained in the prescribed position. Another advantage is that the position is not as likely to prove reinforcing to an individual as other forms of restraint because it is relatively uncomfortable and limits the degree that the individual can see what is going on around him or her.

Rolider and Cummings (1988) employed the momentary movement restraint procedure to reduce SIB in two mentally retarded clients. The treatment procedure was first introduced during brief sessions while teaching functional skills. The introduction of the momentary movement restraint procedure was also associated with a large reduction of SIB and an increase in performance on each of the functional skills. Figure 7.1 shows the number of times per hour that one of the clients, a 5-year-old profoundly retarded boy, banged his head against plate glass windows at home prior to and after the implementation of the momentary movement restraint procedure. The momentary movement restraint procedure produced a rapid and sustained reduction in SIB.

## Treatments Combining Restraint with Compliance Training

### *Overcorrection*

One treatment strategy based in part on teaching compliance is overcorrection. SIB has been reduced and, at times, successfully eliminated by utilizing a variety of overcorrection procedures (Azrin, Gottlieb, Hughart, Wesolowski, & Rahn, 1975; Clements & Dewey, 1979; Conley & Wolery, 1980; DeCatanzaro & Baldwin, 1978; Harris & Romanczyk, 1976; Measel & Alfieri, 1979; Strauss, Rubinoff, & Atkeson, 1983). Although overcorrection procedures vary greatly from one study to the next, there are several common elements worth noting. First, if the environment has been altered, the requirement is to restore surroundings to a better state than its original condition (restitution), and second, the client must practice the correct form of the behavior (positive practice). These two components of overcorrection have been used both in conjunction with one another (Azrin & Wesolowski, 1974) and alone (Decatanzaro & Baldwin, 1978; Foxx & Azrin, 1973). When considering SIB, restitutional overcorrection is rarely involved because there is no environmental effect. In the majority of studies on the use of overcorrection for the treatment of SIB, researchers have employed positive practice overcorrection alone.

Most programs that employ overcorrection incorporate the following basic protocol. Contingent upon each occurrence of SIB, the therapist: (a) delivers a firm reprimand, (b) requests performance of the positive practice behavior, (c) verbally requests repetition of the positive practice, and (d) provides "graduated guidance" upon noncompliance to requests. *Graduated guidance* consists of applying sufficient manual assistance to ensure that the behavior occurs while reducing the amount of guidance as the client begins to perform the behavior independently.

Azrin and Foxx (1971) postulated several elements that may be responsible for reductions of behavior produced by overcorrection. These elements include compliance training, punishing noncompliance, negative reinforcement, time-out, and feedback. In addition, Azrin and Wesolowski (1974) claimed that the procedure had an "educative" component because it involved practicing a positive action.

One of the first attempts at elimination of SIB using overcorrection methodology was by Measel and Alfieri (1976). They used a combination of differential reinforcement of incompatible behavior and positive practice overcorrection to reduce head-slapping. Upon introduction of the reinforcement and overcorrection procedure, SIB dropped almost immediately to near-zero levels. The initial success of overcorrection led to a great increase in its use by practitioners. Interest mounted regarding which of the many components were key to the success of the procedure.

The questions addressed by research have been (a) whether the positive practice procedure has to be topographically similar to the SIB, (b) whether overcorrection has an educative component, (c) how long the procedure should be employed following each instance of the behavior, (d) whether the effects of overcorrection generalize, (e) whether overcorrection produces positive or negative side effects, and (f) whether reinforcement is a necessary component.

In the early descriptions of overcorrection, positive practice procedures were selected that were thought to be functionally related to the aberrant behavior (DeCantanzaro & Baldwin, 1978; Foxx & Azrin, 1973; Measel & Alfieri, 1976). Selecting behaviors that were functionally related to the target behavior was thought to have two advantages. First, it was suggested that this requirement enhanced the effectiveness of overcorrection by "topographically matching" unwanted and desired behaviors, and second, it was thought that this topographic similarity would enable the client to learn and acquire alternative adaptive behaviors (Marholin, Luiselli, & Townsend, 1980). However, in most studies using overcorrection to treat SIB, the positive practice procedure employed was *functional movement training*, which involved moving the part of the body involved in emitting the behavior in accordance with a series of commands (Foxx & Bechtel, 1983). For example, a person who struck her head with her hand would be required to hold her hands out in front of her, above her head, or at her sides on command. If these behaviors were considered to be competing responses, one might expect to see the person spending the day with her hands variously extended at her sides, out in front of her, or over her head. This rationale for the use of positive practice would appear on the surface to be tenuous (Axelrod, Brantner, & Meddock, 1978).

Topographical similarity may also reinforce the idea that there is a direct benefit from the client practicing correct forms of behavior rather than a behavior selected for reasons of convenience. The elimination of the requirement of topographically similar behavior leads to the conceptualization of overcorrection as a punishment procedure based upon compliance training and contingent effort. There are, however, several examples that demonstrate that overcorrection can be effective when topographically dissimilar behaviors are employed (Carey & Bucher, 1981; Daniel, 1982; Luiselli, Suskin, & McPhee, 1981; Savie & Dickie, 1979; Tarnowsky & Drabman, 1985). The results of these experiments indicate that it does not make any difference whether the behavior selected for positive practice is related to the target behavior. Furthermore, Secan and Egel (1986) demonstrated that making children who engaged in stereotypic clapping perform rapid clapping contingent upon inappropriate clapping was very effective as a response deceleration technique (negative practice). In this example, the practiced behavior was topographically identical to the target behavior and was, therefore, nonfunctional as an alternative response. The most important implication of these findings is that one need not weigh the relationship between the behavior selected for practice behavior and the target behavior heavily when selecting the behavior to be required for overcorrection. This leaves one free to select target behaviors based on the criterion of how easy it would be to apply guidance if the client does not exhibit compliance with the overcorrection procedure. For example, one might conclude that it would be easier to use manual guidance to get someone to stand up and sit down a number of times on command following the target behavior than to get him to engage in behavior that requires more elaborate arm and hand movements. This is not an unimportant consideration because the selection of a difficult behavior to prompt could lead to injury or unrealistic staffing requirements (Kelly & Drabman, 1977b; Zehr & Theobald, 1978).

Early in the development of overcorrection, the procedure was described as being educative (Azrin & Wesolowski, 1974). The educative nature of overcorrection describes a product rather than a process. This product can be as simple as the teaching instruction following behavior to a person with a history of noncompliance. Increases in the general level of compliance have been reported in several studies (Foxx & Azrin, 1973a; Foxx & Azrin, 1973b), and increases in compliance during the overcorrection interval also have been recorded (Azrin & Wesolowski, 1974; Duker & Seys, 1977; Kissel & Whitman, 1977; Matson, Stephens, & Smith, 1978; Wells, Forehand, & Hickey, 1977). Overcorrection may be educative in another way, by teaching the client to perform a new behavior through positive practice training. This can be accomplished by introducing or shaping behavior that has previously not been emitted spontaneously (Carey & Bucher, 1981; Luiselli & Rice, 1983; Tarnowski & Drabman, 1985; Wells, Forehand, Hickey, & Green, 1977). For example, Tarnowski and Drabman (1985) described an overcorrection procedure in which they taught a child that was previously confined to a wheelchair to walk while concomitantly reducing self-stimulatory behavior.

The use of overcorrection as an educative tool may be a very important factor determining the acceptance of overcorrection, but it need not be considered essential to the success of the procedure. Many persons with SIB have severe limitations behaviorally, and as such, they may require more effort to implement a procedure that would be educative. Furthermore, in several instances, the behaviors taught or practiced during positive practice may not be spontaneously emitted upon removal of the overcorrection contingencies. This may be interpreted as the absence of an educative effect. The obvious solution to this problem is to plan for generalization and maintenance of the behavior that was taught.

A related concern has been that some clients never perform the positive practice behavior without guidance. This indicates that they may not have learned either the behavior or compliance. It is clear, however, that these same individuals are responsive to the contingencies that were enforced during overcorrection procedures, as indicated by the reduction and/or elimination of the targeted behavior.

The duration of the positive practice portion of the overcorrection procedure has varied from 20 minutes (Foxx & Azrin, 1973) to as little as 2 or 3 seconds (Richmond, 1983). The duration of positive practice is not directly comparable across all studies, due to the diverse practice routines that have been devised. Generally, it has been reported that increasing the duration of positive practice following brief-duration applications has direct effects on the aversiveness of the procedure (Holburn & Dougher, 1985), with the effectiveness of the procedure being increased by extending the duration of positive practice (Maag, Rutherford, Wolchik, & Parks, 1986). If short durations of positive practice are not achieving the desired results, then increasing the duration may bring about a better response to the intervention. Conversely, increases in duration and response requirement also may lead to negative side effects, such as aggression and resistance.

Recent overcorrection studies that have addressed SIB ranged in duration from 5 seconds (Holburn & Dougher, 1985; Singh, Watson & Winton, 1986) to 15 minutes (Fleming & Nolley, 1981; Singh & Bakker, 1984). Most studies used positive practice procedures that lasted approximately 5 minutes. The efficacy of any specific duration cannot be judged without reference to the specific positive practice routine. It must be realized that longer durations require more staff attention, thereby compromising the time available to reinforce alternative behaviors (Luiselli, 1984a). Another related concern is that if the duration is too long from the onset, there may be more resistance to the procedure.

In any program utilizing overcorrection as a means for reducing SIB, it must be recognized that it is a punishment procedure. Although overcorrection has been utilized in the guise of an educative program, it should be noted that the reductions in behavior observed are primarily the result of punishment. Gibbs and Luyben (1985), for example, demonstrated that positive practice training was only effective in reducing the frequency of self injury when it was made contingent upon its occurrence. When positive practice training was administered in a noncontingent manner, it had no effect on the frequency of self-injury. However, this is not an adequate control for the role of compliance training in overcorrection because the client did not receive reprimands following incidents of SIB during the noncontingent overcorrection condition. Though the client may have learned to comply with the therapist's request, the client had no way to discriminate that the therapist did not wish him to engage in SIB because this was not directly or indirectly requested.

Several studies have noted that the reduction of SIB during overcorrection did not generalize to other settings or behaviors (Czyzewsky, Barrera, & Sulzer-Azaroff, 1982; Matson, & Stephens, 1981,). Furthermore, once the contingencies were removed, the SIB returned to baseline levels. When using overcorrection and any other behavior modification procedure, efforts to promote generalization should be part of the overall treatment plan. In studies where generalization and maintenance have been programmed, effects of the treatment typically endure. Due to the nature of SIB, in some cases, even low levels of behavior are unwanted. With this in mind, several studies have left overcorrection procedures in effect without terminating the program (Gibbs & Luyben, 1985; Singh & Winton, 1985).

The positive features of overcorrection are that it often produces rapid effects, can reduce SIB to near-zero levels, can be effective in teaching compliance to verbal commands, and may teach new behavior. The procedure also may produce positive side effects, such as improved affect (Matson & Stephens, 1981), increased social responsiveness (Singh & Winton, 1985; Wesolowski & Zawlocki, 1982), and more appropriate play (Watson et al., 1986). However, negative side effects have been reported. These include aggression (Carey & Bucher, 1986; Foxx, McMorrow, Bittle, & Bechtel, 1986) and physical resistance to the positive-practice procedures (Holborn, & Dougher, 1985). The possibility of negative side effects must be taken into consideration prior to the administration of any overcorrection program.

The role of reinforcement in overcorrection has not been extensively researched. Foxx and Bechtel (1983) point out the role of negative reinforcement in the form of graduated guidance when enforcing compliance with requests. They caution further against the use of positive reinforcement during overcorrection because it might make the overcorrection activity reinforcing to the client. However, the limited research available has indicated that reinforcing alternative behaviors enhances the process substantially while concomitantly decreasing the negative side effects. One study in particular addressed the issues of reinforcing compliance during positive practice training (Carey & Bucher, 1986). Carey and Bucher (1986) found that reinforcing unprompted responses during positive practice lead to more rapid reductions in self-stimulatory behavior and faster acquisition of compliance during positive practice training than the use of the same procedure without reinforcement. In another experiment, Tierney (1986) reduced the frequency of SIB through positive practice of appropriate sitting behavior, maintained by graduated guidance and positive reinforcement for compliance during positive practice training.

It should be noted that the function of target behavior may influence the effects of reinforcement during positive practice training. When a client engages in SIB to escape demands rather than to produce sensory stimulation, it is possible that the introduction of reinforcement into the overcorrection procedure might have the negative effects that Foxx and Bechtel (1983) suggest. On the other hand, reinforcement is frequently employed successfully, along with graduated guidance related to the use of abrupt prompts when teaching proper sitting and other compliance-related behaviors to autistic children whose noncompliant behavior is frequently escape related (Lovaas, 1981).

Reinforcement during the training phase has been shown on several occasions to be an integral part of the treatment package. The inclusion of reinforcement in this procedure does not reduce or eliminate the need for referring to the overcorrection component as a punishment procedure.

## Contingent Exercise

Another punishment procedure that is based on producing compliance is contingent exercise (Luce, Delquadri, & Hall, 1980; Luce & Hall, 1981; Savie & Dickie, 1979). Following a target behavior, the person is required to engage in vigorous activity such as standing up and sitting down several times or running a specified distance. Graduated guidance is provided, as necessary, in order to obtain compliance with requests. Essentially, contingent exercise is a form of overcorrection employing topographically dissimilar behaviors. The major difference between contingent exercise and overcorrection is the selection of behavior that involves a fair amount of physical exercise in the former case.

Borreson (1980) employed contingent exercise that consisted of forced running to eliminate SIB. Luiselli (1984b) employed a contingent exercise procedure that consisted of physically stopping a behavior followed by 30 seconds of arm movements to reduce hand biting. Following a baseline condition, the introduction of a DRI procedure that involved providing praise for incompatible behavior was ineffective in reducing SIB. The addition of the physical effort procedure was associated with a slow decline in the daily frequency of SIB. In another study, Singh, Watson, and Winton (1986) followed self-abusive ear rubbing with forced guided-arm exercise. The results showed that the forced guided-arm exercise procedure produced a greater reduction in SIB than a contingent water-mist procedure.

## Movement Suppression

Another procedure that involves teaching compliance is movement suppression (Rolider & Van Houten, 1985a, 1985b; Van Houten & Rolider, 1988). This technique consists of telling the client to go to a corner while guiding him or her into the corner with accompanying physical assistance. The corner is padded in order to reduce the likelihood of an injury being produced if the client resists or engages in head-banging while in the corner. The client is positioned with his or her chin against the corner, both hands behind his or her back, with one hand on top of the other and both feet close together and touching the wall. Whenever the client moves or makes a verbalization, the mediator gives a firm loud reprimand (either "Don't move" or "Don't talk") while pressing the client's back into the corner by placing one hand against the upper back between the shoulder blades. The pressure is not forceful but it is very abrupt, like a nudge. If the person attempts to turn his or her head or bend the knees, the mediator says "Face the corner" while guiding the head back or "Straighten up and don't move" while abruptly pressing the person's body back into the corner. This procedure is applied even if the person only moves a small amount, such as wiggling a finger or shifting weight from one leg to the other. It is essential that the mediator stand directly behind the person so that the aforementioned procedure can be applied very rapidly following any movement. The procedure is typically carried out for 1–4 minutes following each instance of the target behavior. Rolider and Van Houten (1985a) completely suppressed the SIB of two children with the movement suppression procedure used in conjunction with a reinforcement program. Matson and Keyes (1990) reported reducing SIB in two mentally retarded adults using the movement suppression procedure. Although the movement suppression procedure appears to offer promise in the treatment of self-injury, further research is required before firm conclusions can be drawn.

There are several advantages offered by the movement suppression procedure. First, it is difficult to engage in SIB or self-stimulatory behaviors while the procedure is being applied. Second, the behavior involves producing compliance by stopping the behavior rather than forcing it to occur. This greatly reduces the need for extra staff and reduces the likelihood of an injury occurring. Third, the procedure can be applied for a short period of time to be effective. Fourth, the procedure may result in a high degree of personal stimulus control over the client's behavior. As the person learns to stand motionless in the corner, there can be an increase in compliance with requests when the person is outside of the corner (Rolider, 1989).

Although movement suppression, like overcorrection and contingent exercise, appears to offer hope in reducing or eliminating SIB, these procedures should only be employed as part of a balanced treatment plan that includes a careful functional analysis of controlling variables and the extensive use of positive reinforcement.

## The Role of Compliance in the Treatment of SIB

All situations that involve compliance are characterized by an instruction to respond, to cease responding, or not to respond in a particular way. Overcorrection and contingent exercise represent treatment techniques that require the client to respond to various requests. An example of a treatment technique that requires the client to inhibit responding is the movement-suppression procedure. Alternatively, one could conceptualize the procedure as teaching a client to comply with an implied request to stand in a rigid position.

One reason why it may be important to teach compliance is that several studies have reported an inverse relationship between compliance and inappropriate behavior such that the reinforcement of compliant behavior produced both an increase in compliance and a decrease in inappropriate behavior, and the punishment of inappropriate behavior produced both a decrease in inappropriate behavior and an increase in compliance (Johansson, 1971; Parrish, Cataldo, Kolko, Neef, & Egel, 1986; Russo, Cataldo, & Cushing, 1981). In the Russo et al. (1981) study, an increase in compliance in two children was associated with a decrease in self-injury.

Furthermore, their are several reasons why it may be beneficial to teach individuals who are exhibiting SIB to comply with requests. First, if a person learns consistently to follow requests to initiate, terminate, or avoid behaviors, problems potentially can be brought under instructional control. Once a history of following a request in a particular circumstance has been developed, it is possible that the behavior requested will occur more consistently in the absence of a verbal request.

Second, improved compliance makes it easier to teach incompatible alternative behaviors to the self-injurious client. In general, the higher the incidence of compliance, the more likely the client will follow an instruction designed to prompt a desirable behavior. To the degree that clients do not respond to instructions, it is difficult to get them to initiate new behavior.

All of the procedures that are based on compliance require that a high level of compliance be obtained in order for the procedures to be carried out effectively. Therefore, it is essential that clinicians are skilled in producing compliance. This section examines some of the more important factors that influence whether persons will comply with a request.

Many factors have been shown to be related to the level of compliance with requests. One important factor is whether the mediator demands eye contact prior to making the request (Hamlet, Axelrod, & Kuerschner, 1984). Hamlet et al. (1984) had parents and teachers make standard requests to children with and without demanding eye contact. Demand for eye contact consisted of saying the child's name and waiting 2 seconds. If the child did not make eye contact, the mediator requested eye contact by saying the child's name, followed by "look at me" in a moderately firm tone of voice. Any time the child broke eye contact while an instruction was being given, the mediator again demanded eye contact. The results of this study indicated that demanding eye contact prior to making a request more than doubled the incidence of compliance in children who showed low initial levels of compliance.

Another factor that has been demonstrated to influence the probability of complying with a request is the sequence of instructional demands. Mace, Hock, Lalli, West, Belfiore, Pinter, and Brown (1988) demonstrated that giving several instructions that had a high probability of compliance prior to making a low-probability request increased the probability that the low-probability request would be complied with. Mace et al. (1988) explained this phenomenon in terms of "behavioral momentum." An alternative explanation might be that the entire behavioral sequence represents a chain of behavior that is likely to be completed after the first component has been initiated. If this explanation is correct, another way to increase compliance would be to break the request into its component parts or at least to initiate the first component of the behavior with a separate request. An example might be to instruct a person to stand up before asking him to turn off a television or asking someone to pick up a toothbrush before asking her to brush her teeth. Within the context of overcorrection or contingent exercise, it should be possible to obtain better compliance by first requesting a relatively easy behavior that typically gains compliance before asking for more difficult or effortful responses.

Still another factor influencing compliance is the tone of voice used by the person making the request. In general, people are less likely to respond to a request that involves a questioning inflection (an increase in pitch on the last word) than one that employs a more assertive inflection (a decrease in pitch on the last word). In addition reinforcing compliance with requests (Bernhardt & Forehand, 1975; Goetz, Holmberg, & Leblanc 1975) and punishing noncompliance with requests (Forehand, Roberts, Doleys, Hobbs, & Resick, 1976; Scarboro & Forehand, 1975) have also been shown to influence the probability that a client will comply with a request.

It is important that practitioners are aware of the aforementioned factors because they could clearly influence the likelihood that the client would comply with requests made as part of an overcorrection or contingent-exercise program. Failure to make use of these variables could easily mean the difference between success and failure.

## Potential Problems Associated with the Use of Physical Restraint

The most important thing to remember when discussing the use of punishment procedures that involve the use of physical restraint is that punishment should only represent one aspect of the total treatment package. A well designed intervention should also include components designed to teach and maintain more adaptive behaviors. In order to determine which behaviors the client needs to learn, it is essential to perform a complete functional analysis of the target behavior. Once the functions of the target behavior have been determined, this information can be employed in order to design a structured setting where the person can be taught to respond in a more appropriate manner in the presence of the stimuli that control the occurrence of SIB. One advantage of employing punishment procedures that involve compliance training is that any increase in the level of compliance produced by these procedures can be of great assistance in teaching new behavior.

The function of the inappropriate behavior should be considered when selecting behaviors to be taught. For example, if one of the functions of self-injury is to escape specific demands, a punishment procedure involving the use of contingent restraint can be made contingent upon any instance of self-injury, first in the presence of demands that only sometimes lead to self-injury and later in the presence of demands more likely to trigger self-injury. If self-injury is more likely when the person has to wait for a reinforcer, that person can be reinforced for waiting longer and longer periods of time. Again, a procedure involving the use of contingent restraint can be employed on those trials when self-injury occurs. If the person is more likely to engage in self-injury upon the termination of reinforcement, the treatment can be first applied following self-injury following the termination of a reinforcer under a low level of deprivation and later when higher levels of deprivation are in effect. If the function of self-injury is the production of sensory reinforcement, the person can be taught to engage in other behaviors that can produce stimulation while self-injury is punished. By gradually decreasing the motivation for self-injury in each of the preceding examples, one may be able to minimize the need to employ punishment. If the results of a functional analysis suggest that a less intrusive procedure would probably prove effective, the use of more restrictive forms of punishment should not be included into the treatment plan unless the less intrusive procedure has proven unsuccessful.

It is also essential that the overall treatment plan include the provision of frequent reinforcement. One of the advantages of the contingent physical restraint procedure employed in the Azrin et al. (1988) study was the use of frequent reinforcement in the context of a teaching program. Although the use of positive reinforcement for compliance during overcorrection is less common, the results of Carey and Bucher (1986) suggest that reinforcing unprompted responses during positive practice should lead to more rapid reductions in SIB and fewer side effects.

Even if a funtional analysis has been performed and the treatment package includes a good deal of reinforcement for appropriate behavior, the use of procedures that require brief restraint could lead to injury with strong combative clients unless adequate staffing is employed to allow for the safe administration of the procedures. In this regard, movement suppression offers an advantage over procedures such as overcorrection or contingent exercise because it is easier and safer to restrain a client in a padded corner than to compel him or her to repeat a series of movements. It is also important to consider the adequacy of staffing. In doing so, it is necessary to take into account the number of staff and the ability of the staff to carry out the various procedures. Factors that need to be considered are strength, quick reaction times, and skill level. It is also important to arrange the physical environment in such a manner as to facilitate ease of implementation. For example, initial treatment sessions should be conducted in close proximity to a corner when using movement suppression.

Finally, it is wise to carry out initial treatment during brief treatment sessions where the procedure can be carefully and precisely implemented. The program should not be carried out over the entire day until good results have been obtained first under more carefully controlled conditions. It certainly makes little sense to carry out a more restrictive procedure over the course of an entire day if it has not yet been determined whether the procedure has a good chance of being effective. Indeed, one can be relatively confident that a procedure will not prove effective in an individual's living environment if it cannot be made effective during a better controlled session under more ideal conditions.

## Summary

Several procedures that involve physical restraint have proven useful in the treatment of SIB. Contingent restraint and contingent momentary movement restraint are examples of two such procedures that do not involve compliance training. Overcorrection, movement suppression, and contingent exercise are three punishment procedures that involve physical restraint, which also teach the client to comply with requests. An advantage offered by these procedures is that they may reduce unwanted behaviors in two ways. First, they are aversive and can directly reduce the frequency of a behavior that they are made contingent upon. Second, they teach compliance, and increased levels of compliance have been demonstrated to negatively co-vary with undesirable behavior.

In order to apply restraint procedures that involve compliance training effectively, the clinician should understand the various factors that influence compliance with requests and should be able to employ them in order to increase the efficacy of treatment. Several factors that have been demonstrated to influence the likelihood that someone will comply with a request are demanding eye contact, first requesting behavior that the client is more likely to comply with, a firm tone of voice and inflection, and reinforcement for following requests and punishment for failing to following requests.

Because the use of physical restraint is relatively restrictive, it is essential that the environment be arranged in such a manner as to reduce the risk of injury. In addition, it is essential that a functional analysis is carried out in order to ensure that the client is taught more effective ways to respond to factors influencing the occurrence of SIB. In teaching adaptive behavior and compliance, it is also important that adequate reinforcement is provided.

## References


Axelrod, S., Brantner, J. P., & Meddock, T. D. (1978). Overcorrection: A review and critical analysis. *Journal of Special Education*, *12*, 367–391.

Azrin, N. H., Besalel, V. A., Jammer, J. P., & Caputo, J. N. (1988). Comparative study of behavioral methods of treating self-injury. *Behavioral Residential Treatment*, *3*, 119–152.

Azrin, N. H., & Foxx, R. M. (1971). A rapid method of toilet training the institutionalized retarded. *Journal of Applied Behavior Analysis*, *4*, 89–99.

Azrin, N. H., Gottlieb, L., Hughart, L., Wesolowski, M. D., & Rahn, T. (1975). Eliminating self-injurious behavior by educative procedures. *Behaviour Research and Therapy*, *13*, 101–111.

Azrin, N. H., & Wesolowski, M. D. (1974). Theft reversal: An overcorrection procedure for eliminating stealing by retarded persons. *Journal of Applied Behavior Analysis*, *7*, 577–581.

Bernhardt, A., & Forehand, R. (1975). The effects of labeled and unlabeled praise upon lower and middle class children. *Journal of Experimental Child Psychology*, *19*, 536–543.

Bitgood, S. C., Crowe, M. J., Suarez, Y., & Peters, R. D. (1980). Immobilization: Effects and side effects on stereotyped behavior in children, *Behavior Modification*, *4*, 187–208.

Borreson, P. M. (1980). The elimination of self-injury avoidance responding through a forced running consequence. *Mental Retardation*, *18*, 73–77.

Carey, R. G., & Bucher, B. (1981). Identifying the educative and suppressive effects of positive practice and restitutional overcorrection. *Journal of Applied Behavior Analysis*, *14*, 71–80.

Carey, R. G., & Bucher, B. (1983). Positive practice overcorrection: The effects of duration of positive practice on acquisition and response reduction. *Journal of Applied Behavior Analysis*, *16*, 101–109.

Carey, R. G., & Bucher, B. D. (1986). Positive practice overcorrection: Effects of reinforcing correct performance. *Behavior Modification*, *10*, 73–92.

Clements, J., & Dewey, M. (1979). The effects of overcorrection: A case study. *Behavior Research and Therapy*, *17*, 515–518.

Conley, O. S., & Wolery, M. R. (1980). Treatment by overcorrection of self-injurious eye gouging in preschool blind children *Journal of Behavior Therapy and Experimental Psychiatry*, *11*, 121–125.

Czyzewski, M. J., Barrera, R. D., & Sulzer-Azaroff, B. (1982). An abbreviated overcorrection program to reduce self-stimulatory behaviors. *Journal of Behavior Therapy & Experimental Psychiatry*, *13*, 55–62.

Daniel, W. H. (1982). Management of chronic rumination with a contingent exercise procedure employing topographically dissimilar behavior. *Journal of Behavior Therapy & Experimental Psychiatry*, *13*, 149–152.

DeCatanzaro, D. A., & Baldwin, G. (1978). Effective treatment of self-injurious behavior through a forced arm exercise. *American Journal of Mental Deficiency*, *82*, 433–439.

Duker, P. C., & Seys, D. M. (1983). Long-term follow-up effects of extinction and overcorrection procedures with severely retarded individuals. *The British Journal of Subnormality*, *29*, 74–80.

Epstein, L. H., Doke, L. A., Sajwaj, T. E., Sorrell, S., & Rimmer, B. (1974). Generality and side effects of overcorrection. *Journal of Applied Behavior Analysis*, *7*, 385–390.

Favell, J. E., McGimsey, J. F., & Jones, M. L. (1978). The use of physical restraint in the treatment of self-injury and as a positive reinforcement. *Journal of Applied Behavior Analysis*, *11*, 225–241.

Fleming, A., & Nolley, D. (1981). A comparison of techniques for the elimination of self-injurious behavior in a mildly retarded woman. *Journal of Behavior Therapy & Experimental Psychiatry*, *12*, 81–85.

Forehand, R., Roberts, M. W., Doleys, D. M., Hobbs, S. A., & Resick, P. A. (1976). An examination of disciplinary procedures with children. *Journal of Experimental Child Psychology*, *21*, 109–120.

Foxx, R. M., & Azrin, N. H. (1973a). Dry pants: A rapid method of toilet training children. *Behaviour Research and Therapy*, *11*, 435–442.

Foxx, R. M., & Azrin, N. H. (1973b). The elimination of autistic self-stimulatory behavior by overcorrection. *Journal of Applied Behavior Analysis*, *6*, 1–14.

Foxx, R. M., & Bechtel, D. R. (1983). Overcorrection: A review and analysis. In S. Axelrod & J. Apsche (Eds.), *The effects of punishment on human behavior* (pp. 133–220). New York: Academic Press.

Foxx, R. M., McMorrow, M. J., Bittle, R. G., & Bechtel, D. R. (1986). The successful treatment of a dually-diagnosed deaf man's aggression with a program that included contingent electric shock. *Behavior Therapy*, *17*, 170–186.

Gibbs, J. W., & Luyben, P. D. (1985). Treatment of self-injurious behavior: Contingent versus non-contingent positive practice overcorrection. *Behavior Modification*, *9*, 3–21.

Goetz, E. M., Holmberg, M. C., & Leblanc, J. M. (1975). Differential reinforcement of other behavior and non-contingent reinforcement as control procedures during the modification of a preschooler's compliance. *Journal of Applied Behavior Analysis*, *8*, 77–82.

Griffin, J. C., Locke, B. J., & Landers, W. F. (1975). Manipulation of potential punishment parameters in the treatment of self-injury. *Journal of Applied Behavior Analysis*, *8*, 458.

Hamlet, C. C., Axelrod, S., & Kuerschner, S. (1984). Eye contact as an antecedent to compliant behavior. *Journal of Applied Behavior Analysis*, *17*, 553–557.

Harris, S. L., & Romanczyk, R. G. (1976). Treating self-injurious behavior of a retarded child by overcorrection. *Behavior Therapy*, *7*, 235–239.

Holburn, C. S., & Dougher, M. J. (1985). Behavioral attempts to eliminate air-swallowing in two profoundly mentally retarded clients. *American Journal of Mental Deficiency*, *89*, 524–536.

Johansson, S. (1971). *Compliance and noncompliance in young children.* Unpublished doctoral dissertation. University of Oregon.

Kelly, J. A., & Drabman, R. S. (1977a). Generalizing response suppression of self-injurious behavior through an overcorrection punishment procedure: A case study. *Behavior Therapy*, *8*, 468–472.

Kelly, J. A., & Drabman, R. S. (1977b). Overcorrection: An effective procedure that failed. *Journal of Clinical Child Psychology*, *6*, 38–40.

Kissel, R. C., & Whitman, T. L. (1977). An examination of the direct and generalized effects of a play-training and overcorrection procedure upon the self-stimulatory behavior of a profoundly retarded boy. *American Association for the Education of the Severely/Profoundly Handicapped Review*, *2*, 131–146.

Lovaas, O. I. (1981). *Teaching developmentally disabled children: The me book.* Baltimore, MD: University Park Press.

Luce, S. C., Delquadri, J., & Hall, R. V. (1980). Contingent exercise: A mild but powerful procedure for suppressing inappropriate verbal and aggressive behavior. *Journal of Applied Behavior Analysis*, *13*, 583–594.

Luce, S. C., & Hall, R. V. (1981). Contingent exercise: A procedure used with differential reinforcement to reduce bizarre verbal behavior. *Education and Treatment of Children*, *4*, 309–327.

Luiselli, J. K. (1984a). Effects of brief overcorrection on sterotypic behavior of mentally retarded students. *Education and Treatment of Children*, *7*, 125–138.

Luiselli, J. K. (1984b). Therapeutic effects of brief contingent effort on severe behavior disorders in children with developmental disabilities. *Journal of Clinical Child Psychology*, *13*, 257–262.

Luiselli, J. K., & Rice, D. M. (1983). Brief positive practice with a handicapped child: An assessment of suppressive and reeducative effects. *Education and Treatment of Children*, *6*, 241–250.

Luiselli, J. K., Suskin, L., & McPhee, D. F. (1981). Continuous and intermittent application of overcorrection in a self-injurious autistic child: Alternating treatments design analysis. *Journal of Behavior Therapy & Experimental Psychiatry*, *12*, 355–358.

Maag, J. W., Rutherford, R. B., Wolchik, S. A., & Parks, B. T. (1986). Brief report: Comparison of two short overcorrection procedures on the stereotypic behavior of autistic children. *Journal of Autism and Developmental Disorders*, *16*, 83–87.

Mace, F. C., Hock, M. L., Lalli, J. S., West, B. J., Belfiore, P., Pinter, E., & Brown, D. K. (1988). Behavioral momentum in the treatment of noncompliance. *Journal of Applied Behavior Analysis*, *21*, 123–141.

Marholin, D., II, Luiselli, J. K., & Townsend, N. M. (1980). Overcorrection: An examination of its rationale and treatment effectiveness. *Progress in Behavior Modification*, *9*, 49–80.

Matson, J. L., & Keyes, J. B. (1990). A comparison of DRO to movement suppression time-out and DRO with two self-injurious and aggressive mentally retarded adults. *Research in Developmental Disabilities*, *11*, 111–120.

Matson, J. L., & Stephens, R. M. (1981). Overcorrection treatment of stereotyped behaviors. *Behavior Modification*, *5*, 491–502.

Matson, J. L., Stephens, R. M., & Smith, C. (1978). Treatment of self-injurious behaviour with overcorrection. *Journal of Mental Deficiency Research*, *22*, 175–178.

Measel, J. C., & Alfieri, P. A. (1979). Treatment of self-injurious behavior by a combination of reinforcement for incompatible behavior and overcorrection. *American Journal of Mental Deficiency*, *81*, 147–153.

Parrish, J. M., Cataldo, M. F., Kolko, D. J., Neef, N. A., & Egel, A. L. (1986). Experimental analysis of response covariation among compliant and inappropriate behavior. *Journal of Applied Behavior Analysis*, *19*, 241–254.

Rapoff, M. A., Altman, K., & Christophersen, E. R. (1980). Reducing aggressive and self-injurious behavior in institutionalized retarded blind child's self-hitting by response-contingent brief restraint. *Education and Treatment of Children*, *3*, 231–236.

Richmond, G. (1983). Evaluation of a treatment for a hand-mouthing stereotypy. *American Journal of Mental Deficiency*, *87*, 667–699.

Roberts, P., Iwata, B. A., McSween, T. E., & Desmond, Jr., E. F. (1979). An analysis of overcorrection movements. *American Journal of Mental Deficiency*, *83*, 588–594.

Rolider, A. (1989, Sept). *Side-effects of punishment: A fine grained analysis of assumed side-effects of therapeutic punishment.* Paper presented at the ninth annual meeting of the Florida Association for Behavior Analysis, Tampa, FL.

Rolider, A., & Cummings, A. (1988). The effects of momentary movement restriction on self-injury. Paper presented at the 14th annual convention of the Association for Behavior Analysis, Philadelphia, Penn.

Rolider, A., & Van Houten, R. (1985a). Movement suppression time-out for undesirable behavior in psychotic and severely developmentally delayed children. *Journal of Applied Behavior Analysis*, *18*, 275–288.

Rolider, A., & Van Houten, R. (1985b). Suppressing tantrum behavior in public places through the use of delayed punishment mediated by audio recording. *Behavior Therapy*, *16*, 181–194.

Russo, D. C., Cataldo, M. F., & Cushing, P. J. (1981). Compliance training and behavioral covariation in the treatment of multiple behavior problems. *Journal of Applied Behavior Analysis*, *14*, 209–222.

Saloviita, T. (1988). Elimination of self-injurious behaviour by brief physical restraint and DRA. *Scandinavian Journal of Behaviour Therapy*, *17*, 55–63.

Savie, P., & Dickie, R. F. (1979). Overcorrection of topographically dissimilar autistic behaviors. *Education and Treatment of Children*, *2*, 177–184.

Scarboro, M. E., & Forehand, R. (1975). Effects of two types of response-contingent time-out on compliance and oppositional behavior of children. *Journal of Experimental Child Psychology*, *19*, 252–264.

Secan, K. E., & Egel, A. L. (1986). The effects of a negative practice procedure on the self-stimulatory behavior of developmentally disabled children. *Education and Treatment of Children*, *9*, 30–39.

Singh, N. N., & Bakker, L. W. (1984). Suppression of pica by overcorrection and physical restraint: A comparative analysis. *Journal of Autism and Developmental Disorders*, *14*, 331–341.

Singh, N. N., Dawson, M. J., & Manning, P. J. (1981). The effects of physical restraint on self-injurious behaviour. *Journal of Mental Deficiency Research*, *25*, 207–216.

Singh, N. N., Watson, J. E., & Winton, A. S. W. (1986). Treating self-injury: Water mist spray versus facial screening or forced arm exercise. *Journal of Applied Behavior Analysis*, *19*, 403–410.

Singh, N. N., & Winton, A. S. W. (1985). Controlling pica by components of an overcorrection procedure. *American Journal of Mental Deficiency*, *90*, 40–45.

Strauss, C. C., Rubinoff, A., & Atkeson, B. M. (1983). Elimination of nocturnal headbanging in a normal seven-year-old girl using overcorrection plus rewards. *Journal of Behavior Therapy & Experimental Psychiatry*, *14*, 269–273.

Tarnowski, K. J., & Drabman, R. S. (1985). The effects of ambulation training on the self-stimulatory behavior of a multiply handicapped child. *Behavior Therapy*, *16*, 275–285.

Tierney, D. W. (1986). The reinforcement of calm sitting behavior: A method used to reduce the self-injurious behavior of a profoundly retarded boy. *Journal of Behavior Therapy & Experimental Psychiatry*, *17*, 47–50.

Underwood, L. A., Figueroa, R. G., Thyer, B. A., & Nzeocha, A. (1989). Interruption and DRI in the treatment of self-injurious behavior among mentally retarded and autistic self-restrainers. *Behavior Modification*, *13*, 471–481.

Van Houten, R., & Rolider, A. (1988). Recreating the scene: An effective way to provide delayed punishment for inappropriate motor behavior. *Journal of Applied Behavior Analysis*, *21*, 187–192.

Van Houten, R., & Rolider, A. (1989, May). *The side effects of punishment: Does it matter how well punishment is applied? You bet it does*! Paper presented at the 15th annual convention of the Association for Behavior Analysis, Milwaukee, WI.

Watson, J., Singh, N. N., & Winton, A. S. (1986). Suppressive effects of visual and facial screening on self-injurious finger-sucking. *American Journal of Mental Deficiency*, *90*, 526–534.

Wells, K. C., Forehand, R., Hickey, K., & Green, K. D. (1977). Effects of a procedure degived from the overcorrection principle or manipulated and non-manipulated behaviors. *Journal of Applied Behavior Analysis*, *10*, 679–687.

Wesolowski, M. D., & Zawlocki, R. J. (1982). The differential effects of procedures to eliminate an injurious self-stimulatory behavior (digito-ocular sign) in blind retarded twins. *Behavior Therapy*, *13*, 334–345.

Zehr, M. D., & Theobald, D. E. (1978). Manual guidance used in punishment procedure: The active ingredient in overcorrection. *Journal of Mental Deficiency Research*, *22*, 263–272.

# 8
# Facial Screening and Visual Occlusion

JOHANNES ROJAHN and ELAINE C. MARSHBURN

## Introduction

Vision is one of the most essential and powerful faculties of organisms, and it seems intuitively plausible that interfering with it and denying it, even if only temporarily, must have a profound impact on a person's behavior. Systematically blocking a client's vision has played a small but important role in the treatment of behavior problems in persons with mental retardation particularly their self-injurious behavior (SIB). Visual occlusion as a mechanism of behavioral intervention can be used in two functionally different modes: Either it is administered contingent upon the target behavior, as in *facial or visual screening*, or independent of the target behavior, as in *sensory extinction*. Both application modes are covered in this chapter. A literature review uncovered a total of 12 papers[1] on the treatment of SIB utilizing visual occlusion. In order to base our conclusions regarding visual occlusion techniques on a large enough sample, studies focusing on behavior problems other than SIB were included as well. This increased the number of articles to 31. Of these, 29 papers involved contingent visual occlusion, and only two employed visual sensory extinction. Naturally, the emphasis of this chapter is on contingent visual occlusion.

## Contingent Visual Occlusion Procedures

Response-contingent visual occlusion was originally developed as a mild, nonnoxious aversive stimulus. The first report of such a procedure was published by Giles and Wolf (1966; cited in Lutzker & Wesch, 1983), who

[1] A computerized literature search was conducted using ERIC, MEDLINE, and Psych Abstracts. In addition, review articles on screening by Lutzker and Wesch (1983) and Singh (1981) were consulted, and the reference sections from articles were screened for unpublished work and presented material.

TABLE 8.1. Standardized breakdown of relevant characteristics of research studies involving contingent visual occlusion procedures [1974–1989].

| Authors | Subjects | Topography | Setting | Treatment | Design | Interobserver agreement | Generalization | Follow-up | Results |
|---|---|---|---|---|---|---|---|---|---|
| Lutzker & Spencer (1974) | (see Lutzker & Wesch, 1983) | | | | | | | | |
| Zegiob, Jenkins, Becker, & Bristow (1976) | 7-yr.-old nonverbal schizophrenic boy | Hand-clapping | Classroom | Facial screening with terrycloth bib 10 sec., with release contingency and verbal command vs. Positive reinforcement for appropriate behavior | A-B-A-C-D-C Reversal design | Independent observer; 100% for hand-clapping, 96% for appropriate behavior | None | Posttreatment observational data 1 day at 2 mos. and 3 days at 6 mos. | Facial screening suppressed hand-clapping without negative side effect on verbal responding |
| Apsche, Bacevich, Axelrod, & Keach (1978) | 17-yr.-old mildly retarded girl | Aggression, noncompliance, running away | Residential area; classroom in institution | Contingent physical restraint vs. Contingent physical restraint plus eyescreen (opaque green cloth, 2 in. wide) | Multiple baseline across behaviors | One primary observer; average agreement <95% on observations 5 day wk. by staff | None | None | Physical restraint did not decrease target behavior; addition of visual screening virtually eliminated all three problem behaviors instantly |

TABLE 8.1. (Continued)

| Authors | Subjects | Topography | Setting | Treatment | Design | Interobserver agreement | Generalization | Follow-up | Results |
|---|---|---|---|---|---|---|---|---|---|
| *Lutzker (1978) | 20-yr.-old profoundly retarded male with PKU | Face- and head-slapping and -hitting | 3 special educ. classrooms | Facial screening with terrycloth bib (60 cm × 53 cm) 3 sec., with release contingency and verbal command | Multiple baseline across settings | 2 observers; 83–100% agreement | Programmed across settings and therapists | Informal observation | Facial screening rapidly reduced SIB to low rates in three settings |
| *Zegiob, Alford, & House (1978) | 13-yr.-old profoundly retarded and deaf boy | SIB—striking objects, biting self, hand-flapping | Classroom | Facial screening with terrycloth bib 10 sec., with release contingency | A-B-A-B-B′-C-A-C″ Partial component analysis | 2 observers; 90–100% agreement on 40% of sessions | Response generalization observed; programmed across other activities | None | Facial screening decelerated high-rate SIB (target behavior) without eliminating entirely; a simultaneous decrease in non-consequated behavior was observed |

| | | | | | | | | | |
|---|---|---|---|---|---|---|---|---|---|
| *Demetral & Lutzker (1980) | *Experiment 1* 14-yr.-old severely retarded boy | Hand-biting | Experimental setting; classroom; home | Facial screening with terrycloth bib (42 cm × 38 cm) 10 sec., with release contingency and verbal command vs. Noncontingent facial screening VI (variable interval) 5 minutes | Multiple baseline across settings | Independent observer; 83–98% agreement on 8 occasions | Programmed across settings; some generalization of treatment with contingent facial screening | 9 mos. follow-up without bib | Facial screening was found to be most effective when contingently employed |
| | *Experiment 2* 12-yr.-old severely retarded nonambulatory boy | Chest-hitting | Experimental setting; classroom | Facial screening with sheer black nylon bib for 10 sec. and verbal command vs. Facial screening with opaque bib for 10 sec. and verbal command | A-B-A-C-C′-C″-C-A Component analysis reversal design | 80–94% agreement on 6 occasions | Programmed across therapists | None | Facial screening was found to be most effective when employed with an opaque screen |

TABLE 8.1. (Continued)

| Authors | Subjects | Topography | Setting | Treatment | Design | Interobserver agreement | Generalization | Follow-up | Results |
|---|---|---|---|---|---|---|---|---|---|
| *Singh (1980) | 11-mo.-old microcephalic boy with cerebral palsy | Thumb-biting | Home | Facial screening with terrycloth bib (30 cm × 25 cm) 3 sec., and verbal command | Multiple baseline across settings | 2 observers; 100% agreement | Programmed across settings; parents trained as therapists | Posttreatment observation 1/mo. for 12 mos. | Facial screening gradually reduced and eliminated thumb-biting |
| Barmann & Murray (1981) | 14-yr.-old severely retarded boy | Sexual behavior (rubbing crotch) | Classroom; school bus; home | Facial screening with bib (64 cm × 58 cm) 5 sec., with release contingency and verbal command | Multiple baseline across settings | 2 observers; 84–100% agreement on 18 occasions across conditions | Programmed across settings and therapists | Posttreatment observation 1/mo. for 6 mos. | Facial screening reduced inappropriate sexual behavior by over 98%, 88%, and 92% from baseline condition in each of the 3 settings, respectively |
| Barrett, Matson, Shapiro, & Ollendick (1981) | 5-yr.-old nonverbal, behaviorally disturbed, moderately retarded girl<br><br>9-yr.-old nonverbal, behaviorally disturbed, moderately retarded boy | Finger-sucking, tongue protrusion | Laboratory setting; classroom | Visual screening 5 sec., with release contingency vs. DRO | Alternating treatment with multiple baseline across settings | 83–100% agreement with independent observer at least twice per phase | Programmed across setting | Posttreatment observation 5 consecutive days 1/mo. for 6 mos. | Visual screening was more effective for suppressing stereotypic behavior in both subjects than was DRO |

| | | | | | | | | | |
|---|---|---|---|---|---|---|---|---|---|
| *Singh, Beale, & Dawson (1981) | 18-yr.-old severely retarded girl | Face and jaw hitting | Residential ward | Facial screening with terrycloth bib (30 cm × 25 cm) vs. Various durations of facial screening (3 sec., 1 min., and 3 min.) | Alternating treatments | 4 observers; 86.4–93.7% agreement on 15% of total observations | 30 min. posttreatment of each 1 hr. session; programmed across ward settings | None | Facial screening implemented for 1 min. was found to be more effective in terms of immediate response suppression and short-term generalization than 3 sec. or 3 min |
| *Barmann & Vitali (1982) | 5-yr.-old developmentally disabled girl<br>9.5-yr.-old developmentally disabled girl<br>3-yr.-old developmentally disabled boy | Trichotillomania (hair-pulling) | Home; care facility | Facial screening with bib (64 cm × 48 m) 5 sec. and verbal command | Modified reversal design | 2 observers; 85–100% agreement on 15 occasions across conditions for each subject | Programmed across therapists | Posttreatment observation 1 mo. for 7 mos. | Facial screening gradually but completely and lastingly suppressed hair-pulling in 3 subjects |
| *Gross, Farrar, & Liner (1982) | 4-yr.-old mildly retarded boy with cerebral palsy | Trichotillomania (hair-pulling) | Classroom | Facial screening with terrycloth bib (55 cm × 50 cm) 15 sec. & DRO vs. Overcorrection & DRO | Modified reversal design | 2 observers; 89–100% agreement on 9 occasions | Programmed across time of day | 4 consecutive days 6 wks. posttreatment | Combination of DRO and overcorrection substantially decreased hair-pulling; DRO and facial screening completely suppressed the behavior |

TABLE 8.1. (Continued)

| Authors | Subjects | Topography | Setting | Treatment | Design | Interobserver agreement | Generalization | Follow-up | Results |
|---|---|---|---|---|---|---|---|---|---|
| *McGonigle, Duncan, Cordisco, & Barrett (1982) | *Experiment 1* 9-yr.-old moderately retarded girl and boy | Visual stereotypic behavior (waving hands and objects, vocalizations) | Free play in classroom | Visual screening 5 sec. | Multiple baseline across subjects and behaviors | 6 observers; 95–100% agreement on 32–47% of observations with independent observers | Observed across behaviors | Posttreatment observations at 6, 12, & 18 mos. for 5 consecutive days | Facial screening gradually reduced and completely suppressed different types of stereotyped behaviors |
| | *Experiment 2* 13-yr.-old profoundly retarded girl and boy | SIB (ear bending); fabric pulling | Community residence | Same as Experiment 1 | Same as Experiment 1 | Same as Experiment 1 | Observed across behaviors | Posttreatment observations at 2, 3, & 6 mos. for 5 consecutive days | Facial screening completely suppressed stereotyped behaviors; SIB was eliminated after 1 session without recovery at treatment withdrawal |
| Singh, Winton, & Dawson (1982) | *Experiment 1* 20-yr.-old microcephalic profoundly retarded woman | Screaming | Residential ward (lobby, courtyard, dayroom) | Facial screening with terrycloth bib (30 cm × 25 cm) 1 min. or if resistance | Multiple baseline across settings | 6 observers; 85–93% agreement on 25% of sessions by second observer | Programmed across settings | 6-mo. maintenance; posttreatment observational data 1 mo. for 6 mos. | Facial screening resulted in complete suppression of screaming, with very low levels maintained 6 mos. later |

| | | | | | | | | |
|---|---|---|---|---|---|---|---|---|
| | *Experiment 2* 2.5-yr.-old developmentally normal girl | Screaming | Home | Facial screening with terrycloth bib (30 cm × 25 cm) 1 min., 30 sec., 3 sec. | Alternating treatments design | 100% agreement on 25% of sessions by second observer | Programmed across time of day | 7-mo. maintenance; posttreatment observational data 1/mo. for 6 mos. | Facial screening (FS) resulted in complete suppression of screaming; other FS durations resulted in partial suppression |
| Barrett, Staub, & Sisson (1983) | 4.5-yr.-old mildly retarded boy | Compulsive rituals & repetitive behavior (related to shoes) | Laboratory; classroom; residential home | Visual screening 30 sec., with release contingency and verbal command vs. Treatment withdrawal using only verbal warning | Multiple baseline across settings, with partial withdrawal procedure | Independent rater 3–5 times each phase; 69–100% agreement across settings | Programmed across settings and therapists | Posttreatment observations at 3, 6, 9, & 12 mos. in home | Visual screening gradually and completely suppressed compulsive rituals |
| Dick & Jackson (1983) | 4-yr.-3-mos.-old severely retarded boy | Stereotypic loud screaming | School; home | Visual screening (1 min. decreased to 15–20 sec.) and verbal command vs. Treatment withdrawal | Alternating treatments and multiple baseline across settings | 1 primary observer in each setting; 100% agreement with independent observer on 18% of sessions | Programmed across settings and therapists | Posttreatment observations at 1, 3, & 6 mos. | Visual screening gradually suppressed stereotypic screaming and maintained its effectiveness across a 6-mos. period; social validation: Behavior was rated as less frequent and less annoying than before |

TABLE 8.1. (Continued)

| Authors | Subjects | Topography | Setting | Treatment | Design | Interobserver agreement | Generalization | Follow-up | Results |
|---|---|---|---|---|---|---|---|---|---|
| *Lutzker & Wesch (1983) | 20-yr.-old profoundly retarded man with PKU<br><br>9-yr.-old severely retarded boy with Down syndrome | Head slapping | Experimental setting in residential facilities<br><br>Positive reinforcement for appropriate behavior throughout sessions | Facial screening with terrycloth bib (61 cm × 53 cm) 3 sec., with release contingency and verbal command vs. Facial screening with bib 3 sec., 15 sec., and verbal command vs. Verbal command vs. Bib around neck | Multiple baseline across subjects and subsequent component analysis | 83–100% (mean 95.1%) | None | None | Facial screening was effective in reducing SIB rapidly in one subject and gradually in another to low levels; increasing the duration of the screen from 3 to 15 sec. increased suppressing properties |

| | | | | | | | | | |
|---|---|---|---|---|---|---|---|---|---|
| St. Lawrence & Drabman (1984) | 15-yr.-old microcephalic male with congenital rubella and partial vision | Spitting | Class in nonresidential setting | Facial screening with towel held in front of face 4 sec., with release contingency vs. DRO vs. Facial screening and positive reinforcement vs. Positive reinforcement | Multiple baseline across situations and within-subjects Reversal | 1 primary observer; 94% agreement across conditions on 23% of sessions by 2 additional raters | Programmed across settings and teachers | Telephone follow-up 1-yr. posttreatment | Facial screening plus DRO more completely suppressed spitting behavior than either one of the treatments alone |
| *Singh & Winton (1984) | 24-yr.-old right hemiplegic profoundly retarded woman | Pica (collateral behaviors observed) | Residential ward (dayroom, TV room, outside) | Screening with blindfold 1 min., with release contingency | Multiple baseline across settings | 5 observers; 84–92% agreement on pica; 81–97% agreement on collateral behaviors | Programmed across settings; decrease in collateral behaviors observed | 8-wk. maintenance; posttreatment observational data 1 mo. for 6 mos. | Screening rapidly suppressed pica and reduced it to near-zero levels; untreated collateral problem behaviors also decreased |

TABLE 8.1. (Continued)

| Authors | Subjects | Topography | Setting | Treatment | Design | Interobserver agreement | Generalization | Follow-up | Results |
|---|---|---|---|---|---|---|---|---|---|
| *Winton, Singh, & Dawson (1984) | *Experiment 1* 19-yr.-old profoundly retarded girl, also deaf | Face-slapping; head-hitting | Residential unit | Facial screening with terrycloth bib (30 cm × 25 cm) 1 min., with release contingency vs. Facial screening with bib modified with 15 cm × 10 cm transparent plastic center | Alternating treatments design | 6 observers; 91–97% agreement with independent observers on 12 sessions | Programmed across time of day and staff in maintenance | Maintenance data weekly for 5 wks.; posttreatment observations 1 mo. for 6 mos. | Standard facial screening with opaque screen gradually reduced SIB; only a slight decrease occurred with a transparent screen |
| | *Experiment 2* 15-yr.-old profoundly retarded boy due to PKU | Face-slapping | Dayroom of residential ward | Facial screening with bib 1 min., with release contingency vs. Facial screening modified with transparent center | Alternating treatments with reversal component | 2 observers, 85% agreement prior to baseline; 86–97% agreement with independent observer on 24% of sessions | Programmed across time of day and staff in maintenance | 5-wk. maintenance | Standard facial screening with opaque screen gradually reduced SIB; only a slight decrease occurred with a transparent screen |

| | | | | | | | | | |
|---|---|---|---|---|---|---|---|---|---|
| | *Experiment 3* 12-yr.-old profoundly retarded and emotionally disturbed boy | Face-hitting | Dayroom & training room of residential ward | Facial screening with bib 1 min., with release contingency vs. Blindfold (eye screen) | Alternating treatments | 2 observers; 85% agreement prior to baseline; 89–97% agreement with independent observer on 25% of sessions | Programmed across time of day and ward staff in maintenance | 10-wk. maintenance; posttreatment observations 1 mo. for 12 mos. | Standard facial screening and blindfold screening were equally effective in suppressing SIB |
| McGonigle (1986) | Four developmentally delayed boys, 3–4 yrs. old, with social, emotional, and behavioral problems | Stereotyped behaviors (hand-flapping, jumping, gazing, vocalizations, mouthing, posturing, etc.) | Classroom | Visual screening 5 sec. vs. DRO | Alternating treatments combined with multiple baseline and withdrawal phases | 3 observers 63–100% agreement on occurrence; 50–100% for agreement on nonoccurrence; 26% of all sessions | Programmed across settings | None | Visual screening was more effective than DRO; transitory negative side effects appeared in two subjects; on-task behavior increased as stereotypic behavior decreased in three subjects |

TABLE 8.1. (continued)

| Authors | Subjects | Topography | Setting | Treatment | Design | Interobserver agreement | Generalization | Follow-up | Results |
|---|---|---|---|---|---|---|---|---|---|
| Singh, Watson, & Winton (1986) | *Experiment 1* 17-yr.-old profoundly retarded girl | Face-slapping | Residential dayroom | Facial screening with terrycloth bib (30 cm × 35 cm) 5 sec., with release contingency vs. Water mist spray | Alternating treatments | 2 observers; 87–100% agreement with independent observer on 25% of sessions | Programmed across time of day | None | Facial screening and water mist were both effective in reducing SIB in similar rates with FS achieving slightly lower levels of suppression |
| | *Experiment 2* 17-yr.-old profoundly retarded girl | Finger-licking (observation of collateral behaviors) | Residential dayroom | Facial screening with terrycloth bib 5 sec., with release contingency vs. Water mist spray | Alternating treatments | 4 observers; 81–91% agreement across all behaviors | Programmed across therapists and time of day; observed generalization of treatment to collateral behaviors | 6mo. maintenance | Facial screening was significantly more effective than water mist in reducing SIB rapidly to near-zero levels |
| Watson, Singh, & Winton (1986) | *Experiment 1* 18-yr.-old profoundly retarded boy confined to wheelchair | Sucking fingers (observed collateral behavior— toy play) | Experimental room in residential ward | Visual screening 5 sec., with release contingency vs. Facial screening with terrycloth bib (45 cm × 30 cm, same duration) vs. Treatment withdrawal | Alternating treatments | 4 observers; 92–98% agreement on 28% of observations | Programmed across staff in maintenance | 30wk. maintenance | Visual screening was slightly more effective than facial screening |

| | | | | | | | | | |
|---|---|---|---|---|---|---|---|---|---|
| | *Experiment 2* 19-yr.-old profoundly retarded boy | Same as Experiment 1 | Same as Experiment 1 | Same as Experiment 1 | Alternating treatments | 3 observers; 92–98% agreement on 16% of observations | Same as Experiment 1 | 18-wk. maintenance | Visual and facial screening were more effective in reducing SIB than no treatment |
| Zlomke, Smith, & Piersel (1986) | 32-yr.-old moderately retarded male | Excessive verbalizations | Residential facility (training room, class, vocational workshop)<br>Ongoing DRI procedure throughout study | Visual blocking with opaque card 4 in. in front of subject's eyes 15 sec., with release contingency | Multiple probe variation of multiple baseline across settings | Independent observer 1 wk. across settings | Hourly interval sampling procedure 1 wk. | Observational data once a week following criterion level in each setting; posttreatment observations 1 wk. for 8 wks. | Visual blocking gradually reduced excessive verbalization to zero levels in two of three settings |
| Horton (1987a) | 8-yr.-old severely retarded microcephalic girl | Spoon-banging at meal time | Experimental classroom setting | Facial screening with terrycloth bib 5 sec., with release contingency and verbal command | A-B-A-B replicated in two settings | 2 observers; 80–90% agreement for procedure and response | Programmed across classroom settings | Posttreatment observations at 6, 10, 15, & 19 mos. | Facial screening rapidly decelerated spoon-banging behavior to near-zero levels |
| Horton (1987b) | 4.5-yr.-old moderately retarded boy with cerebral palsy | Mouthing objects | Classroom (closed and open space) | Facial screening with towel (30 cm × 30 cm) 3 sec., an verbal command | A-B-A-B | 2 observers; 87–100% agreement on 23–33% of sessions | Programmed across settings | Posttreatment observations at 6, 12, & 18 mos. | Facial screening rapidly decelerated mouthing behavior to near-zero levels |

TABLE 8.1. (Continued)

| Authors | Subjects | Topography | Setting | Treatment | Design | Interobserver agreement | Generalization | Follow-up | Results |
|---|---|---|---|---|---|---|---|---|---|
| McGonigle, Rojahn, Dixon, & Strain (1987) | *Experiment 1* 3-yr.-8-mos.-old severely retarded boy with seizure disorder | Mouthing objects and fingers | Special educ. classroom in psychiatric care facility | Visual screening 5 sec., with release contingency Verbal prompt/ interruption vs. DRO vs. Extinction | Alternating treatments with change in ICI and withdrawal component | 2 observers; 88–100% agreement with independent observers on 18 occasions | Programmed across time of day | None | Extinction reduced mouthing to lower levels than visual screening, DRO, and interruption/ redirection |
| | *Experiment 2* 3-yr.10-mos.-old moderately retarded boy | Noncompliant behaviors (whining, screaming, spitting, out-of-seat) | Special educ. classroom in psychiatric care facility | Visual screening vs. DRO | Alternating treatments with withdrawal component | 2 observers; 81–99% agreement on 18 sessions | Programmed across time of day | None | Visual screening was more effective in reducing the rate of disruptive noncompliance as compared to DRO |

| | | | | | | | | | |
|---|---|---|---|---|---|---|---|---|---|
| Dixon, Helsel, Rojahn, Cipollone, & Lubetsky (1989) | 6-yr.-8-mos.-old severely retarded nonambulatory boy | Aggression (assault & throwing), destruction, loud screeching | Psychiatric hospital classroom | Visual screening with hand over eyes & contingent hands down 10 sec., with release contingency and verbal command vs. Visual screening & contingent hands down & aromatic ammonia Also phenytoin & carbamzepine mainipulations | B-A-B-C-B-C-B Partial multiple baseline across behaviors | 1 primary rater; 50–100% agreement with independent observer across all target behaviors on 25% of sessions | Programmed across behaviors | None | Visual screening, which reduced rates of aggressive and destructive behaviors and loud screaming, was combined with aromatic ammonia to decelerate these behaviors to near-zero rates |
| Jordan, Singh, & Repp (1989) | 21-yr.-old profoundly retarded man<br>28-yr.-old profoundly retarded man | Stereotypic behavior (mouthing, hand flapping) | Therapy room in MR residential facility | Operant task training (OT) vs. OT & visual screening 5 sec., with release contingency vs. Gentle teaching | Alternating treatments design + no treatment control | 1 primary rater; 73–100% agreement for stereotyped behavior in 25% of the sessions | Programmed across therapists | None | Visual screening was the most effective treatment for reduction of stereotypic behavior; gentle teaching reduced stereotypic behavior in two of three subjects |

Articles with an asterisk describe clients with SIB.

used a mask with eye holes to punish toilet accidents of residents with mental retardation. However, Lutzker and Spencer (1974) were the first to systematically investigate facial screening with SIB.

After the early demonstrations of successfully controlling SIB with aversive stimuli such as electric shock (e.g., Corte, Wolf, & Locke, 1971; Lovaas & Simmons, 1969; Tate & Baroff, 1966); alternate aversive stimuli were explored. Among them were slaps (Birnbrauer, 1968), citric acid (e.g., Sajwaj, Libet, & Agras, 1974), aromatic ammonia (e.g., Tanner & Zeiler, 1975), Tabasco sauce (Murray, Keele, & McCarver, 1977), restraint (Favell, McGimsey, & Jones, 1978), water mist (e.g., Dorsey, Iwata, Ong, & McSween, 1980), and forced running (Borreson, 1980). Despite the undeniable success of punishment, resentment started to build up against it as a treatment paradigm for humans. People began to question the ethics of these procedures, and many service delivery agencies for people with mental retardation prohibited their use. Because punishment was still considered by many clinical researchers to be the most effective treatment paradigm to control severe behavior problems, other ethically more acceptable punishers were explored (Lutzker, 1978). They had to be nonnoxious, easy to implement, inexpensive, and without danger for the client (Demetral & Lutzker, 1980). Contingent visual occlusion appeared to fulfill most of these prerequisites.

Response-contingent visual occlusion procedures are typically known as facial screening (Zegiob, Jenkins, Becker, & Bristow, 1976), visual screening (Barrett, Matson, Shapiro, & Ollendick, 1981), or blindfold screening (Singh & Winton, 1984). These procedures differ from one another primarily in terms of the devices used to cover the client's eyes. These different covers, however, also require slightly different therapist manipulations. *Facial screening*, for example, the earliest form of visual occlusion, is performed with a terry-cloth bib that is secured around the neck and hangs down the client's chest. Bib size has varied, ranging from 30 cm × 25 cm (e.g., Singh, Beale, & Dawson, 1981) to 64 cm × 58 cm (Barmann & Murray, 1981). Contingent upon the occurrence of a target behavior, the therapist, usually positioned in front of the client, grabs the bib and pulls it over the face of the client for a short period of time. In an effort to improve the screening technique, Barrett et al. (1981), and later McGonigle, Duncan, Cordisco, and Barrett (1982), introduced *visual screening*, in which the therapist, usually approaching the client from behind, covers the client's eyes with the palm of the therapist's hand. The other hand is used to hold the client's head back for stabilization and to prevent the client from getting free. The hold is necessary because some clients initially attempt to resist the intervention (e.g., McGonigle, 1986).

Other screening techniques have included fastening felt spectacles with an elastic band around the head (Singh & Winton, 1984), using a 2-inch opaque cloth (Apsche, Bacevich, Axelrod, & Keach, 1978), and holding an *opaque card* in front of the subject's eyes to block visual input

(Zlomke, Smith, & Piersel, 1986). Other eye covers, such as bibs with a transparent plastic center, have been made for experimental purposes.

As Table 8.1 shows, most contingent visual occlusion procedures were accompanied by verbal commands, pointing out the target behavior and a command to stop. Screening procedures also usually included release contingencies in order to avoid incidental reinforcement of inappropriate behaviors, such as struggling or screaming.

The following contains a discussion of the literature on contingent visual occlusion, according to critical study characteristics.

## Subjects

Contingent screening has been used with individuals from a broad range of age and intellectual functioning. In the 12 SIB studies, 19 clients participated. Their mean age was 12.9 years, with a range from 11 months to 24 years, and the majority (12) of them were male. Nine individuals were diagnosed as having profound, four severe, and one mild mental retardation; in five cases, level of mental retardation was not reported. In the 17 non-SIB studies, 26 individuals participated as clients. Their mean age was 10.8 years; 20 clients were male, and 6 were female. Seven subjects had either no or an undisclosed level of mental retardation, two had mild, five moderate, seven severe, and five profound mental retardation.

## Settings

One of the criticisms raised against the punishment technology has been its insignificant value for community and social integration (LaVigna, 1987). A review of the literature does not support this claim, as far as contingent visual occlusion is concerned. Contingent visual occlusion was evaluated in simulated laboratory settings, in the clients' natural environment, and in institutions. However, there were also several others that were performed in community settings, such as in the home (Barmann & Murray, 1981; Barmann & Vitali, 1982; Barrett, Staub, & Sisson, 1983; Demetral & Lutzker, 1980; Singh, 1980; Singh, Winton, & Dawson, 1982); in the clients' natural classrooms (Barmann & Murray, 1981; Demetral & Lutzker, 1980; Gross, Farrar, & Liner, 1982; McGonigle, 1986; St. Lawrence & Drabman, 1984), and even on the school bus (Barmann & Murray, 1981). This suggests that contingent visual occlusion can be integrated relatively easily into natural settings.

## Topographies

Contingent visual occlusion has been used on many different types of aberrant behavior, ranging from rather benign forms of stereotypy to serious aggression and SIB, such as head- or face-striking and biting.

Other behaviors treated included property destruction, inappropriate sexual activities, compulsive rituals, out-of-seat behavior, spitting, running away, and noncompliance.

## Efficacy

*Efficacy* refers to the quickness and degree of response suppression achieved by a treatment procedure. The literature review revealed a fairly consistent response deceleration pattern across different types of subjects and behaviors. Most importantly, contingent visual occlusion has a quick impact. If the procedure is effective with a given client, one can expect as early as in the first session to see the response rate drop to levels 50% or less as compared to baseline. From then on, the response rate tends to decline in a steady and gradual fashion, reaching near-zero levels after 5–10 treatment sessions. However, total elimination of behaviors occurs rarely when only contingent visual occlusion is utilized. This raises the question of the usefulness of contingent visual occlusion for high-intensity behaviors, where serious damage can be caused even by a rare occurrence.

As Table 8.1 indicates, maintaining treatment effects over a long period of time seems possible. Some studies reported successful maintenance for over a year.

Unfortunately, very little research has been conducted to investigate how visual/facial screening might be affected by simultaneous pharmacological treatment. The only study that came close to such a project was one in which unanticipated seizure medication changes that happened to occur while an evaluation of a visual screening program was in progress were closely monitored (Dixon, Helsel, Rojahn, Cipollone, & Lubetzky, 1989). The timing of the drug manipulations was dictated by medical considerations rather than experimental planning so that strong inferences regarding interaction between medication and behavioral intervention were not possible. The data suggested that neither discontinuation of carbamazepine nor introduction and titration of phenytoin appeared to have an impact on problem behaviors (aggression, destruction, screaming), while visual screening did.

## Comparative Efficacy of Contingent Visual Occlusion

Several researchers have attempted to compare contingent visual occlusion procedures with other treatment techniques in terms of their efficacy.

### *Facial Screening Versus Overcorrection*

Gross et al. (1982) compared facial screening and overcorrection for the treatment of hair-pulling in a 4-year-old boy with mild mental retardation. Both treatments were accompanied by a 10-second DRO schedule of social reinforcement. Fifteen-second facial screening was performed with a terry-cloth bib. Overcorrection consisted of 2-minute exercises of extended arms, alternating with arms over the client's head and perpendicular to his body. The data indicated that overcorrection plus DRO substantially decreased hair pulling, but without achieving clinically acceptable levels. The introduction of facial screening almost instantly eliminated hair-pulling to zero levels. These results were maintained 6 weeks later, and observations indicated that they also generalized across the entire school day.

## *Facial Screening Versus Water Mist Spray*

Singh, Watson, and Winton (1986) compared 5-second facial screening with water mist spray in two clients. Both were 17-year-old girls with profound mental retardation who resided in an institution. The first client exhibited face-slapping and the other excessive finger-licking. In the first client, facial-screening and water spray mist had an immediate impact, resulting in a response decrease of about 50% in the first treatment session. From then on, face-slapping gradually decreased to very low levels. Response rate had reached zero for the first time in the ninth treatment session. Water-mist spraying showed a very similar downward trend and similar, although somewhat higher, frequencies of responding. The results were clearer in the second subject, were facial screening was shown to be more effective than water mist.

## *Blindfold Screening Versus Physical Restraint*

In one of the earlier studies, Apsche et al. (1978) looked at the effect of a time-out with physical restraint procedure on three different target behaviors (aggression, noncompliance, and running away) in an institutionalized 17-year-old girl with mild mental retardation. The procedure consisted of contingent directing of the client to a corner of the room. If the client refused to comply, a fall-back contingency consisting of 10 minutes of physical restraint followed. This had virtually no beneficial effect on the frequency of these behaviors. The addition of a blindfold immediately eliminated all three high-frequency behaviors to near-zero levels. Unfortunately, it was not investigated as to what effect the blindfold alone had on these behaviors.

## *Visual Screening Versus DRO*

Barrett et al. (1981) compared differential reinforcement of other behavior (DRO) and visual screening. Subjects were two children with moderate mental retardation and high rates of stereotyped SIB. The results clearly indicated that visual screening reduced SIB in the typical fashion: a quick reduction beginning with the first session and a gradual decline to near-zero rates of responding. DRO administered by itself, on the other hand, did not have a clinically significant impact on stereotyped behavior. McGonigle (1986) conducted a similar study involving four children and came to the same conclusion: Visual screening was effective in decreasing stereotyped behavior, while it was not possible to achieve clinically satisfactory results with DRO.

## *Visual Screening Versus Gentle Teaching*

As a result of the aforementioned sentiment against the use of aversive treatment procedures, treatment packages based primarily on positive reinforcement have been proposed (e.g., Carr & Durand, 1985). One of the more prominent alternative approaches has been "gentle teaching" (McGee, 1986; Menolascino & McGee, 1983). Gentle teaching utilizes positive operant conditioning techniques, emphasizes the importance of the humanizing bond between therapist and client, and, above all, rules out any type of punishment. Jordan, Singh, and Repp (1989) put gentle teaching to an empirical test by systematically evaluating its impact on stereotyped behavior. They also compared it to visual screening. Three low-functioning subjects participated in the study; two adults and a 7-year-old boy. Visual screening was the more effective procedure in reducing stereotyped behavior. Interestingly, behaviors that were representative of human bonding, such as smiling and approaching the therapist, did not differ as a result of the type of treatment.

Overall, contingent visual-occlusion procedures have been shown each time to be more effective than the contrasted treatment that consisted of standard behavioral interventions or gentle teaching. It must be pointed out, however, that the evidence provided for the superiority of visual/facial screening over other interventions must be viewed with some caution. These comparisons were all limited to one or two single-subject design studies, involving a maximum of four clients per study. Evidently, replications are needed to draw firmer conclusions about relative effectiveness. For instance, it is conceivable that changing some parameters in some of the other procedures could have changed the results. Nevertheless, it seems as if contingent visual occlusion procedures are quite effective in reducing SIB and other maladaptive behaviors when compared to other behavioral interventions.

# Comparative Efficacy Among Contingent Visual Occlusion Techniques

For clinical and theoretical reasons, it is important to assess what variations of contingent visual occlusion are most effective. A few of the studies found in the literature included comparative investigations of different types of screening.

### *Facial Screening Versus Visual Screening*

Watson, Singh, and Winton (1986) compared the efficacy of facial and visual screening applied for the same duration (5 seconds minimum) in two adolescent boys with profound mental retardation. Both exhibited high rates of finger-sucking behavior. It was found that visual screening was more effective in rapidly decreasing finger-sucking in one of the clients, while no differences were found in the second client.

### *Facial Screening Versus Blindfold Screening*

Winton, Singh, and Dawson (1984) compared the effects of two contingent visual-occlusion techniques, one involving a bib, the other a blindfold made of soft black felt. The screening procedures achieved very similar results in decreasing SIB from a mean rate of approximately 13 responses per hour to 3. The effects were compared by using an alternating-treatments design. Obviously, both treatments clearly suppressed SIB, but it could not be decided unequivocally, on the basis of response deceleration, which technique was the most effective. However, given the design, multiple treatment interference cannot be ruled out as possibly exaggerating the efficacy of one of the procedures.

### *Contingent Versus Noncontingent Facial Screening*

Demetral and Lutzker (1980) investigated whether the schedule of punishment was a relevant variable for facial screening. Screening was first presented on a variable interval 5-minutes schedule, independent of the occurrence of the target behavior (biting). Next, the standard contingent schedule was introduced. As expected, noncontingent screening did not decrease biting behavior, while contingent facial screening quickly reduced it to near-zero levels. The authors concluded that the schedule of punishment was an important treatment variable.

## Component Analyses

There are several components involved in visual and facial screening that may contribute to its effects on behavior. For instance, screening is likely to contain unconditioned aversive properties, such as response interruption, blocking of visual input, and physical immobilization (see Winton et al., 1984). There also might be a response cost component involved by temporarily being forced to surrender control over the environment (restricted sensory input and motor movement). Finally, nonexclusionary time-out from reinforcement is in effect and might contribute to the overall response-suppressive properties.

Some researchers attempted to test experimentally the role of certain characteristics of contingent screening on reducing target behaviors.

## Blocking of Visual Input

The term *visual screening* implies that the withdrawal of visual input is a major treatment component. Two studies have investigated this theory. Demetral and Lutzker (1980) tested whether a bib had to be opaque in order to be effective or whether a translucent bib also would suppress behavior. They found that facial screening with an opaque bib immediately reduced SIB to comparatively low rates, while a translucent bib did not seem to have an impact on reducing the behavior. This study provided evidence that (a) blocking of the visual input might be the major treatment component, and (b) screening without visual blocking does not suppress behavior. Winton, Singh, and Dawson (1984) compared the standard facial screening with a transparent screen in two single-case studies. In both cases, the transparent screen minimally reduced SIB, while standard screening showed the typical decrease to total suppression. In a third subject, facial screening, as well as opaque blindfolding, were very effective. The available evidence supports the notion that blocking a client's vision is indeed one of the more potent ingredients of facial screening.

## Physical Restraint

One could argue that contingent visual occlusion procedures involve varying amounts of physical restraint, which may contribute to the success of screening procedures. In an early study, Zegiob, Alford, and House (1978) conducted a partial component analysis that consisted of a sequence of reversal phases implemented in two settings. They investigated the effects of both facial screening and restraint. Due to the number of variables involved and the variability in the behavior, neither presenting the bib without screening nor restraining the head alone were sufficient to substantially reduce self-hitting.

## Duration of Screening

The duration of contingent visual-occlusion procedures discussed in the literature ranged from 3 seconds to 3 minutes, with a median of between 5 and 10 seconds. Two obvious questions are (1) How long does screening have to be implemented to be effective? and (2) What is the relationship between length of screening and suppressive effect? Only three studies directly addressed either of these questions. Lutzker and Spencer (1974; cited in Lutzker & Wesch, 1983) implemented a 15-second facial screening after a 3-second screening failed to eliminate SIB completely. It was found that the 15-second screening was more suppressive than the 3-second procedure. Similarly, Singh, Winton, and Dawson (1982) compared 1-minute, 3-second, and 30-second screening, with regard to the suppression of screaming behavior of a developmentally normal child with severe behavior problems. The 1-minute duration of screening was reported to be more effective than either of the other two durations. It appears that, within a limited range, a linear relationship existed between efficacy and duration of screening. Singh et al. (1981) addressed the limit of this range. Using an alternating-treatments design, the authors found that 1-minute screening decreased SIB to significantly lower levels than either a 3-second or a 3-minute screening procedure. Thus, 1-minute screening might be close to an efficacy plateau, which within limits of therapeutic feasibility cannot be easily surpassed by simply extending the screening duration.

## *Discriminative Stimuli and Aversive Conditioning*

In an effort to move toward less intrusive and more normalized forms of behavior control, some researchers have investigated to what extent relatively neutral stimuli, such as verbal commands, could be conditioned to assume properties of the screening procedure. The idea was that verbal commands could eventually replace screening in maintaining the target behavior at low levels. Several kinds of conditioned aversive stimuli were found in the reviewed literature. Most frequently used were verbal statements. The typical procedure was that during the original treatment phases, the stimuli would consistenly precede visual occlusion. For instance, the therapist used a command such as "No, don't do . . . ," or "(*Name*), stop. . . ."

Only a handful of studies systematically investigated the effect of conditioned aversive stimuli. Lutzker and Spencer (1974) combined facial screening with a "No" command during the first treatment phase, reducing SIB to much lower levels than during baseline. During a subsequent return to baseline, the behavior quickly recovered to pretreatment levels. When, in the following three sessions, the verbal command was used without screening, a reduced rate was only visible in the first session. The verbal stimulus apparently had not achieved strong enough control over SIB.

In another study, Barrett et al. (1983) began to use only verbal cues after the target behavior had been eliminated by a combination of verbal commands and screening. The verbal warning program required that visual screening be withheld if the client stopped engaging in the target behavior after the verbal cue was given. In this way, the verbal warning procedure maintained target behavior responding at near-zero levels for several days and in different settings. However, no long-term effects were reported. It is also unclear how often screening had to be implemented as a back-up during the verbal-cue phase.

Zegiob et al. (1978) investigated stimulus-control properties of the bib after successful suppression of self-hitting. In a period subsequent to the initial treatment phase, the bib was put on the subject without actual screening. After initial reduction of the target behavior to low levels, the behavior slowly recovered and soon reached baseline rates. Similarly, Demetral and Lutzker (1980) found that the bib and the noncontingent implementation of contingent screening had acquired some controlling properties outside the treatment setting only as long as active treatment was going on.

In summary, existing data suggest that conditioned stimuli will fail to become potent enough in maintaining low response levels by simply pairing them with visual/facial screening unless the stimuli can be backed up by screening. However, as is the case with most other issues discussed in this paper, strong and replicated empirical evidence is unavailable.

Aversive conditioning was also used in an opposite direction—namely, to increase the suppressive properties of visual screening. In that case, screening was the conditioned (CS), rather than the unconditioned stimulus (UCS), as in the preceding examples. Dixon et al. (1989) investigated whether the efficacy of a previously effective visual screening program could be recharged by aversive conditioning with a noxious stimulus. This maneuver was a desperate attempt to save a previously effective visual screening procedure that had lost its suppressive effects in the natural environment. The client had severe and high-frequency aggressive behavior, as well as several other behavior problems. Aversive conditioning involved a trial of continuous pairing of visual screening (CS) with aromatic ammonia (UCS) in a classroom treatment setting. According to expectation, the data showed that the addition of ammonia was more effective than screening alone. When ammonia was discontinued and visual screening was implemented alone, screening maintained its strong suppressive effect for only several days before slowly and gradually losing it again. There was not enough time, however, to investigate the clinical utility of such conditioning procedures in order to restore the suppressive effects of visual-screening procedures.

## Side Effects

There has been great concern that punishment procedures have negative side effects, such as the client's avoidance of and escape from the therapist, the emergence of aggressive behavior, and undesirable emotional states (cf. Matson & DiLorenzo, 1984). Technically, side effects are changes (or the lack thereof) in untreated behavior that result from the treatment of the target behavior.

## *Undesirable Side Effects*

Undesirable side effects in this population can occur as a collateral increase of existing or emergence of new problem behaviors, or as a decrease of appropriate behaviors not targeted in the treatment procedure. Only a few studies addressed this issue openly. One of them was a study conducted by McGonigle (1986), who systematically collected data on side effects, upon visual screening implemented for stereotyped behavior. He found that two of the four young clients initially tried to resist visual screening by screaming, having tantrums, and falling to the floor. These behaviors, however, were soon extinguished after only a few sessions. Extinction was facilitated by the fact that the clients were 4-year-old children. There is no question that it would have been a more serious problem with physically strong individuals. Zegiob et al. (1976), on the other hand, who also made explicit efforts to identify specific adverse effects in the form of a decrease in appropriate verbal behavior, failed to find any. In the many papers that did not mention side effects, it would be misleading to conclude that none had occurred. It appears that negative side effects may occur with some individuals, particularly in those who have a history of escape and avoidance behaviors.

## *Desirable Side Effects*

Positive secondary treatment effects can occur either as an unintended decrease of inappropriate behaviors (other than the target behavior) or as an increase in desirable behaviors. There are a few accounts in the literature showing that contingent visual occlusion procedures can generalize in a positive fashion to nontargeted problem behaviors. For instance, Singh and Winton (1984) found that stereotypic, aggressive, and self-injurious behaviors decreased (after an initial slight increase) following the implementation of blindfold screening for pica (Singh & Winton, 1984); and Singh et al. (1986) reported that collateral jaw-hitting and finger-rubbing had decreased, while facial screening was focused on excessive finger-licking.

Likewise, the observation has been made that suppression of targeted problem behavior also can be accompanied by a collateral increase of desirable behavior (Koegel, Firestone, Kramme, & Dunlap, 1974). In the case of visual screening, McGonigle et al. (1982) observed that while stereotyped behavior was suppressed, self-initiated play behavior increased. In another study, parents and other care givers reported gains of positive behaviors following the elimination of hair-pulling by facial screening (Barmann & Vitali, 1982). McGonigle (1986) demonstrated that on-task behavior increased as stereotypic behavior was decreased by visual screening, and Singh et al. (1986) found an increase of appropriate social interaction during facial screening and water-mist punishment. It was reported that facial screening achieved higher levels of desirable social behavior than did water mist. Positive side effects are not unlikely to occur in some clients while inappropriate behaviors are being reduced by facial/visual screening.

## Practicality, Acceptability, and Social Validity

The fact that behavioral procedures can be very effective in reducing SIB and other problem behaviors has been demonstrated in hundreds of articles, but if programs are difficult to use or are unacceptable for other reasons, chances are they will not become very popular in the real world. A few studies addressed the feasibility of contingent visual-occlusion programs.

Barmann and Vitali (1982) had parents and other caregivers rate facial screening on four scales: difficulty in administering the procedure, acceptability, perceived efficacy, and the degree of improvement of the children's behaviors. The data indicated that contingent visual occlusion was very well received in all of these areas. In addition, facial screening training was found to be easy. Barmann and Murray (1981) reported that the average training of parents, teachers, and school-bus aides lasted about 1 hour. Dick and Jackson (1983) assessed the social validity of the treatment results achieved with visual screening and received very positive feedback. In comparing facial and blindfold screening, Winton et al. (1984) noted that all of their therapists who were involved in the treatment had expressed a preference for facial screening over blindfolding for practical reasons. Visual screening, however, was rated by therapists to be even more convenient to use than facial screening (McGonigle et al., 1982; Watson et al., 1986). Winton et al. (1984) found that teachers, parents, and nurses preferred facial screening over other more aversive techniques.

In summary, the available evidence seems to indicate that contingent visual occlusion has been fairly well received in terms of practicality, efficacy, and acceptability. It should be pointed out, however, that the reported evaluations were performed with a potentially biased group of informants: first of all, the informants were a natural preselection of people who presumably had consented to contingent screening in the first place, and, second, they were questioned after successful implementation of screening programs. These data, therefore, do not indicate how acceptable visual and facial screening might be among the general population of parents, teachers, service agencies' staff, and advocates for people with mental retardation.

## Sensory (Visual) Extinction

Sensory extinction works under the assumption that some behaviors are maintained by stimulating sensory reinforcement produced by the act itself (Lovaas, Newsome, & Hickman, 1987). Withholding that stimulation would consequently extinguish the behavior. Research on *visual* sensory extinction was first described by Rincover (1978), who investigated whether different forms of sensory stimulation had functional relevance for stereotyped behavior. The study included three psychotic, low-functioning children (one of whom had a visual impairment) with different forms of stereotypies. Rincover found that masking of proprioceptive and auditory stimuli reduced stereotyped behavior in two subjects, but he failed to provide such evidence for visual blocking.

Table 8.2 presents the only two research articles to date that have dealt with visual sensory extinction and SIB. The researchers used either a handkerchief (Rincover, 1978) or switching off the light (Rincover, Cook, Peoples, & Packard, 1979) to achieve visual blocking.

Visual sensory extinction programs have never become popular for the treatment of SIB. This state of affairs is not surprising, however, for several reasons. First, extinction is characterized by a slow response deceleration rate, which is usually a prohibiting quality for an SIB treatment due to the risk of severe damage. In addition, SIB, like most other behaviors, only rarely has only one single functional purpose (Iwata, Dorsey, Slifer, Bauman, & Richman, 1982), which makes extinction even less feasible. However, even if self-stimulation were identified as a main reinforcer, sensory extinction hardly would be the most preferred treatment option. There are other more feasible procedures available. For instance, Repp, Felce, and Barton (1988) successfully used an active training procedure to engage subjects in sensorially stimulating activities to avoid understimulation. Finally, blindfolding a person for a long period of time would be considered restrictive and counterproductive from a developmental point of view. In summary, visual sensory sxtinction appears to be more useful for the functional analysis of SIB than for intervention.

## Conclusions

Contingent visual-occlusion procedures have been shown to be generally very effective response-decelerating procedures. Response suppression usually sets in quickly, and it is not uncommon to see the response rate drop to levels 50% or lower as compared to baseline in the very first treatment session. From there on, response rate reduction takes place in a gradual fashion, usually reaching near-zero levels within 10 treatment

TABLE 8.2. Standarized breakdown of relevant characteristics of research studies involving visual sensory extinction procedures [1974–1989].

| Authors | Subjects | Topography | Setting | Treatment | Design | Interobserver agreement | Generalization | Follow-up | Results |
|---|---|---|---|---|---|---|---|---|---|
| Rincover (1978) | 7-yr.-old mute, psychotic and autistic girl (IQ untestable)<br><br>10-yr.-old psychotic and autistic boy (IQ untestable)<br><br>14-yr.-old psychotic profoundly retarded boy | Stereotypic behavior (twirling objects, finger flapping) | Experimental classroom | Sensory extinction with blindfold (handkerchief placed over eyes) vs. Sensory extinction (mask auditory or proprioceptive feedback) | Multiple treatments across subjects with treatment withdrawal | 2 observers, 73–100% agreement on 18 sessions | None | Posttreatment observations as long as 37 wks. after analysis | Noncontingent blindfolding did not reduce stereotypic behaviors in any of the three subjects |
| Rincover, Cook, Peoples, & Packard (1979) | 8- & 9-yr.-old autistic boys 8- & 9-yr.-old autistic girls | Stereotypic behavior (echolalia, flapping hands, twirling objects) | Laboratory & classroom | Sensory extinction with handkerchief blindfold or turning out lights vs. Sensory extinction (mask auditory & proprioceptive feedback) | A-B-A-B & multiple baseline across subjects | 2 observers, 71–100% agreement for all behaviors on 27 occasions | Response generalization informally observed | Posttreatment observation at least twice between 1 & 13 mos. | Noncontingent removal of visual consequences reduced self-stimulatory behavior in two subjects |

sessions. However, persistent and total elimination of the target behaviors was not consistently achieved. Contingent visual occlusion also fared well when compared to other aversive behavioral procedures, such as overcorrection and water-mist punishment.

Although it is important to judge behavioral treatment procedures according to their efficacy, variables related to their social validity also must be considered (Kazdin, 1977; Kazdin & Matson, 1981). Wolf (1978) suggested that *acceptability* may be a particularly important form of social validity. It refers to judgments by nonprofessional people, laypersons, and clients as to whether a treatment is appropriate, fair, reasonable or overly intrusive for a given problem (Kazdin, 1980). There have been two acceptability studies that dealt specifically with treatment procedures for SIB (Pickering & Morgan, 1985; Tarnowski, Rasnake, Mulick, & Kelly, 1989), but, unfortunately, none of them explicitly investigated contingent visual occlusion, nor did any of the other acceptability studies, for that matter. The essential finding of those acceptability studies was that response-accelerating techniques were rated as being more acceptable than response-decelerating procedures. However, it also was found that these ratings were not independent of the severity of the behavior; decelerating interventions (overcorrection, contingent restraint) became more acceptable with greater severity of SIB (Tarnowski et al., 1989). The information that has been gathered and reported in the treatment studies reviewed in this chapter indicated that contingent visual occlusion procedures generally seem to be well received by therapists, parents, and teachers who had been exposed to successful implementations.

One of the most appealing aspects of visual occlusion techniques is that they are *simple* to implement and can be easily adopted by teachers and parents in a variety of settings. They are also versatile regarding client characteristics. Studies have shown that visual screening can be successfully implemented with young children, adolescents, or adults. The majority of the clients were in the lower ranges of mental retardation. These are important prerequisites for a successful transfer of a treatment program to the natural setting. A cautionary note, which is based on the authors' clinical experience rather than the reviewed literature, is warranted, however. Therapists would be well advised to carefully consider whether visual screening is advisable with physically strong, combative clients, who might strongly resist screening and thereby force the therapist into undesirable struggles.

A frequently voiced concern with punishment procedures is that they cause negative side effects (e.g., LaVigna, 1987). With regard to contingent visual occlusion, this has not been a major concern. In fact, one of the more noteworthy conclusions of this review was that contingent visual occlusion showed positive collateral effects on several occasions. Positive side effects appeared as a concurrent increase in appropriate behavior rates (e.g., McGonigle, 1986) and as a decline of untreated maladaptive behaviors (Singh & Winton, 1984; Zegiob et al., 1978). Of course, it can not be ruled out that in some clients, new problem behaviors may appear or that old ones may become worse. A case in point was the escape behavior displayed by two of the four clients in the investigation by McGonigle (1986), who initially resisted the implementation of visual screening. However, if one can afford to treat these newly emerging problem behaviors by extinction, they are likely to vanish soon.

Also, there was some evidence in the literature that contingent visual occlusion can lose its efficacy to suppress a target behavior (Dixon et al., 1989). This in itself would be a trivial finding if it were not for the symptomatic circumstance that the visual-occlusion program ceased to be effective in a community program after the client had been released from a treatment facility. However, problems of maintenance and stimulus generalization are not germane to contingent visual occlusion but are a common issue among all behavior programs.

As in all other areas of behavioral research, one has to wonder to what extent these conclusions about contingent visual occlusion might be distorted by the selective control exerted by editorial boards of scientific journals that allow primarily positive results to appear in print. In this case, however, we hasten to add that our own clinical experience with contingent visual-occlusion techniques has been very similar to the positive conclusions drawn on the basis of the literature review.

Overall, if the limited number of studies hold their promise, contingent visual-occlusion techniques—and visual screening in particular—can be regarded as effective, user-friendly, mild punishment procedures for SIB and other challenging behaviors in persons with mental retardation. Much more research should be done, however, to corroborate and extend the existing body of evidence.

Visual sensory extinction, on the other hand, does not seem to be particularly practical and feasible as a treatment technique that deserves to be broadly recommended. Its main contribution probably has been in the area of experimental and functional analysis of problem behaviors.

*Acknowledgments.* Preparation of this chapter was supported by grants from the United States Office of Human Development Services Grant 07 DD 0270/16) and the Maternal and Child Health Service (Training Project 922) awarded to the Nisonger Center for Mental Retardation and Developmental Disabilities, The Ohio State University.

## *References*

Apsche, J., Bacevich, R., Axelrod, S., & Keach, S. (1978, April). *Use of an Eyescreen (Blindfold) as a Timeout Procedure*. Paper presented at the 11th annual Gatlinburg Conference on Mental Retardation, Gatlinburg, TN.

Barmann, B. C., & Murray, W. J. (1981). Suppression of inappropriate sexual behavior by facial screening. *Behavior Therapy*, *12*, 730–735.
Barmann, B. C., & Vitali, D. L. (1982). Facial screening to eliminate trichotillomania in developmentally disabled persons. *Behavior Therapy*, *13*, 735–724.
Barrett, R. P., Matson, J. L., Shapiro, E. S., & Ollendick, T. H. (1981). A comparison of punishment and DRO procedures for treating stereotypic behavior of mentally retarded children. *Applied Research in Mental Retardation*, *2*, 247–256.
Barrett, R. P., Staub, R. W., & Sisson, L. A. (1983). Treatment of compulsive rituals with visual screening: A case study with long-term follow-up. *Journal of Behaviour Therapy and Experimental Psychiatry*, *14*, 55–59.
Birnbrauer, J. S. (1968). Generalization of punishment effects—A case study. *Journal of Applied Behavior Analysis*, *1*, 201–211.
Borreson, P. M. (1980). The elimination of a self-injurious avoidance response through a forced running consequence. *Mental Retardation*, *18*, 73–77.
Carr, E., & Durand, V. M. (1985). Reducing behavioral problems through functional communication training. *Journal of Applied Behavior Analysis*, *18*, 111–126.
Corte, H. E., Wolf, M. M., & Locke, B. J. (1971). A comparison of procedures for eliminating self-injurious behavior of retarded adolescents. *Journal of Applied Behavior Analysis*, *4*, 201–213.
Demetral, G. D., & Lutzker, J. R. (1980). The parameters of facial screening in treating self-injurious behavior. *Behavior Research in Severe Developmental Disabilities*, *1*, 261–277.
Dick, D. M., & Jackson, H. J. (1983). The reduction of stereotypic screaming in a severely retarded boy through a visual screening procedure. *Journal of Behaviour Therapy and Experimental Psychiatry*, *14*, 363–367.
Dixon, J. M., Helsel, W. J., Rojahn, J., Cipollone, R., & Lubetzky, M. J. (1989). Aversive conditioning of visual screening with aromatic ammonia for treating aggressive and disruptive behavior in a developmentally disabled child. *Behavior Modification*, *13*, 91–107.
Dorsey, M. F., Iwata, B. A., Ong, P., & McSween, T. E. (1980). Treatment of self-injurious behavior using water mist: Initial response suppression and generalization. *Journal of Applied Behavior Analysis*, *13*, 343–354.
Favell, J. E., McGimsey, J. F., & Jones, M. L. (1978). The use of physical restraint in the treatment of self-injury and as positive reinforcement. *Journal of Applied Behavior Analysis*, *11*, 225–241.
Giles, D. K., & Wolf, M. M. (1966). Toilet training institutionalized, severe retardates: An application of operant behavior modification techniques. *American Journal of Mental Deficiency*, *70*, 766–780.
Gross, A. M., Farrar, M. J., & Liner, D. (1982). Reduction of trichotillomania in a retarded cerebral palsied child using overcorrection, facial screening, and differential reinforcement of other behavior. *Education and Treatment of Children*, *5*, 133–140.
Horton, S. V. (1987a). Reduction of disruptive behavior by facial screening. *Behavior Modification*, *11*, 53–64.
Horton, S. V. (1987b). Reduction of maladaptive mouthing behavior by facial screening. *Journal of Behavior Therapy and Experimental Psychiatry*, *18*, 185–190.

Iwata, B. A., Dorsey, M. F., Slifer, K. J., Bauman, K. E., & Richman, C. S. (1982). Toward a functional analysis of self-injury. *Analysis and Intervention in Developmental Disabilities*, *2*, 3–21.

Jordan, J., Singh, N. N., & Repp, A. C. (1989). An evaluation of gentle teaching and visual screening in the reduction of stereotypy. *Journal of Applied Behavior Analysis*, *22*, 9–22.

Kazdin, A. E. (1977). Assessing the clinical or applied importance of behavior change through social validation. *Behavior Modification*, *1*, 427–452.

Kazdin, A. E. (1980). Acceptability of time out from reinforcement procedures for disruptive child behavior. *Behavior Therapy*, *11*, 329–344.

Kazdin, A. E., & Matson, J. L. (1981). Social validation in mental retardation. *Applied Research in Mental Retardation*, *2*, 39–53.

Koegel, R. L., Firestone, P. B., Kramme, K., W., & Dunlap, G. (1974). Increasing spontaneous play by suppressing self-stimulation in autistic children. *Journal of Applied Behavior Analysis*, *7*, 521–528.

LaVigna, G. W. (1987, May 25–28). *The case against aversive stimuli: A review of the clinical and empirical evidence*. Invited paper presented at the 13th annual convention of the Association for Behavior Analysis, Nashville, TN.

Lovaas, O. I., Newsome, C., & Hickman, C. (1987). Self-stimulatory behavior and perceptual reinforcement. *Journal of Applied Behavior Analysis*, *20*, 45–68.

Lovaas, O. I., & Simmons, J. Q. (1969). Manipulation of self-destruction in three retarded children. *Journal of Applied Behavior Analysis*, *2*, 143–157.

Lutzker, J. R. (1978). Reducing self-injurious behavior by facial screening. *American Journal of Mental Deficiency*, *82*, 510–513.

Lutzker, J. R., & Spencer, T. (1974, September). *Punishment of self-injurious behavior in retardates by brief application of a harmless face cover*. Paper presented at the meeting of the American Psychological Association, New Orleans.

Lutzker, J. R., & Wesch, D. (1983). Facial screening: History and critical review. *Australia and New Zealand Journal of Developmental Disabilities*, *9*, 209–223.

Matson, J. L., & DiLorenzo, T. M. (1984). *Punishment and its alternatives*. New York: Springer-Verlag.

McGee, J. J. (1986). *Gentle approach: A four part video series on gentle teaching*. Omaha, NE: Media Resource Center, Meyer Children's Rehabilitation Institute.

McGonigle, J. J. (1986). *An experimental comparison of visual screening and differential reinforcement of other behaviors on the reduction of stereotyped acts in preschool handicapped children*. Unpublished doctoral dissertation, University of Pittsburgh (University Microfilms No. 87–01, 975).

McGonigle, J. J., Duncan, D., Cordisco, L., & Barrett, R. P. (1982). Visual screening: An alternative method for reducing stereotypic behavior. *Journal of Applied Behavior Analysis*, *15*, 461–467.

McGonigle, J. J., Rojahn, J., Dixon, J., & Strain, P. S. (1987). Multiple treatment interference in the alternating treatment design as a function of the intercomponent interval length. *Journal of Applied Behavior Analysis*, *20*, 171–178.

Menolascino, F. J., & McGee, J. J. (1983). Persons with severe mental retardation and behavioral challenges: From disconnectedness to human engagement. *Journal of Psychiatric Treatment and Evaluation*, *5*, 187–193.

Murray, M. E., Keele, D. K., & McCarver, J. W. (1977). Treatment of ruminations with behavioral techniques: A case report. *Behavior Therapy*, *8*, 999–1003.

Pickering, D., & Morgan, S. B. (1985). Parental ratings of treatments of self-injurious behavior. *Journal of Autism and Developmental Disorders*, *15*, 303–314.

Repp, A. C., Felce, D., & Barton, L. E. (1988). Basing the treatment of stereotypic and self-injurious behaviors on hypotheses of their causes. *Journal of Applied Behavior Analysis*, *21*, 281–289.

Rincover, A., (1978). Sensory extinction: A procedure for eliminating self-stimulatory behavior in developmentally disabled children. *Journal of Abnormal Child Psychology*, *6*, 299–310.

Rincover, A. Cook, R., Peoples, A., & Packard, D. (1979). Sensory extinction and sensory reinforcement principles for programming multiple adaptive behavior change. *Journal of Applied Behavior Analysis*, *12*, 212–233.

Rincover, A., & Devany, J. (1982). The application of sensory extinction procedures to self-injury. *Analysis and Intervention in Developmental Disabilities*, *2*, 67–81.

Sajwaj, T., Libet, J., & Agras, S. (1974). Lemon juice therapy: The control of life-threatening rumination in a six-month old infant. *Journal of Applied Behavior Analysis*, *7*, 557–563.

Singh, N. N. (1980). The effects of facial screening on infant self-injury. *Journal of Behavior Therapy and Experimental Psychiatry*, *11*, 131–134.

Singh, N. N. (1981). Current trends in the treatment of self-injurious behavior. In L. A. Barness (Ed.), *Advances in pediatrics* (Vol. 28, pp. 377–440). Chicago: Year Book Publishers.

Singh, N. N., Beale, I. L., & Dawson, M. J. (1981). Duration of screening and suppression of self-injurious behavior: Analysis using an alternating treatments design. *Behavioral Assessment*, *3*, 411–420.

Singh, N. N., Watson, J. E., & Winton, A. S. W. (1986). Treating self-injury: Water mist spray versus facial screening or forced arm exercise. *Journal of Applied Behavior Analysis*, *19*, 403–410.

Singh, N. N., & Winton, A. S. W. (1984). Effects of a screening procedure on pica and collateral behavior. *Behavior Therapy and Experimental Psychiatry*, *15*, 59–65.

Singh, N. N., Winton, A. S. W., & Dawson, M. J. (1982). Suppression of antisocial behavior by facial screening using multiple baseline and alternating treatments designs. *Behavior Therapy*, *13*, 511–520.

St. Lawrence, J. S., & Drabman, R. S. (1984). Suppression of chronic high frequency spitting in a multiply handicapped and mentally retarded adolescent. *Child and Family Behavior Therapy*, *6*, 45–55.

Tanner, B. A., & Zeiler, M. (1975). Punishment of self-injurious behavior using aromatic ammonia as the aversive stimulus. *Journal of Applied Behavior Analysis*, *8*, 53–57.

Tarnowski, K. J., Rasnake, L. K., Mulick, J. A., & Kelly, P. A. (1989). Acceptability of behavioral interventions for self-injurious behavior. *American Journal of Mental Retardation*, *93*, 575–580.

Watson, J., Singh, N. N., & Winton, A. S. W. (1986). Suppressive effects of visual and facial screening on self-injurious finger-sucking. *American Journal of Mental Deficiency*, *5*, 526–534.

Winton, A. S. W., Singh, N. N., & Dawson, M. J. (1984). Effects of facial screening and blindfold on self-injurious behavior. *Applied Research in Mental Retardation*, *5*, 29–42.

Wolf, M. M. (1978). Social validity: The case for subjective measurement or how applied behavior analysis is finding its heart. *Journal of Applied Behavior Analysis*, *11*, 203–214.

Zegiob, L., Alford, G. S., & House, A. (1978). Response suppressive and generalization effects of facial screening on multiple self-injurious behavior in a retarded boy. *Behavior Therapy*, *9*, 688.

Zegiob, L. E., Jenkins, J., Becker, J., & Bristow, A. (1976). Facial screening: Effects on appropriate behaviors. *Journal of Behavior Therapy and Experimental Psychiatry*, *7*, 355–357.

Zlomke, L., Smith, P., & Piersel, W. C. (1986). Visual blocking: Suppression of excessive verbalizations. *Education and Training of the Mentally Retarded*, *21*, 138–143.

# 9
# Protective Equipment

JAMES K. LUISELLI

Protective equipment has been utilized for many decades with developmentally disabled persons displaying self-injurious behavior (SIB). Unfortunately, the application of protective devices in such cases often times has involved continuous mechanical restraint. For many individuals, the image of protective equipment is that of the self-injurer physically immobilized at the arms, wrapped in a bodyjacket, wearing a helmet, and unable to participate in meaningful habilitation activities due to restriction of movement. It is distressing that this impression lingers because it represents a very narrowly defined focus and the least therapeutic utilization of protective equipment. In fact, recent years have witnessed many advances in the *multiple* uses of protective equipment for the *therapeutic management* of SIB.

This chapter is a review of various treatment strategies that incorporate protective equipment and devices. Specific methods of intervention are explained, including the conceptual basis for each technique and procedural format. Research studies that document the clinical effectiveness of these approaches are then described and evaluated. Throughout the review, the rationale for selecting a particular treatment method and its respective advantages and disadvantages are addressed. Finally, recommendations for clinical application and experimental research are presented.

## Classification of Protective Equipment

Richmond, Schroeder, and Bickel (1986) describe the use of protective equipment in treating SIB as a method of *tertiary prevention*. They state that, "Tertiary methods attempt to prevent further tissue damage from SIB but do not focus on habilitating the problem" (p. 99). The types of protective equipment cited by Richmond et al. (1986) include camisoles, arm splints, and various helmets with and without face-shields. It is important to note that in discussing devices such as these, the authors actually focus on only two methods of application. First, the wearing of camisoles and arm splints represents mechanical restraint, the intent of which is to physically restrict self-injurious responding. As discussed subsequently, restraint interventions of this type have the least therapeutic value and are associated with numerous deleterious effects. The second method includes the wearing of helmets and similar headgear that do not restrain movement but rather, serve primarily as a response-prevention tactic.

Richmond et al. (1986) state further that, "Having to resort to the sole use of a device is tantamount to failing to treat the behavior" (p. 106). In effect, the implication is that the incorporation of protective equipment with a self-injurious client should be considered as an intervention of "last resort." They acknowledge, however, that certain clinical situations may arise that warrant use of protective devices. One such utilization is to protect the client from physical injury during the course of day-to-day habilitative programming. An example would be the case of an individual who engages in very severe and high-rate face-punching. Due to the intensity and frequency of this behavior, staff are required to block and redirect SIB responses continuously. This demand interferes seriously with, and may preclude totally, instructional interactions and the ability to reinforce alternative behaviors. If this client could be protected by wearing some form of equipment (e.g., padded gloves), habilitation efforts may be enhanced significantly.

Another potential application of protective equipment cited by Richmond et al. (1986) is when therapeutic effects from a treatment program either are not immediate or lasting. In such a context, the equipment would protect the client during the gradual extinction of self-injurious responding or would provide ongoing protection from SIB that is greatly reduced but not eliminated. An additional possible role for protective devices cited by the authors is when resources are not available to maintain a systematic treatment program "around the clock." Some self-injurious clients, for example, may be exposed to a carefully implemented intervention plan during portions of the day but due to staffing shortages and other practical exigencies, that plan cannot be instituted consistently at other times. In order to ensure the client's well-being during "out of program" time, protective equipment could be considered. Finally, when there is an absence of skilled clinicians, administrative support, and therapy personnel, protective devices may be the only readily available strategy to ensure a client's safety.

In a rejoinder to Richmond et al. (1986), Griffin, Ricketts, and Williams (1986) contend that the assumption that mechanical restraint and protective devices represent "last resort" measures for managing SIB should be examined more closely. They cite incidence data from a survey of 13 state schools for mentally retarded persons in Texas, indicating that 27.2% of 1352 self-injurious clients were restrained at least once during a specified 12-month period. For 120 clients identified as being the most self-injurious, mechanical restraint has been used at least once during a 12-month period for 52% of these persons. Griffin et al. (1986) conclude that, "The data support the contention that behavioral programming often is either not effective enough or cannot be implemented with sufficient speed to completely disallow the use of restraints while maintaining acceptable levels of physical safety for the clients" (p. 111). Therefore, protective devices and restraint methods should not be viewed as tertiary prevention but rather, "as techniques that can and should be used for the benefit of the clients" (p. 113). Once again, this discussion seems to define protective equipment synonymously with mechanical restraint. To reiterate, restraint is but one modality that incorporates protective equipment and devices.

Table 9.1 presents different methods for treating SIB with protective equipment. These techniques can be distinguished by a particular topography (i.e., how the equipment is worn and/or applied) and specific therapeutic intent. For certain methods, the actual topography may be similar, although the intended purpose and conceptual foundation may be quite different. Thus, both response-prevention and sensory-extinction procedures entail the noncontingent wearing of devices, although different sources of control are assumed with each intervention. In the following section, each method and its respective research findings are reviewed.

## Review of Clinical and Experimental Research

### *Mechanical Restraint*

Earlier, it was stated that restriction of movement through mechanical restraint devices represents the poorest therapeutic application of protective equipment. The primary disadvantage in this regard is that simply restraining the client does not take into account those medical, interpersonal, and environmental variables that are maintaining the SIB. Having a client wear a restrictive device may prevent tissue damage, but because the intervention is not based upon a careful behavioral analysis, self-injury will be unaffected once the equipment in removed. Therefore, other than ensuring immediate safety for the client, continuous restraint cannot be regarded as therapeutic on a long-term basis.

There are numerous detrimental effects that can occur as a result of chronic mechanical restraint. Because movement is restricted, range of motion is reduced and at times impeded totally. This, in turn, can produce problems such as muscle atrophy, shortening of tendons, and bone demineralization. Also, the client's participation in essential instructional activities is usually compromised. Because most self-injurious

TABLE 9.1. Treatment methods utilizing protective equipment.

| Method | Description/therapeutic intent |
|---|---|
| Mechanical restraint | Physically impedes SIB through complete restriction of movement |
| Mechanical restraint with Restraint Fading | Physically impedes SIB with attempts to eliminate gradually the protective equipment |
| Response interruption | Physically blocks SIB but only restricts SIB movement |
| Response prevention | Allows SIB to occur but prevents physical damage |
| Adapted clothing | Allows occurrence of "acceptable" topographies of self-restraint |
| Sensory extinction | Removes, blocks, or masks purported sensory reinforcing effects from SIB |
| Contingent application | Protective equipment is applied for specified duration, contingent upon SIB (equipment may interrupt or prevent SIB) |

persons who receive mechanical restraint are afflicted with severely handicapping conditions (e.g., severe-to-profound mental retardation), training methodologies for those persons typically include some form of physical prompting, graduated guidance, and similar "hand-over-hand" procedures. These methods, of course, cannot be implemented if the client is unable to move freely because hands, arms, and body are immobilized.

Clients who are maintained in mechanical restraint may also receive little social stimulation and constructive interactions from significant others. For many persons with chronic SIB, the decision to institute mechanical restraint is tantamount to an existence of social isolation. This is so because once a client is protected physically via restraint, the tendency for staff is to leave that person alone. As already mentioned, because continuous restraint prohibits training efforts, there is even a greater reluctance by staff to initiate interactions. Add to this the fact that most self-injurers who become candidates for protective restraint reside in large, extended-care facilities where staff-to-client ratios are poor and the frequency of naturally occurring social interactions is minimal. Therefore, the client in restraint can be easily forgotten or, in fact, actively avoided. As reviewed in a later section, some empirical evidence exists showing the potential interrelationships that can develop between the wearing of protective equipment and the social behavior of client and staff (Mace & Knight, 1986; Rojahn, Schroeder, & Mulick, 1980).

The choice to place a self-injurer in protective equipment, whether to establish mechanical restraint or to perform any of the other functions listed in Table 9.1, also must be considered with regard to self-restraining behavior. As discussed in Chapter 6 of this volume, self-restraint refers to the purposeful restriction of movement displayed by some persons with SIB. For these individuals, contingent physical restraint and other forms of immobilization serve as functional reinforcement (Favell, McGimsey, & Jones, 1978; Favell, McGimsey, Jones, & Cannon, 1981). If self-restraint is displayed by a client, then the application of protective equipment to prohibit movement simply perpetuates the problem. When the equipment is removed, these clients engage in high-rate and severe SIB while actively seeking to have it reapplied. Most clinicians who have been confronted by a self-injurious client with self-restraining behavior and a chronic history of mechanical restraint are aware of the extreme difficulties when attempting to eliminate the protective devices. To illustrate, the well-known case of "Harry" reported by Foxx and Dufrense (1984) represents an innovative clinical program in which access to restraint was actually programmed as reinforcement for increasingly longer durations of time spent out of protective equipment in a self-injurious man who had been restrained continuously prior to intervention.

The deleterious features of mechanical restraint also are highlighted by litigation that emanated in the early-to-mid-1970s (see White & Morse, 1988). Some court decisions ruled that certain types of restraint (camisoles, enclosed cribs, binding of extremities) and excessive and improper use violates a client's Eighth Amendment rights of freedom from cruel and unusual punishment (*Pena. v. New York State Division for Youth*, 1976; *Welsch v. Likins*, 1974). Other decisions allowed restraint for the purpose of stopping self-inflicted injury but only after less-intrusive methods were proposed and/or evaluated (*Wyatt v. Stickney*, 1972). Additional guidelines stemming from these and other rulings require application of restraint only following a physician's order, systematic monitoring by qualified staff, maximum duration of application, adherence to prewritten procedures, and ongoing review by an independent treatment team. It is noteworthy, of course, that the adoption of mechanical restraint is still encountered with regularity in institutions despite these court-mandated regulations and notable improvements in overall habilitative care.

## *Mechanical Restraint and Restraint Fading*

The preceding discussion focused on the many problems associated with continuous mechanical restraint. Given the protracted periods of time many clients spend in restraint, it is usually impossible to remove their equipment abruptly without experiencing an extensive course of high-frequency, intense, and, at times, near-continuous SIB. The possible occurrence of severe physical abuse as a result of such injury demands alternative methods to either reduce the amount of time in restraint or eliminate it completely.

*Restraint fading* is a method of intervention that is based upon a *transfer-of-stimulus-control* paradigm. The purpose of this approach is to maintain mechanical restraint so that the client's SIB remains under control and then to gradually reduce (fade out) the restrictive properties of the equipment. During the fading process, positive reinforcement is delivered for relevant alternative behaviors and/or the absence of self-injury. The eventual goal of restraint fading is to alter the function, size, and appearance of the physical equipment without obtaining concomitant increases in SIB. If fading is successful, the client ends up wearing some stimulus that no longer restricts movement but continues to exert control over self-injurious responding. In effect, the inhibiting function of the original mechanical restraint equipment is transferred to the nonrestrictive stimulus.

Ball, Campbell and Barkemeyer (1980) reported on the use of inflatable air-splints in a restraint fading program with a 22-year-old, profoundly retarded woman. Her SIB consisted of chronic finger-sucking, the effects of which had produced salivary dermatitis and skin infections. The air-splints were constructed of thick, transparent plastic and were inflated through rubber tubing attached to a sphygmomanometer inflation bulb. When deflated, they measured 37.5 × 17 cm. To prevent removal, a string was tied to each splint and connected across the upper back. The maximum inflation was set at 60 mm/Hg pressure on flexion; with arms extended, the pressure ranged from 0 to 20 mm/Hg. Restraint was induced by having the client wear the splints at maximum pressure. Over time, the pressure was reduced in 10 mm/Hg decrements. In comparison to baseline phases in which the splints were not worn, the results demonstrated that control over SIB was established up to a reduction to 50 mm/Hg. Beyond this point, finger-sucking increased toward baseline levels. Thus, fading was only marginally successful with this client.

In a second phase of evaluation, Ball et al. (1980) combined pressure fading with a DRO procedure (differential reinforcement of other behavior). A mercury sensor switch that responded to changes in orientation was attached to the client's shirt cuffs. As long as she did not raise her wrists above her elbows, the circuit of the switch remained closed. The absence of these behaviors every 15 seconds produced an audible tone (buzzer) which, in turn, signalled the experimenter to deliver social praise and a small amount of ice cream. With the DRO procedure in effect, it was possible to refuce the air-splint pressure on flexion to zero. Although limited to only one person, these results suggest that restraint fading may progress more successfully when reinforcement contingencies are applied concurrently.

Pace, Iwata, Edwards and McCosh (1986) extended the restraint fading approach to two self-injurious adolescents who also engaged in self-restraint behavior. One client was an 18-year-old, profoundly retarded male who had been institutionalized since he was 3 years of age. His SIB included biting of the hand, biceps, and shoulder, plus scratching of hands and legs. Previous treatments consisted of medication, differential reinforcement, extinction, and various forms of protective equipment, such as wrist restraint, a neck collar, and a football helmet with a plastic face-guard. At the time of the study, he wore rigid arm tubes, 47 cm in length, that extended from his shoulders to his hands. These devices restrained his movement and the possibility of self-biting. He self-restrained "24 hours a day" by grasping the bottom portion of each tube with his hands.

The study was performed within a specialized hospital program. During baseline phases of a multiple baseline across settings design, the client remained in restraint and was provided with praise and physical contact upon engagement with toys. Next, he was prompted to remove the restraints, and reinforcement was presented for their absence approximately every 60 seconds. Restraint fading was implemented by reducing the length of the arm tubes from 47 cm to 5 cm in a series of eight steps over 22 days. Prompts for restraint removal and contingent reinforcement remained in place up to a length of 5 cm. At this dimension, they were allowed to remain in place, were covered with fabric, and faded eventually to tennis wristbands. During baseline, high but variable rates of self-restraint were recorded with corresponding low levels of SIB. A 1-day baseline probe without restraint revealed 100% occurrence of self-injury. Self-restraint decreased following the introduction of prompts plus reinforcement, but SIB also increased. During restraint fading, both behaviors decreased to low levels up through and including the wearing of wristbands. Another 1-day probe, this time without the bands, resulted in 100% occurrence of SIB. The absence of restraint and low rates of SIB were maintained 2 years following discharge. During follow-up assessment, the client continued to wear the tennis wristbands, indicating that stimulus control over SIB had been established successfully with these items.

The second client treated by Pace et al. (1986) was a 15-year-old, profoundly retarded male who engaged in scratching his skin behind each ear. His topography of self-restraint included placement of hands into pockets, under thighs, and behind neck. When the study began, he was restrained in elbow splints that prevented arm flexion. Baseline sessions were conducted while the client remained out of the splints, and adult praise and touch were contingent upon contact with toys. The findings were that during baseline, self-restraint was continuous and SIB rarely occurred. Under treatment conditions, inflatable air-splints similar to those described by Ball et al. (1980) were worn. Pressure was set initially at 30 mm/Hg, which prevented arm flexion. Self-restraint was eliminated immediately, and toy play increased during the course of air-splint fading. Fading was accomplished by reducing the pressure in 5 mm/Hg decrements, from 30 to 0 mm/Hg, over a period of 63 days. During fading, a 1-day probe was scheduled in which the air-splints were removed. The 1-day probe without the splints resulted in a 100% occurrence of self-restraint. Also, continuous self-restraint was encountered as soon as the air pressure in the splints was reduced to 0 mm/Hg. Pressure was subsequently inflated and faded to less than 1 mm/Hg to maintain an absence of both self-restraint and SIB.

Programs that incorporate restraint fading procedures offer a distinct advantage over continuous mechanical restraint because they include a deliberate attempt to withdraw and ultimately eliminate the wearing of protective equipment. The research to date indicates that in some cases, equipment can be faded totally, with controlling effects transferred to an essentially inconspicuous stimulus (Pace et al., 1986, Study 1). Other studies demonstrate that fading may only be partially completed (Ball et al., 1980; Pace et al., 1986, Study 2). However, even incomplete fading can be considered a therapeutic success when dealing with a client who has been restrained on a continuous basis. For example, splint pressure reduced to a near-zero reading would still permit full range of motion of arms and enable the client to benefit from active therapeutic programming.

How to conduct restraint fading depends largely on the physical characteristics of the protective devices. Equipment such as arm tubes, elbow restraints, and the like lend themselves to a gradual reduction in length, width, and/or thickness. In a study described in a subsequent section of this chapter, Luiselli (1991a) faded the large padded mittens worn by a self-injurious woman along a sequence of (a) leather batter's gloves, (b) thin latex gloves, (c) latex gloves with two fingers removed, (d) latex gloves with all five fingers removed, and (e) no gloves. Pace et al. (1986) suggest that, "when choosing protective equipment for a self-injurious client, one should consider a restraint that may be systematically eliminated" (p. 387). Recall that in their research, air-splints were used with one clinet who self-restrained by putting hands in pockets, under thighs, and behind the back. The splints were choosen because they provided a more "acceptable" topography of restraint that could then be faded very systematically overtime. Therefore, in cases where low rates of SIB are correlated with high levels of self-restraint, the induction of restraint via devices that can be gradually reduced or eliminated represents a potentially efficacious therapeutic strategy.

## *Response Interruption*

Like mechanical restraint, a response interruption approach to SIB requires the noncontingent wearing of protective equipment. However, the devices employed in response interruption do not restrict a client's range of movement. Instead, movement is possible *up to* the actual self-injurious response. At this point, the equipment blocks or interrupts completion of the response and possible physical damage.

Rojahn, Schroeder, and Mulick (1980) evaluated the therapeutic effects from self-protective equipment with three profoundly retarded adults. An interesting feature of this research was the assessment of collateral social and adaptive behaviors while clients were in and out of the equipment. For two of these clients, a fencing mask was worn to stop behaviors such as pica, object insertion into the nose, and coprophagy. The third client was placed in a camisole to immobilize arm movements and as such, this method does not qualify as response interruption, as defined. With masks in place, the target behaviors were virtually eliminated in both clients. However, side effects included a decrease in social interaction between clients and staff, reduced positive instructions, and for one client, a decrement in work and play behaviors. To reiterate a point made earlier in this chapter, the potential detrimental effects on socialization patterns associated with the wearing of protective devices must be carefully considered with severely handicapped persons, "whose learning development and skill acquisition depend on consistent and structured attention of supervising adults" (Rojahn et al., 1980, p. 65).

Another response interruption device applied to the management of SIB is the flexible arm-splint (flex-splint). Ball, Datta, Rios, and Constantine (1985) described two variations of the flex-splint in treatment programs with chronically self-injurious, institutionalized clients. The first device was made of two 15.5- and 9.5-cm sections of 2-mm-thick PVC (polyvinyl chloride—plastic) pipe with an 8.26 cm inside diameter. Ends of each segment were cut at an angle and joined by a hinge that was riveted in place. When closed (flexed), the two sections formed an angle of 110 degrees. Treatment with the splints was conducted with an 11-year-old, nonambulatory boy with Lesch–Nyhan disease. He displayed finger-biting and before intervention was kept in soft-tie restraints. Daily observation sessions were conducted during baseline (no splints) and treatment (flex-splint) phases of an A-B-A-B reversal design. During all sessions, an experimenter interacted with the boy and blocked his movement whenever his hands approached his mouth. The rate of SIB attempts was reduced dramatically from an average of 30.3 responses during baseline phases to an average of 2.4 responses under treatment conditions.

The second apparatus evaluated by Ball et al. (1985) consisted of metal arms that extended from an adjustable arm-hinge (Universal Polycentric Elbow Hinge, Poly-Med, Inc., 109 Industry Lane, Cockeysville, MD 21030). The arms were attached with screws to 10.5-cm long leather cuffs. In contrast to the first device, this apparatus permitted adjustment of the degree of flexion. It was evaluated with a 38-year-old profoundly retarded man who inserted fingers into his mouth. Using an A-B-A-B reversal design, daily sessions were conducted with and without the splints. Similar to the first study, the splint device produced significant suppression of the target SIB.

Because response-interruption methods permit motor responding but do not allow SIB to occur, the practitioner is able to prompt and reinforce many alternative behaviors. The flex-splints described by Ball et al. (1985), as an example, enable the client to move his or her arms and hands instead of remaining in a rigid position characteristic of mechanical restraint. These devices obviously remain in place to achieve therapeutic effects and, therefore, efforts to eventually fade and discontinue their use should be a priority.

## *Response Prevention*

Equipment utilized as a response prevention tactic allows SIB to occur but provides protection from physical injury. To illustrate, a client who engages in face-slapping with the hands might be required to wear a football helmet with a face-guard. With this equipment in place, the slapping behavior could still be performed, but the completed response would be a slap against the helmet/guard rather than the face. Although a client who displays pica behavior may also wear similar headgear, the response of placing a nonedible object into the mouth would be blocked and left uncompleted, thereby qualifying as a method of response interruption. Thus, both methods protect the self-injurer but differ with regard to how much of the self-injurious response can be completed.

Parrish, Aguerrevere, Dorsey, and Iwata (1980) evaluated the effects from a foam-padded football helmet with plastic face-shield on the SIB of a 17-year-old, profoundly retarded male. The targeted SIB included hitting of the head with hands and striking of the head against a wall, floor, or object. Daily assessment sessions lasting from 5 to 15 mimutes in duration were conducted within an inpatient hospital setting. Each day, the boy participated in two baseline and treatment sessions. Under baseline conditions, he was placed alone in a room without furniture or play materials. Treatment sessions were identical except that the participant wore the protective helmet throughout. The study was performed for 5 days and revealed an overall average of 60 self-injurious responses per minute during baseline sessions and 5 responses per minute during treatment sessions. An interesting finding was that on three days in which baseline rates of SIB were extremely high, a rapid suppression effect was achieved when the helmet was applied. On 2 days when the baseline frequencies were low, the helmet had no effect or was associated with a slight increase in SIB. Such findings suggest that the rate of responding may be influential in determining the controlling effects exerted by protective equipment, at least when employed for the purpose of response prevention.

Wurtele, King, and Drabman (1984) also incorporated self-protective devices in a clinical treatment program for severe SIB. Their client was a 13-year-old, nonambulatory boy with a diagnosis of Lesch–Nyhan syndrome. He engaged in thumb-biting and upon placement in a residential treatment facility, he presented with deep lacerations on both thumbs, infection, and finger abrasions. His parents attempted to manage biting behavior by wrapping his thumbs in gauze and elastic bandages during the day and wrapping his hands in towels in the evening. This boy also engaged in self-restraint by sitting in his wheelchair with both arms folded behind his back. Observation indicated that his self-biting increased when he was not receiving direct attention from staff, suggesting that the behavior was reinforced and maintained by contingent social responses (i.e., admonishments to stop biting). Because the staff was reluctant to ignore SIB, given the potential for physical damage, a program of social extinction was instituted, with the addition of a protective device. It consisted of a plastic, athletic mouthguard with a built-in air hole that prevented the boy from inserting his thumb into his mouth. Although the mouthguard provided necessary protection, it had to be discontinued because several biting incidents occurred when the boy learned he could move it around in his mouth and expose his teeth. In its place, a soft acrylic mouthguard was made in two separate pieces to cover the upper and lower arches. This device allowed the boy to place thumb into mouth without damage. In addition, it could not be removed like the former device, did not interfere with his expressive language, and was essentially inconspicuous in his mouth. During activities when the mouthguard had to be removed (meals), the boy wore fingerless, nylon mesh and leather bicycling gloves composed of thick padding in the thumb area. The combined use of the mouthguard and gloves provided total protection from biting and by the authors' account, eliminated SIB within the residential setting.

It was noted previously that the distinction between response prevention and response interruption methods is that with the former technique, the equipment allows the self-injurious response to be completed, while the latter technique stops the response before completion is possible. It is noteworthy that at least two studies have documented control over SIB even though the intended response prevention or response interruption function was not actually realized. Because of the detail of each study, the methodologies and results are described separately as follows.

In the first study, Mace and Knight (1986) treated the long-standing pica behavior of a 19-year-old profoundly retarded male. Before the study, a physician had prescribed the use of a helmet with face-shield to prevent placement of nonedible objects into the mouth. Of significance in this case was the fact that the equipment *did not entirely interrupt* the occurrence of pica (e.g., the client could wedge items between his face and the face-shield). Pica responses (completed and attempted) were recorded in two settings within a residential facility. During an initial baseline phase, the client wore the protective helmet, and staff delivered a mild reprimand, followed by object removal, whenever a pica response was detected.

The second phase of the study consisted of an analysis of social interaction conditions because it appeared that the client "was less likely to engage in pica during periods of interaction with staff" (p. 413). The interaction analysis was conducted using an alternating-treatments design and included three situations: (a) *frequent interaction* (near-continuous eye contact and task instructions provided by staff), (b) *limited interaction* (staff conversed with client for 15–30 seconds approximately every 3 minutes), and (c) *no interaction* (staff did not look at or converse with client).

The final phase was an analysis of helmet conditions in which the client either wore the helmet with face-shield, wore the helmet without face-shield, or did not wear the helmet. All helmet conditions were evaluated during the situation of limited interaction. The results from these analyses were that decreased rates of pica were associated with conditions of frequent and limited interaction, as compared to near-baseline rates when there was no interaction. Paradoxically, the *lowest* rates of pica were recorded when the client did not wear the helmet. Given these findings, a treatment program that combined limited social interaction with no helmet

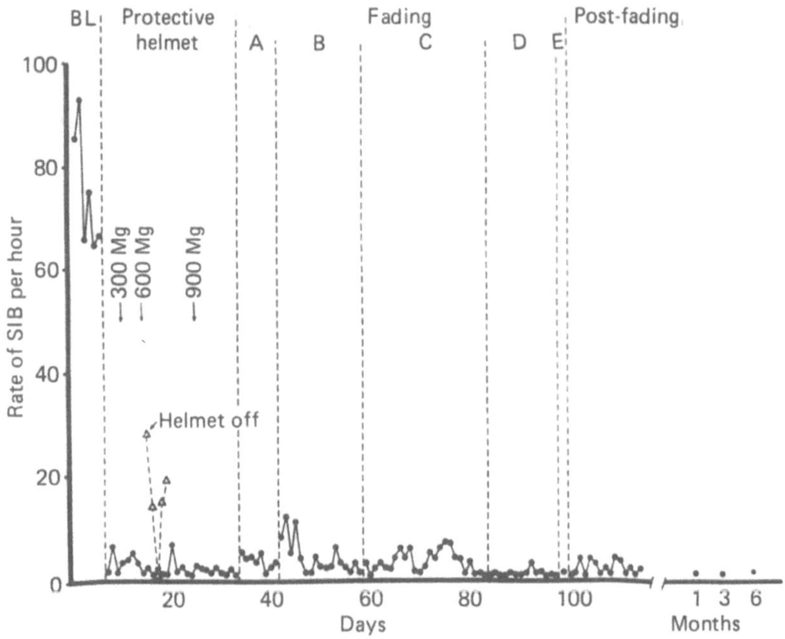


FIGURE 9.1. Rate of SIB (face-slapping) per hour displayed by a 22-year-old, deaf, visually impaired woman with moderate-to-severe mental retardation. Treatment included the noncontingent wearing of a protective helmet and gradual elimination of this device during successive fading steps (A–E). Arrows indicate introduction and dosage levels of lithium. (From Luiselli, 1991b.)

was prescribed and shown subsequently to maintain reduced rates of pica.

Mace and Knight (1986) interpreted their results by suggesting that under natural conditions, staff interaction with the client was greater when he was not wearing the helmet, in order to manitain sufficient supervision to prevent pica responses and as a result, "a consequence of closer supervision may have been that a higher proportion of pica responses resulted in punishment (i.e., reprimands)" [p. 414]. When wearing the helmet, less supervision was provided and, therefore, resulted in a lower probability of pica-contingent reprimands. According to the authors, "a plausible hypothesis appears to be that both interaction and the protective equipment may influence pica by enhancing discrimination of the consequences for the behavior" (p. 415). The very interesting results attained in this study attest to the stimulus-control functions possible when protective equipment is utilized. For this client, it appears that therapeutic control was established due to the discriminative features of the equipment in relation to different patterns of social interaction and not the intended prevention/interruption effect.

Luiselli (1991b) also employed a helmet with face-shield in a treatment program with a 22-year-old, deaf, visually impaired woman with moderate-to-severe mental retardation. Her topography of SIB was a very forceful slap to the face with the open palm of her hands. Upon referral, she presented with inflamation around her face and several open sores on her upper left cheekbone. Prior to the introduction of formalized assessment procedures, the woman was seen by two physicians in an effort to detect or rule out possible physical causes for the behavior. These diagnostic evaluations failed to reveal any such conditions.

The study was carried out in a day habilitation program within a community prevocational workshop. Rate of face-slapping was recorded 6 hours a day throughout all workshop activities. Given the severity of the problem, the client received one-to-one supervision within activities. During a baseline phase, staff used physical blocking and redirection procedures in an effort to prevent face-slapping. The initial phase of treatment consisted of having the client wear a bicycle helmet with plastic face-shield, noncontingently throughout the day. As shown in Figure 9.1, the rate of SIB decreased immediately and substantially following introduction of the helmet. Interestingly, when the client slapped her face, she did so by lifting the helmet away from her face, delivering a slap, and returning the helmet to its proper position. Therefore, the reduction in slapping occurred even though the helmet did not provide full protection.

Five days after the helmet was introduced, the client began receiving lithium as prescribed by a consulting psychiatrist. The medication was initiated at 300 mg daily and was increased to 900 mg daily over the course of the study. While still receiving the medication, the stimulus control features of the helmet were evaluated by having the client out-of-helmet for 1 randomly determined hour each day. These data revealed higher rates of SIB although they did not approach the levels recorded during the initial baseline phase. Over time, the helmet was faded gradually across the following sequence: (a) absence of face-shield, (b) absence of chin strap, (c) absence of frontal portion of helmet while client wears headband, (d) headband with stocking cap on top of head, (e) headband alone, and (f) no headband (postfading). Throughout fading, frequency of SIB remained low, with results maintained at follow-up.

The findings obtained by Luiselli (1991b) are difficult to interpret and, like those by Mace and Knight (1986), suggest that therapeutic control can be established even though the equipment does not provide protection or interruption of responding. It is noteworthy that in this study, reduced rates of SIB were achieved *before* medication was prescribed and that during the probe assessments without the helmet, SIB increased. One explanation might be that the client's SIB was escape-motivated and that when the protective equipment was in place, staff spent less time with her and made fewer demands. However, systematic observations indicated that staff did not vary their interactions or training requirments with the client across experimental phases. Another interpretation is that the blocking and physical interruption procedures operative during baseline were reinforcing. With the protective helmet, the same physical intervention was not required, and once control was acquired, it was possible to transfer effects to an alternative stimulus (headband) and ultimately, to its absence. Another possibility is that the "response cost" of lifting the helmet to perform SIB may have been sufficiently burdensome to inhibit high-rates of the behavior, with effects again maintained via fading. Finally, the medication may have helped stabilize the client's behavior following the introduction of the helmet and subsequently facilitated the progressive fading and elimination of equipment.

Because equipment utilized as a response-prevention tactic allows SIB to occur, it differs significantly from the approaches reviewed previously. Recall that mechanical restraint, restraint-fading, and response-interruption procedures are intended to restrict and impede self-injurious responding. Because SIB cannot be emitted and/or completed when such methods are employed, it is difficult to attribute therapeutic control within a strictly operant framework. With response prevention, on the other hand, the actual topography of SIB is free to occur, but the equipment ensures safety from self-inflicted abuse. Therefore, when control over responding is produced in this manner, it must be a function of changing one or more *consequence effects*. Procedurally, the equipment must somehow alter the response-contingent reinforcement for SIB such that the behavior is extinguished or greatly diminished.

One way in which protective equipment can affect the reinforcing consequences for SIB is to enable significant others to withold social attention that may be maintaining the unwanted behavior (cf. Wurtele et al., 1984). Thus, if the hand-biting of a mentally retarded child appeared to be reinforced by contingent staff attention, the witholding of attention through planned ignoring would be difficult to implement because the child could inflict substantial injury during the process of extinction. However, if the child's hands could be protected with equipment such as padded gloves, the program of social extinction could be implemented properly, knowing that the child would be fully protected. Another means by which a response-prevention procedure exerts operant control is that the equipment removes response-elicited *sensory reinforcement* of SIB. This treatment approach is classified as sensory extinction and is reviewed extensively in a later section. Third, the consequence of exhibiting SIB when wearing equipment may be aversive and in this manner may function as response-contingent punishment. As an example, striking the sides of a protective helmet with the hands may be sufficiently unpleasant and, therefore, may reduce the frequency of this form of SIB. Given the multiple sources of control possible when response prevention is implemented, it is clear that one or more of these sources may be operating when therapeutic changes are demonstrated.

## *Adaptive Clothing and Equipment to Establish "Acceptable" Self-restraint*

The section on restraint-fading methods discussed the introduction of mechanical devices (e.g., air-splints) to establish physical immobilization in clients who display self-restraint. By inducing restraint via mechanical means, the clinician establishes a condition that is associated with low frequencies of SIB. Over time, the restraint is faded gradually and either eliminated totally or transferred to an alternative stimulus. This approach then, requires that physical restraint be manipulated directly and altered slowly without sacrificing clinical control. Another treatment option is to have the self-injurer wear a piece of adapted clothing that permits a more "acceptable" topography of self-restraint. In this manner, self-restraint is always accessible to the client and is performed on his or her own initiative.

Rojahn, Mulick, McCoy and Schroeder (1978) studied two self-injurious persons who engaged in frequent self-restraining behavior. The first participant was a 30-year-old man who was blind, nonambulatory, and profoundly mentally retarded. His SIB included slapping the head with the palms of his hands, hitting his forehead/eyebrows with his knuckles, and striking the side of his head against his shoulders. These behaviors were recorded during daily assessment sessions within a specialized residential treatment program for self-injurious persons. Inappropriate self-restraint (wrapping up arms and hands in clothing, locking his arms under chair rests) and appropriate self-restraint (keeping hands in pockets) were also recorded during sessions. Treatment phases consisted of recording frequencies of SIB and self-restraint while the client was wearing various types of adaptive clothing and equipment: (a) a jacket with large side pockets, (b) a foam-rubber neckbrace, and (c) the jacket and neckbrace simultaneously. When contrasted to baseline (no equipment) phases, head-slapping and knuckles-to-head hitting decreased markedly when the participant was wearing the jacket. These topographies of SIB were not affected when only the neckbrace was worn; instead, head-to-shoulder striking was reduced with this piece of equipment in place. The most pronounced clinical effect was obtained when the participant wore both the jacket and the neckbrace. The data for self-restraint indicated that appropriate restraint was evinced at near-100% levels when the participant was dressed in the jacket and that inappropriate restraint only occurred when the jacket was not worn. Because head-striking behavior was incompatible with appropriate self-restraint, the reductions in this SIB were a direct result of allowing the client to restrain his hands freely in the jacket pockets.

The second participant studied by Rojahn et al. (1978) was a 26-year-old blind, severely retarded man. His topography of SIB was slapping of the head with hands. He had a protracted history of self-restraint that entailed wrapping up his hands in the T-shirt he was wearing. Baseline sessions were conducted, during which time the participant wore either the T-shirt or a jumpsuit that prevented inappropriate self-restraint. A treatment condition was then introduced, consisting of a 30-second immobilization time-out procedure contingent upon SIB, again while the T-shirt or jumpsuit was worn. The findings were that under baseline conditions, the rate of SIB was 52% higher with the jumpsuit, as contrasted to sessions with the T-shirt. The time-out procedure effectively reduced SIB under both clothing conditions. Self-restraint remained elevated when the T-shirt was worn but most significantly, self-injury continued to be displayed. The authors concluded that for this person, the ability to engage in self-restraining behavior was contratherapeutic because it was not correlated consistently with reduced rates of SIB and occurred so often that it interfered with instructional efforts.

Although it is appealing conceptually, the actual practice of shaping "appropriate" self-restraint in self-injurious clients who demonstrate restraining behavior is not common, nor has sufficient experimental research been conducted on this topic. The equivocal results reported by Rojahn et al. (1978) indicate that self-restraint is a complex clinical phenomenon that is not easily understood or categorized. In responding to this research, Murphy (1978) commented that the differentiation between appropriate and inappropriate self-restraint is, in itself, problematic. She states, "It is likely that when self-injury is severe and/or its rate is high, then self-restraint (such as putting hands in jacket pockets) is seen as desirable, whereas when the injury is less severe and/or its rate less high, self-restraint is seen as undesirable as it usually involves the client's hands and makes them unavailable for more positive activities" (p. 198).

This appraisal suggests that the covariation between SIB and self-restraint must be assessed empirically and must focus on the topography of self-injury, the manner(s) in which self-restraint is performed, and the impact of self-restraining behavior on skill acquisition and development. Murphy (1978) adds further that, "It must suffice to say that normally the replacement of self-injury by self-restraining behavior is not an ideal long-term solution" (p. 198), a judgment that is acknowledged by Rojahn et al. (1978). If functional self-restraint can be established, then effective restraint fading becomes a critical therapeutic goal. To date, data in support of this position have not been presented.

Protective equipment can also affect the frequency of self-restraint and corresponding SIB even though it does not allow the self-injurer to perform restraining behaviors. An interesting study in this regard was conducted by Silverman, Watanabe, Marshall, and Baer (1984), with a 13-year-old boy who was profoundly retarded and legally blind. His predominant forms of SIB were punching the eyes/chin, kicking his legs, and striking his forearm against hard objects. Two types of protective equipment were evaluated. One was a plastic helmet with clear plastic face-mask and padding on the inside. A 3-cm thickness of foam padding was also placed on the outer surface of the helmet and mask except around the eye and mouth openings. The second piece of equipment was a pair of slippers with a thick forearm pad covering each heel and extending up the back of each leg. The equipment was applied within three daily conditions, assessed randomly, within a multiple schedule design: (a) helmet only, (b) helmet and slippers, and (c) no equipment. Frequencies of arm SIB, leg SIB, arm restraint, and leg restraint were recorded per condition. The results were that when the boy wore the helmet, arm SIB and arm restraint decreased; similarly, leg SIB and leg restraint occurred less frequently when he wore the protective slippers. Following exposure to the helmet condition, a new topography of SIB emerged, consisting of hits to the body other than head and helmet and mainly directed to the legs. The authors concluded that, "Self-restraint showed the selective characteristics that it should if its function were to escape, avoid, hinder, or delay self-injurious behaviors" (p. 551). This interpretation adheres to the commonly accepted view that self-restraint is negatively reinforced by the avoidance of the pain stimulation caused by SIB. Thus, in the study by Silverman et al. (1984), the rates of self-injury and self-restraint decreased simultaneously when the body part involved in both movements (e.g., hitting with arms and restraining arms) was protected with a particular type of equipment.

Silverman et al. (1984) discussed several additional concerns related to the interrelationship between SIB and self-restraint. One is that self-injury could be a discriminative stimulus ($s^d$) for self-restraint rather than a negative reinforcer. There is also a question of whether restraint functions as a reinforcer only when SIB is possible. On a clinical level, the authors emphasize that trying to eliminate self-restraint may leave a client defenseless against SIB. It may be more efficacious, therefore, to target reductions in SIB initially, while assessing corresponding decreases in self-restraint. Also, as mentioned several times in earlier sections, some forms of self-restraint are unusual and idiosyncratic so that, "other more acceptable typographies of self-restraint should be found or developed by caretakers to diminish SIB" (Silverman et al., 1984, p. 552).

## *Sensory Extinction*

This treatment procedure is formulated on the theory that aberrant behaviors can, in some instances, be reinforced by the sensory consequences they produce. Visual, auditory, olfactory, gustatory, and proprioceptive stimulation are sources of sensory reinforcement that can maintain responding. By masking, blocking, or otherwise attenuating response-elicited stimulation, it is purported that the problem behaviors can be eliminated or diminished significantly. The initial research on sensory extinction was reported by Rincover and associates in a series of studies concerning the management of stereotypic behaviors in developmentally disabled children. Rincover (1978), for example, demonstrated that the object-spinning behavior of an autistic child could be decreased by eliminating auditory feedback, in this case, by placing carpet on a table top such that the sound from rotating the objects could not be detected. In another study (Rincover, Newsom, & Carr, 1979b), the sensory reinforcement for light-switch flicking behavior of a child was identified as the resulting photic stimulation. Control over this behavior was established by disconnecting the switch so that the lights could not be illuminated. Rincover, Cook, Peoples, and Packard (1979a) reduced finger and arm stereotypies in two children by having them wear a small vibrating pulsator on the backs of their hands to mask proprioceptive sensory feedback that was produced by finger/arm movements.

The application of sensory extinction to the treatment of SIB was reported initially by Rincover and Devany (1982). The participants were three, 4-year-old children who were multiply handicapped and severely developmentally delayed. Two of the children engaged in head-banging by striking their heads against furniture, walls, and floors. The third child exhibited scratching of the skin on her face and neck. Assessment and intervention procedures were performed within each child's classroom setting at local developmental disabilities centers. Evaluation consisted of recording frequencies of SIB during baseline (no treatment) and sensory-extinction phases. For two of the children, an A-B-A-B reversal design was instituted; for the third child, a simple A-B design was used. Sensory extinction for head-banging was introduced in two ways. One child wore a padded helmet, constructed of synthetic leather, which was strapped under his chin. During sensory-extinction treatment, he wore the helmet throughout the class day. The second method of sensory extinction was to cover the walls and floor of a specified work area with 1-inch thick, foam-filled mats. For the child displaying skin-scratching behavior, intervention consisted of having her wear thin rubber (dish-washing) gloves. All three children responded positively to the treatment programs, evincing rapid and stable reductions in SIB. A significant feature of this research was the introduction of fading procedures to eliminate gradually the protective devices for two of the children (fading with the third child could not be evaluated). The fading sequence entailed having the children remain out of the equipment for increasingly longer durations during the day, until eventually, it was no longer used. Fading was successfully completed with both children, with rates of SIB maintained at near-zero levels at 3 and 7 months posttreatment.

Dorsey, Iwata, Reid, and Davis (1982) extended the application of sensory extinction for SIB to three adolescent clients. They were 14–16 years of age, with severe-to-profound mental retardation and accompanying sensory deficits (impaired hearing and blindness). All three were treated in a state residential facility for developmentally handicapped persons. Targeted forms of self-injury were hand-hitting (striking head with hand), hand-biting (inserting hand into mouth), and eye-gouging (contact with fingers against eye or into eye socket). Prior to sensory-extinction treatment, the clients were exposed to several intervention programs following an initial baseline phase: DRI (reinforcement of toy play), DRI plus verbal reprimand, and a combination of DRI, reprimand, and contingent water mist. These procedures did not produce clinically significant reductions in self-injury. Effective decreases in SIB were established when the clients were required to wear a football helmet and foam-padded gloves continuously throughout assessment sessions. Subsequent to this phase, the equipment was applied for a 2-minute duration *contingent* upon SIB in an effort to reduce the amount of time the clients were exposed to the equipment. Low levels of responding were maintained during the phase of contingent application.

The study by Dorsey et al. (1982) included a comparison of sensory extinction with other decelerative procedures. Comparative analyses of this type are particularly useful because they provide a critical measure of clinical efficacy. Another important topic in this vein is the comparison of different methods of administering sensory extinction. It is likely, for example, that certain types of equipment may mask or block sensory feedback more efficiently than others or that some formats may be equally effective.

Thus far, only one study has examined this issue. Luiselli (1988) reported the case of a 6-year-old boy with multiple developmental disabilities who bit his wrists. Assessment and treatment procedures were implemented at a specialized day school for handicapped children. In this study, two methods of sensory extinction were compared with three

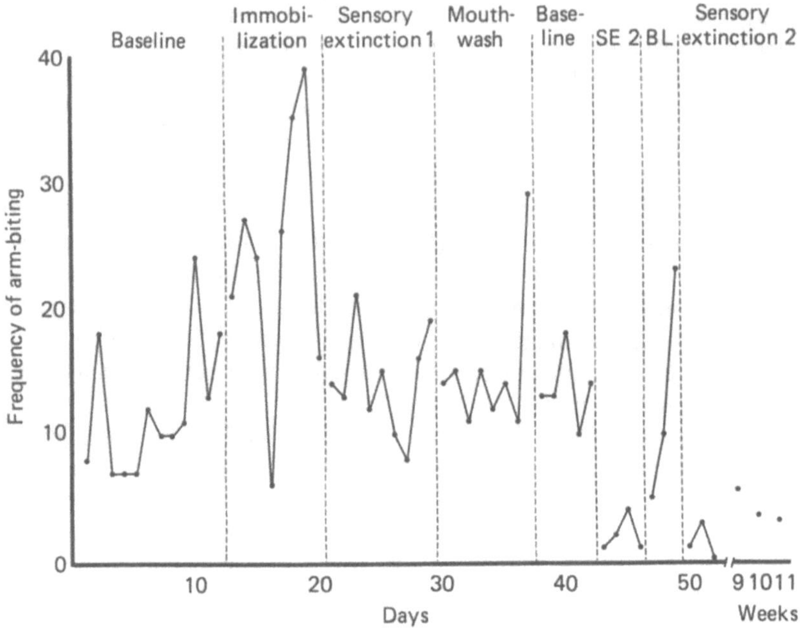


FIGURE 9.2. Frequency of SIB (arm-biting) per day displayed by a 6-year-old boy with multiple disabilities who was treated with two methods of contingency management and two forms of sensory extinction. During sensory extinction phases, he wore either tennis wristbands (sensory extinction 1) or custom-made orthoplas cuffs (sensory extinction 2). (From Luiselli, 1988, reprinted by permission of Clinical Psychology Publishing Co., Inc.).

other conditions in a reversal design: (a) *baseline* (no intervention), (b) *immobilization* (child's hands were held by sides of body for 30-second duration contingent upon bitting), and (c) *mouthwash* (child received 1-second application of diluted mouthwash to lips, contingent upon biting). The first sensory extinction procedure (sensory extinction 1) required the child to wear tennis wristbands on each arm, positioned over the area where biting was directed. The bands were worn continuously throughout the day.

With the second procedure (sensory extinction 2), the child was fitted with pliable plastic cuffs, similar to the wristbands, that were placed over the bitten areas on each arm. The cuffs were composed of pliable plastic ("orthoplas"), measured approximately $\frac{1}{4}$-inch in thickness, and were molded to fit snuggly on the arms without pinching or irritating the skin. Figure 9.2 shows that frequency of arm-biting did not decrease until the orthoplas cuffs were worn during the sensory extinction 2 phases. As with other sensory extinction studies reviewed previously, response reduction was immediate. Slight increases in arm-biting were recorded at 9- to 11-

week follow-up assessments, but these rates were still very low and manageable, as compared to prior experimental phases.

Recall that in the study by Rincover and Devany (1982), treatment fading was accomplished by having children spend increasingly longer durations out of the equipment. Another approach toward fading, and one described with other treatment methods, is to change gradually the physical characteristics of the protective devices. A recent analysis of equipment fading within the context of sensory extinction treatment of SIB was performed by Luiselli (1991a). The participant was an 18-year-old female who was severely mentally retarded, nonambulatory, nonverbal, and afflicted with cerebral palsy. She resided in a pediatric nursing-care facility, where she demonstrated a protracted history of SIB, characterized by pressing her fingers forcefully against her eyes and inserting her fingers into her eye orbits. To physically prevent this behavior, she was maintained in bilateral elbow splints that extended from the upper arm to midforearm. At the time of referral, she had been wearing the splints almost continuously for the preceding $1\frac{1}{2}$ years.

Eye-pressing behavior was recorded during three 1-hour segments from 9:00 A.M. to 12:00 P.M. each weekday. During Phase 1 of the study, the splints were removed for the entire 3-hour period. For two of the 1-hour segments, she wore large padded mittens on each hand; during the third 1-hour segment, mittens were not applied. The order of segments was determined randomly at the start of each day. As a consequence for SIB, the attending staff person stated, "Hands down," and physically directed the participant's hand away from her eyes. This interruption strategy was implemented during all phases of the study, to reduce exposure to physical harm and to ensure that responses were of a uniform duration. The results, depicted in Figure 9.3, were that substantially higher rates of SIB were recorded when the protective mittens were not worn. This outcome suggested that eye-pressing behavior was reinforced by sensory consequences and that the mittens were associated with lower rates of SIB because they altered response-elicited stimulation.

During subsequent phases, equipment fading was introduced, first by having the participant wear leather batting gloves and then by having her wear thin latex gloves. Self-injurious responding continued to decrease throughout the fading process but increased when the gloves were not applied during a 4-day multielement analysis similar to Phase 1 (see Figure 9.3). The final course of fading entailed the gradual cutting back of the latex gloves along five fading steps: (1) bottom of glove pulled up to back of palm, (2) bottom of glove aligned with base of thumb, (3) third, fourth, and fifth fingers of glove cut off, (4) thumb and index finger of glove cut off, and (5) remaining portion of glove removed (postfading). Self-injurious eye-pressing decreased steadily up to the final fading step. At that point, higher rates were recorded and necessitated a return to the previous fading step. Subsequently, it proved possible to eliminate the

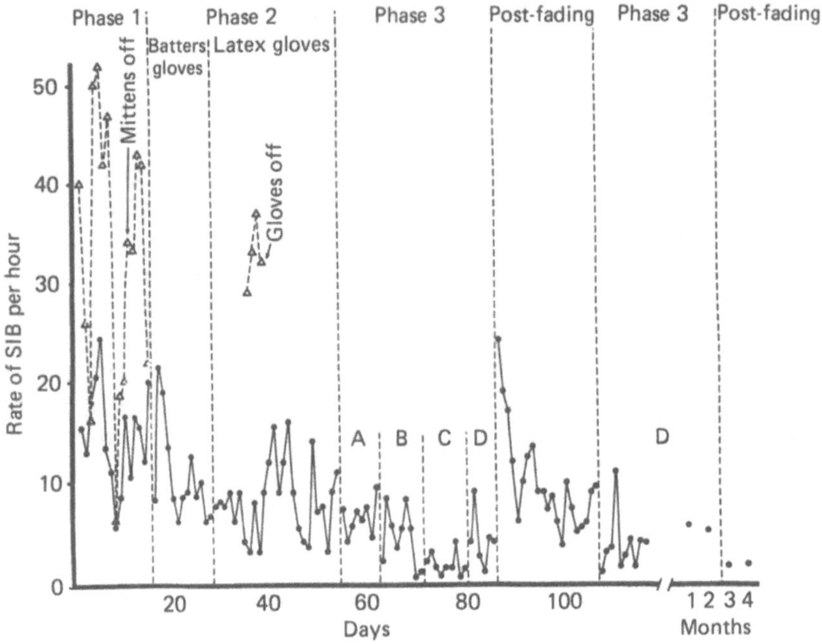


FIGURE 9.3. Rate of SIB (eye-pressing) per hour displayed by an 18-year-old, nonambulatory woman with severe mental retardation. Large padded mittens employed during Phase 1 were faded to latex gloves (Phase 2) that were gradually eliminated across four steps (A–D) during Phase 3. (From Luiselli, 1991a.)

gloves completely and maintain very low rates of SIB during postfading assessments.

One of the primary advantages of sensory extinction as a treatment technique for SIB is that it does not require the delivery of consequences contingently by change-agents. Once a piece of equipment has been identified that effectively blocks sensory reinforcement, the only requirement is that it be worn by the client continuously. Because one does not have to respond to each self-injurious response, the treatment is extremely cost-efficient and less time-intensive in contrast to most operant methods. For reasons of practicality then, sensory extinction has an important clinical advantage.

The issue of treatment efficiency notwithstanding, there are several critical concerns that should be addressed when evaluating sensory extinction. One issue has to do with the *assessment* versus the *treatment* function of the procedure. To illustrate, the purported sensory reinforcement of eye-gouging in a handicapped child could be assessed by having him or her wear a blindfold or large gloves to alter the visual (photic stimulation) and tactile (fingers against eyeball) feedback elicited by the behavior. A decrease in the frequency of self-injury when such equipment is applied would suggest that eye-gouging was sensory motivated. However, the wearing of a blindfold would make it impossible to carry out effective remedial education and habilitation with the child. Similarly, the requirement of wearing large gloves continuously would interfere with meaningful programming. It is significant, therefore, that although some equipment might be utilized advantageously to determine sources of sensory reinforcement, that same equipment may present obstacles when proposed as treatment. A situation such as this would warrant different devices to accomplish assessment and therapeutic objectives.

Response covariation refers to changes that occur in nontargeted behaviors as a result of manipulations directed at target behaviors and represents another concern that has relevance to a better understanding of sensory extinction as a decelerative technique. There are two possible outcomes in this regard. First, the reduction or suppression of one topography of SIB achieved via sensory extinction might result in an emergence or increase in another self-injurious response. Another possibility is that decreases in behaviors exposed to sensory extinction treatment might lead (generalize) to similar reductions in nontreated behaviors. In a study designed to evaluate covariation during the sensory extinction treatment of stereotypic behaviors, Maag, Wolchik, Rutherford, and Parks (1986) found that the masking of sensory consequences reduced a variety of target responses in developmentally disabled children and that generalization occurred with nontargeted, topographically similar behaviors but not those that were topographically dissimilar. This study also demonstrated that nontargeted self-stimulatory behaviors did not increase when targeted behaviors were reduced through sensory extinction.

Unfortunately, research on response covariation has not been conducted with sensory extinction programs for SIB. Luiselli (1984) described the case of a self-injurious boy who engaged in hand-biting until he was fitted with protective mittens. He then started to pull out his hair, a behavior that was suppressed following application of a stocking cap. Subsequent to this change, he began to pick skin from his face. Thus, as each form of sensory feedback was eliminated with protective equipment, another topography of SIB would emerge. However, because these findings were presented as a descriptive case report, it must be acknowledged again that empirical, data-based analyses of covariation are still lacking. Also, it should be emphasized that topographical similarity among responses should not be regarded as the sole predictor of generalization. As noted by Maag et al. (1986), some behaviors may be topographically similar but maintained by different sensory reinforcers. Conceptually, sensory extinction would predict that generalized behavior change would only occur if the application of equipment for one response topography also masked or somehow weakened the sensory effects from other responses.

Finally, the actual pattern of response reduction observed in most studies on sensory extinction raises an interesting question concerning the theoretical basis of the procedure. The majority of research on the sensory extinction treatment of stereotypic behavior, for example, reveals immediate and very stable reductions in responding, upon the introduction of treatment (Maag et al., 1986; Rincover, 1978; Rincover et al., 1979a, Rincover, Newsom, & Carr, 1979b). Similar rapid changes have been recorded when the procedures were used to control SIB (Luiselli, 1988; Rincover & Devany, 1982). Such a pattern, however, does not fit the typical extinction curve. Extinction usually proceeds with an initial burst in responding, associated with the withdrawal of reinforcement, followed by a gradual rate reduction, a brief period of spontaneous recovery, and eventually, complete suppression. Rincover et al. (1979a) pointed out that when rapid and dramatic reductions in responding are evinced, it suggests that some manipulation of stimulus control has occurred. They emphasized that the influence of stimulus control might be, "reliably established and extinguished . . . as a function of the presence versus absence of sensory reinforcers" (p. 231). Rincover and Devany (1982) amended this interpretation further by suggesting that in contrast to the typical social extinction procedure (planned ignoring), sensory extinction includes the presence of conspicuous stimuli that are correlated with the absence of reinforcement. Therefore, when equipment is applied, it acquires stimulus control over nonresponding (Jenkins, 1965; Nevin, 1973) and is responsible for the immediate and sustained rate changes. It can be argued, of course, that the rapid response suppression reported in many sensory extinction studies is achieved operantly through aversive conditioning. At the very least, sensory extinction appears to be an effective intervention for some forms of SIB but one that would benefit from more detailed and systematic experimental analyses.

## *Contingent Application*

With contingent application, the self-injurer is required to wear equipment each time a target response is emitted. The equipment is applied immediately following ISB and remains in place for a predetermined duration (e.g., 2 minutes). The equipment does not restrain or otherwise impede movement but instead, either prevents the self-injurious response from being completed or allows self-injury to occur while affording protection to the client.

Following the reduction of SIB in three mentally retarded residents through continuous wearing of a football helmet and padded gloves, Dorsey et al. (1982) applied the equipment contingently in a second phase of evaluation. Each instance of a target SIB resulted in equipment application for a 2-minute period and the withdrawal of sensory-stimulating toys. Treatment was introduced initially during brief experimental sessions and was effective in maintaining the low rates of SIB achieved during the preceding phase of continuous application. However, two cautions are in order. First, because the condition of contingent treatment followed the use of equipment on a continuous basis, the contingent results are subject to the influence of sequence effects. Second, the contingent application of protective equipment also included the withdrawal of toys, thereby introducing time-out as a possible controlling variable. In a subsequent analysis, the program of contingent application was extended beyond the experimental sessions and into each client's residential living unit. Intervention included access to sensory-stimulating toys and placement of equipment contingent upon SIB in the manner described previously. Once again, control over SIB was demonstrated as a function of the treatment program.

Neufeld and Fantuzzo (1984) described an unusual apparatus for the management of self-injurious hand-biting in a 9-year-old autistic girl. Termed the "bubble helmet," this device, "was a clear plastic sphere which fastened over the child's head, shielding the mouth from contact with the hands and forearms" (p. 80). It measured approximately 30.5 cm in diameter, weighed 1000 g, and was designed to accommodate the child's neck comfortably. To ensure proper ventilation and hearing, small holes were drilled in the top of the helmet. The study was conducted within a community-based, residential treatment facility. After an initial baseline phase, a time-out procedure was programmed in which the child was escorted to a seclusion booth if she did not cease SIB following an initial directive to "stop biting." Duration of time-out was 2 minutes without SIB or vocalizing. Reinforcement on a 30-minute DRO schedule was also combined with time-out. This same reinforcement procedure remained in effect during a second treatment phase except that instead of seclusion time-out, the bubble helmet was applied for a 2-minute duration contingent upon SIB. Interestingly, "Educational and recreational activities, and the directives associated with them, continued while the child wore the Bubble, and she was reinforced for compliance using praise and gentle touch" (p. 81). Although it might be anticipated that a manipulation of this type would establish wearing of the helmet as a pleasurable consequence and hence, produce an increase in SIB, the program of contingent application eliminated biting after only 3 days of implementation. Commenting on these results, the authors emphasized that by maintaining the child within activities with the helmet in place, possible escape-motivated SIB was precluded, and access to positive reinforcement for alternative behaviors was not interrupted. One limitation with this study was that the experimental methodology (A-B-C design) did not permit functional control from the helmet-wearing procedure to be determined unequivocally.

Neufeld and Fantuzzo (1987) expanded treatment with the bubble helmet to three adults with mental retardation who resided in a state hospital. The clients were two males (ages 19 and 30) and one female (age 43), who engaged in face- and head-striking with hands. Treatment evaluation with each client began with a baseline phase wherein staff attempted to reinforce adaptive behaviors and redirected self-injurious responses. Next, appropriate, non-self-injurious behaviors were reinforced with praise, touch, and edible items delivered via DRO or DRI schedules. In the final phase, contingent application of the bubble helmet was programmed in combination with the differential reinforcement strategies. The helmet was applied whenever SIB occurred and remained in place until 30 seconds of nonagitation elapsed. For one client, procedures were introduced in a multiple-baseline design across settings; the two remaining clients were exposed to experimental phases in a sequential A-B-C design. Findings were that baseline rates of SIB persisted during reinforcement conditions but decreased to near-zero levels when the protective helmet was applied contingently. At follow-up assessments 8–18 months from the final treatment phase, very low rates of SIB were recorded, and the clients had made substantial habilitative progress.

Other persons treated effectively with contingently applied protective equipment include mentally retarded adolescents with multiple sensory impairments. Luiselli (1986) evaluated a management program for chronic SIB displayed by a 16.5-year-old male who was deaf and blind as a result of maternal rubella syndrome. His self-injury consisted of striking the face, head, and body with hands and banging head against fixed surfaces, such as a wall, table, or floor. Prior unsuccessful attempts to modify SIB included DRO, overcorrection, immobilization, contingent effort, and water-mist procedures. In this study, all procedures were implemented by direct-care staff in a residential treatment facility. During baseline, ongoing management procedures remained operative. These consisted of a 15-minute DRO strategy (absence of SIB, reinforced with praise and an edible) and protective physical immobilization. The next phase utilized two pieces of equipment that were applied contingently when SIB was exhibited. The first piece was a child-size football helmet with foam padding on the inside and a plastic-coated, wiremesh face-guard. The second device was a pair of cotton padded mittens that extended from the boy's hands, over his forearms, and attached above the elbows, using velcro straps. The equipment remained in place until self-injurious responding ceased for 30 seconds. Throughout treatment with contingently applied protective equipment, the DRO procedure continued to be programmed. Figure 9.4 shows that SIB decreased rapidly with the program in effect. A 1-day baseline probe revealed an increase in responding that was reduced immediately when treatment was reinstated. During this second phase of intervention, the DRO interval

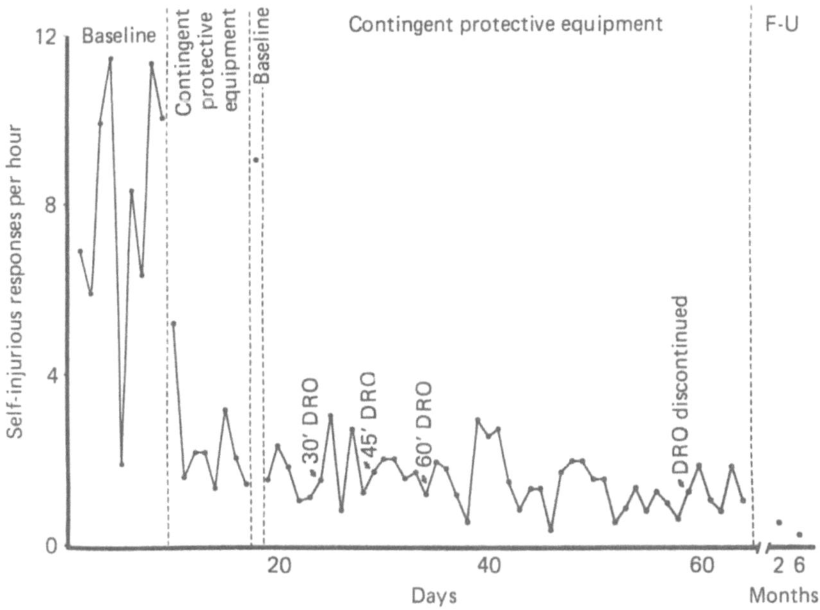


FIGURE 9.4. Frequency of SIB (face- and head-striking) per hour displayed by a 16.5-year-old mentally retarded boy who was deaf and blind. Treatment included a DRO procedure combined with contingent application of a helmet and padded mittens. (From Luiselli, 1986, reprinted by permission of Sage Publications).

was increased gradually from 15 to 60 minutes and eventually discontinued altogether. At 2- and 6-month follow-up assessments, the rate of SIB was below one response per hour.

A second study by Luiselli (1989) was conducted with an 18-year-old deaf, visually impaired male within a residential treatment facility. He engaged in self-inflicted biting and picking of the skin around the cuticles and nails of his fingers. The chronic display of this behavior had produced excoriated sections of skin and small sores on several fingers. Before the study, staff had responded to the SIB with instructions to "Stop picking," with physical redirection, and with the application of antiseptic lotion, but none of these procedures were effective. The treatment program included the application of soft cotton gloves contingent upon the occurrence of self-excoriating behavior. The boy was required to wear the gloves for 1 minute following each application. To establish experimental control, the program of contingent glove-wearing was introduced sequentially in a multiple baseline design across morning and afternon time segments. This simple intervention proved to be highly successful in reducing SIB to manageable levels and maintaining reduced rates at 1- and 3-month follow-ups. It was also extremely practical for staff, in that the average frequency of applying the gloves was less than two times per hour for the duration of the study.

A study by Parrish, Iwata, Dorsey, Bunck, and Slifer (1985) is another example of the clinical utilization of contingently applied equipment and also demonstrates the incorporation of functional assessment methodology to guide treatment selection. The participant was a 17-year-old, severely retarded male who had vision and hearing impairments and had been institutionalized for 9 years. He engaged in SIB by striking his head with his hands and banging his head against fixed objects. In order to identify controlling stimulus conditions, the boy was observed during analogue situations that included escape from academic demands contingent upon SIB (academic demand situation), social attention/physical contact contingent upon SIB (social disapproval situation), an absence of social interaction (alone situation), and access to toys accompanied by praise/physical contact for the absence of SIB (unstructured play situation). These data revealed that SIB was considerably more frequent and intense during the alone situation. Given this finding, it was theorized that the doy's SIB was maintained by sensory reinforcement or the withdrawal of social reinforcement. Therefore, it was decided to evaluate treatment procedures that involved sensory extinction and the differential reinforcement of other behavior (DRO). These included continuous protective equipment, toy play combined with DRO, and both toy play and DRO combined with contingent application of equipment. The most potent treatment effect was produced with the program of contingent application, and it resulted in near suppression of SIB. This program was then transferred successfully outside of the controlled experimental sessions and extended to a hospital setting and, eventually, the boy's residential treatment center.

As gleaned from the studies reviewed in this section, the procedure of contingently applied protective equipment incorporates several therapeutic strategies that may exert operant control over responding. The withdrawal of social interaction and/or materials when the client is placed in the equipment would certainly qualify as a method of time-out. In cases where the equipment is applied while maintaining interaction with the client (cf. Neufeld & Fantuzzo, 1984), it may be that wearing of the equipment is unpleasant and that its removal functions as negative reinforcement for non-SIB. Another possibility is that contingent application by itself may serve as a noxious stimulus much like punishment through aversive stimulation. If the equipment interferes with response-elicited stimulation that is pleasurable, then sensory extinction can influence responding. As with other management techniques (e.g., overcorrection), it is likely that more than one of these influences operates simultaneously. The fact that multiple controlling operations may be at work simply means that the procedure may have wider acceptability and generalized application under diverse clinical conditions (Dorsey et al., 1982).

## Summary and Discussion of Critical Components

This chapter examines the various uses and applications of protective equipment for the treatment of SIB. One conclusion that emerges from this review is that equipment has multiple functions and purposes. Various devices can be used as a primary method of intervention (e.g., sensory extinction), as a means to ensure physical safety while therapeutic strategies are developed, and as an ingredient of multiprocedural treatment packages. Though some techniques have been evaluated more frequently than others and experimental methodologies differ substantially between studies, the overall results from protective equipment interventions have been favorable. Clearly, protective equipment has a role in the comprehensive treatment and management of handicapped persons who are self-injurious. In what follows, several components related to future research and therapy are highlighted.

### *Treatment Selection*

A decision to utilize protective equipment for management of SIB, like other treatment modalities, should follow a careful functional analysis of controlling variables in concert with clinical demands. The study by Parrish et al. (1985) presented an exemplary model of analogue clinical assessment in this regard. Recall that their pretreatment analysis revealed that SIB was most frequent when the participant was left alone in contrast to the academic demand, social attention, and unstructured play conditions. These results suggested that SIB might be maintained by sensory reinforcement or social extinction and, in turn, led to the incorporation of protective equipment on a continuous and contingent basis. Functionally determined treatment such as this ensures that intervention is not chosen randomly or without reference to influential antecedent stimuli or consequent events. When practical exigencies of the clinical environment do not permit the design and implementation of experimentally based, analogue assessment methodologies, various screening inventories and on-line recording instruments can be adopted accordingly. For example, the Motivational Assessment Scale constructed by Durand and Crimmins (1988) requires direct-care providers to respond to specific questions that help pinpoint antecedent, consequent, and setting conditions associated with SIB. This assessment device has been shown to predict responsiveness by children when they were evaluated during experimental, analogue situations similar to those by Parrish et al. (1985). Another method of assessment was presented by Touchette, MacDonald, and Langer (1985) and consists of a scatter-plot recording format that allows stimulus control variables and setting events to be discerned through visual display.

Many of the studies reported in this review relied upon the judgments of clinicians and researchers to identify functionally controlling variables. Rincover and Devany (1982), as an example, selected sensory extinction as a treatment method for SIB because the children in their research, "seemed to prefer being off in a corner or out of sight while self-injuring and seemed to resent any social interruptions while self-injuring" (p. 70). The role of sensory reinforcement as a source of control was suggested further by the fact that, "self-injury had persisted over time in situations where social attention was present as well as when it was not, when demands were present as well as when they were not and, therefore, did not appear to be correlated (positively or inversely) with any obvious social or environmental events in the natural environment" (p. 70). The procedure of contingently applied protective equipment evaluated by Luiselli (1986) was programmed because pretreatment physical-restraint interventions with the client appeared to be reinforcing. The utilization of equipment on a contingent basis enabled staff to withhold physical immobilization while ensuring that the client was afforded protection during the time-out period. Although clinical judgement will probably remain the mainstay of most functional behavior analyses, it bears repeating that standardized, empirically based assessments of motivational variables should be an integral feature of any program that considers protective equipment.

## *Comparative Analysis*

Neufeld and Fantuzzo (1987) commented on the importance of comparing the relative effectiveness of protective equipment procedures (in that case, contingent application) with other management strategies. A number of studies documented therapeutic effects from various protective equipment interventions following unsuccessful modification with other behavioral techniques (Dorsey et al., 1982; Luiselli, 1988; Neufeld & Fantuzzo, 1987). In these and similar cases, it appears that programs incorporating protective equipment were not the initial treatment of choice but instead were instituted sequentially after previous treatment failures. Because such analyses are subject to confounds due to order effects, it would be desirable to conduct systematic evaluations using more methodologically sophisticated formats, such as the alternating treatments design (Barlow & Hayes, 1979). Comparisons of the procedural components that compose treatment packages incorporating protective equipment would be another worthwhile experimental objective.

## *Social Validation*

When a client is required to wear equipment or to have it applied in some systematic manner, that person presents a conspicuous appearance and looks different from his or her peers. It is not uncommon for practitioners to reject a program of protective equipment given these considerations. On other occasions, a program may be implemented reluctantly, thereby leading to inconsistent use or deliberate misapplication. With the present emphasis on community-referenced behavioral intervention (Horner, Dunlap & Koegel, 1988), treatment programs must be developed that have uniform acceptability by clinicians, direct-care providers, and the lay public. Furthermore, these interventions must be adapted to the seriousness of the presenting disorder (i.e., they must be capable of affecting change) while minimizing social stigmatization.

Social validity assessment seeks to elicit information from significant others regarding the quality of the behavior change following treatment (social comparision), the severity of the behavior in question (subjective evaluation), and the acceptance of and satisfaction with the methods of intervention (consumer satisfaction). Social validation yields and additional measure of clinical significance to supplement quantitative changes in behavior. Also, satisfaction ratings by practitioners help identify what characteristics of procedures can be adapted and revised to engender wider acceptance and better marketing of behavioral technology.

Though few in number, recent studies concerned with protective equipment have featured social validation assessment. Luiselli (1986) had direct-care staff judge the effectiveness, acceptability, and level of satisfaction with programming by completing ratings on a brief questionnaire (extremely, very, somewhat, minimally, not at all satisfactory). Staff were also asked whether they would recommend the program for a client with a similar problem (definitely yes, maybe, probably not, definitely not). Results indicated consistently favorable ratings for each questionnaire item. Neufeld and Fantuzzo (1987) used two forms of subjective evaluation within a program of contingently applied equipment (i.e., bubble helmet). First, supervisors and psychologists responsible for the care of the clients were interviewed, to obtain their impressions regarding specific and general changes in behavior. Second, a questionnaire was administered to hospital workers, teachers, and office staff, requesting them to rate the bubble helmet, as compared to two other protective devices (motorcycle helmet, fencing mask) along the criteria of relative effectiveness, comfort, human appearance, treatment selection, and personal choice. Data demonstrated that the bubble helmet was consistently selected as the most acceptable alternative; staff also viewed SIB as a less severe problem for the clients when the helmet procedure was being implemented. The obvious recommendation from these studies is that social validation should be included as a component of multimethod assessment when protective equipment is employed.

## *Fading Strategies*

Once effective control over SIB is established via protective equipment, the next concern should be to withdraw and eventually eliminate such stimuli. In fact, a predetermined equipment-fading sequence should be formulated *before* the actual treatment plan is introduced. Frequently, one encounters a client who has remained in equipment for a protracted length of time, with little or no attempt to remove it. Intervention in such cases must be regarded as incomplete.

Among the studies reviewed, several fading strategies were evaluated empirically. The most common approach is to alter the physical dimensions of the equipment through gradual reduction of size (Ball et al., 1985; Luiselli, (1991a); Pace et al., 1986) or through the substitution of less conspicuous stimuli (Luiselli, 1991b). This approach is most functional when a client must wear equipment noncontingently, for example, with procedures such as sensory extinction, response interruption, response prevention, and restraint procedures. Having the client wear the equipment less frequently is another fading approach but one that has been examined in only one study (Rincover & Devany, 1982). For programs that include contingent application, fading can be accomplished by implementing the procedure on an intermittent basis. Thus, once clinically significant reductions in SIB are achieved with the program, treatment application would be instituted on some predetermined, intermittent schedule. This strategy has yet to be explored and, like other fading approaches, should be studied with the intention of promoting long-term maintenance of treatment gains, improving practicality of program administration, and enhancing acceptability within naturalistic settings.

## References

Ball, T. S., Campbell, R., & Barkemeyer, R. (1980). Air splints applied to control self-injurious finger sucking in profoundly retarded individuals. *Journal of Behavior Therapy & Experimental Psychiatry*, *11*, 267–271.

Ball, T. S., Datta, P. C., Rios, M., & Constantine, C. (1975). Flexible arm splints in the control of a Lesch–Nyhan victim's finger biting and a profoundly retarded client's finger sucking. *Journal of Autism and Developmental Disorders*, *15*, 177–184.

Barlow, D. H., & Hayes, S. C. (1979). The alternating treatments design: One strategy for comparing the effects of two treatments in a single subject. *Journal of Applied Behavior Analysis*, *12*, 199–210.

Dorsey, M. F., Iwata, B. A., Reid, D. H., & Davis, P. A. (1982). Protective equipment: Continuous and contingent application in the treatment of self-injurious behavior. *Journal of Applied Behavior Analysis*, *15*, 217–230.

Durand, V. M., & Crimmins, D. B. (1988). Identifying the variables maintaining self-injurious behavior. *Journal of Autism and Developmental Disorders*, *18*, 99–117.

Favell, J. E., McGimsey, J. F., & Jones, M. L. (1978). The use of physical restraint in the treatment of self-injurious behavior and as positive reinforcement. *Journal of Applied Behavior Analysis*, *11*, 225–241.

Favell, J. E., McGimsey, J. F., Jones, M. L., & Cannon, P. R. (1981). Physical restraint as positive reinforcement. *American Journal of Mental Deficiency*, *85*, 425–432.

Foxx, R. M., & Dufrense, D. (1984). "Harry": The use of physical restraint as a reinforcer, time-out from restraint, and fading restraint in treating a self-injurious man. *Analysis and Intervention in Developmental Disabilities, 4*, 1–14.

Griffin, J. C., Ricketts, R. W., & Williams, D. E. (1986). Reaction to Richmond et al.: Propriety of mechanical restraint and protective devices as tertiary techniques. In K. D. Gadow (Ed.), *Advances in learning and behavioral disabilities* (Vol. 5, pp. 109–116). Greenwich, CT: JAI Press.

Horner, R. H., Dunlap, G., & Koegel, R. L. (Eds.). (1988). *Generalization and maintenance: Lifestyle changes in applied settings*. Baltimore: Paul H. Brookes.

Jenkins, H. M. (1965). Generalization gradients and the concept of inhbition. In D. Mostofsky (Ed.), *Stimulus generalization*. Stanford, CA: Stanford Press.

Luiselli, J. K. (1984). Use of sensory extinction in treating self-injurious behavior: A cautionary note. *The Behavior Therapist, 7*, 2–3.

Luiselli, J. K. (1986). Analysis of contingently applied protective equipment in the modification of self-injurious behavior. *Behavior Modification, 10*, 191–204.

Luiselli, J. K. (1988). Comparative analysis of sensory extinction treatments for self-injury. *Education and Treatment of Children, 11*, 149–156.

Luiselli, J. K. (1989). Contingent glove wearing for the treatment of self-excoriating behavior in a sensory-impaired adolescent. *Behavior Modification, 13*, 65–73.

Luiselli, J. K. (1991a). Application of protective equipment and equipment-fading for the treatment of self-injurious behavior in a pediatric nursing-care resident. *Behavioral Residential Treatment*, in press.

Luiselli, J. K. (1991b) Behavioral–pharmacological treatment of severe self-injury in an adult with dual sensory impairment. *Journal of Behavior Therapy & Experimental Psychiatry* (in press).

Maag, J. W., Wolchik, S. A., Rutherford, R. B., & Parks, B. T. (1986). Response covariation on self-stimulatory behaviors during sensory extinction procedures. *Journal of Autism and Developmental Disorders, 16*, 119–132.

Mace, F. C., & Knight, D. (1986). Functional analysis and treatment of severe pica. *Journal of Applied Behavior Analysis, 19*, 411–416.

Murphy, G. H. (1978). Comment to J. Rojahn, J. A. Mulick, D. McCoy, & S. Schroeder. *Behavioural Analysis and Modification, 2*, 197–199.

Neufeld, A., & Fantuzzo, J. W. (1984). Contingent application of a protective device to treat the severe self-biting behavior of a disturbed autistic child. *Journal of Behavior Therapy & Experimental Psychiatry, 15*, 79–83.

Neufeld, A., & Fantuzzo, J. W. (1987). Treatment of severe self-injurious behavior by the mentally retarded using the bubble helmet and differential reinforcement procedures. *Journal of Behavior Therapy & Experimental Psychiatry, 18*, 127–136.

Nevin, J. A. (1973). Stimulus control. In Nevin, J. A., & Reynolds, G. S. (Eds.), *The study of behavior*. Glenview, IL: Scott, Foresman.

Pace, G. M., Iwata, B. A., Edwards, G. L., & McCosh, K. C. (1986). Stimulus fading and transfer in treatment of self-restraint and self-injurious behavior. *Journal of Applied Behavior Analysis, 19*, 381–389.

Parrish, J. M., Aguerrevere, L., Dorsey, M. F., & Iwata, B. A. (1980). The effects of protective equipment on self-injurious behavior. *The Behavior Therapist, 3*, 28–29.

Parrish, J. M., Iwata, B. A., Dorsey, M. F., Bunck, T. J., & Slifer, K. J. (1985). Behavior analysis, program development, and transfer of control in the treatment of self-injury. *Journal of Behavior Therapy & Experimental Psychiatry*, *16*, 159–168.

Pena, v. New York State Division of Youth, 419 F. Supp. 203 (S.D.N.Y. 1976).

Richmond G., Schroeder, S. R., & Bickel, W. (1986). Tertiary prevention of attrition related to self-injurious behavior. In K. D. Kadow (Ed.), *Advances in learning and behavioral disabilities* (Vol. 5, pp. 97–108). Greenwich, CT: JAI Press.

Rincover, A. (1978). Sensory extinction: A procedure for eliminating self-stimulatory behavior in developmentally disabled children. *Journal of Abnormal Child Psychology*, *6*, 299–310.

Rincover, A., Cook, A. R., Peoples, A., & Packard, D. (1979a). Sensory extinction and sensory reinforcement principles for programming multiple adaptive behavior change. *Journal of Applied Behavior Analysis*,*12*, 221–233.

Rincover, A., & Devany, J. (1982). The application of sensory extinction to self-injury, *Analysis and Intervention in Developmental Disabilities*, *2*, 67–82.

Rincover, A., Newsom, C. D., & Carr. E. G. (1979b). Use of sensory extinction procedures in the treatment of compulsive-like behavior of developmentally disabled children. *Journal of Consulting and Clinical Psychology*, *47*, 695–701.

Rojahn, J., Mulick, J. A., McCoy, D., & Schroeder, S. R. (1978). Setting effects, adaptive clothing, and the modification of head-banging and self-restraint in two, profoundly retarded adults. *Behaviour Analysis and Modification*, *2*, 185–196.

Rojahn, J., Schroeder, S. R., & Mulick, J. A. (1980). Ecological assessment of self-protective devices in three profoundly retarded adults. *Journal of Autism and Developmental Disorders*, *10*, 59–66.

Silverman, K., Watanabe, K., Marshall, A. M., & Baer, D. M. (1984). Reducing self-injury and corresponding self-restraint through the strategic use of protective clothing. *Journal of Applied Behavior Analysis*, *17*, 545–552.

Touchette, P. E., MacDonald, R. F., & Langer, S. N. (1985). A scatter plot for identifying stimulus control of problem behavior. *Journal of Applied Behavior Analysis*, *18*, 343–351.

Welsch v. Likins, 373 F. Supp. 487 (D. Minn. 1974).

White, L. K., & Morse, L. A. (1988). Behavior modification in institutions: The development of legal protections of patients' rights. *Behavioral Residential Treatment*, *3*, 287–314.

Wurtele, S. K., King, A. C., & Drabman, R. S. (1984). Treatment package to reduce SIB in a Lesch–Nyhan patient. *Journal of Mental Deficiency Research*, *28*, 227–234.

Wyatt v. Stickney, 325 F. Supp. 781 (M.D. Ala. 1971); 334 F. Supp. 1341 (M.D. Ala. 1971); enforced by 344 F. Supp. 373, 344 F. Supp. 387 (M.D. Ala. 1973), appeal docketed sub nom. Wyatt v. Aderholt, 503 F. 2d 1305 (5th Cir. 1974).

# 10
# Aversive Stimulation

Thomas R. Linscheid

A major controversy over the use of "aversive treatment procedures" to treat severe behavior disorders in individuals with mental retardation and developmental disabilities has been going on in this country for the past several years. The controversy centers on two main points. First, there is the ethical and humane concern regarding the appropriateness of inflicting pain or discomfort on an individual, especially those with disabilities, for the purpose of therapeutic behavior change (Guess, Helmstetter, Turnbull, & Knowlton, 1987). Second, it has been argued that non-aversive techniques currently exist and have sufficient research backing to negate the need for aversive procedures (cf. LaVigna & Donnellan, 1986). Advocacy organizations for handicapped individuals have adopted position statements against the use of any aversive procedures and have attempted to translate this advocacy position into legal prohibition of aversive procedures via the legislative process. Proponents of the **reasoned** use of aversive procedures generally suggest that there is yet insufficient research on positive alternatives to conclude that aversive procedures are never necessary. Individuals who oppose the categorical banning of aversive procedures are not advocating for the exclusive use of aversive procedures but rather advocate for the right of the trained clinician, parents, and client to choose, based on individual case assessment and review, whether the use of a behavior reductive technique using aversive stimulation is warranted.

As evidence of the intensity and widespread nature of this controversy, the National Institutes of Health (NIH) convened a consensus development conference to discuss this and other treatment issues. The Consensus Development Conference Panel wrote in final its conference statement;

> Behavior reductive procedures should be selected for their rapid effectiveness **only** if the exigencies of the clinical situation require such restrictive interventions and **only** after appropriate review. These interventions should **only** be used in the context of a comprehensive and individualized behavior enhancement treatment package. (NIH, 1989, p. 13)

This conclusion was reached after the panel examined extensive literature reviews prepared for the conference by recognized authorities and heard scientific presentations on various treatment approaches. The panel also heard the testimony of parents, advocacy groups, and other interested parties. The conclusion of the consensus panel in regard to the continued need of behavior reductive procedures (including "aversive procedures") was, of course, questioned by advocacy groups who have proposed a total ban on the use of aversive procedures.

Given that the consensus development panel, after thorough review of the current status of research and treatment on self-destructive behaviors and aggression, felt that there is still a need for these procedures on a limited basis, this chapter reviews what are commonly referred to as aversive procedures and examines factors to be considered in a decision to use the procedures. Because it would be impossible to review all possible "aversive procedures" only a small number which have been used and researched most extensively will be discussed.

## Definitions

There is a great deal of confusion and misunderstanding about terms such as aversive procedures, aversive conditioning, and aversive stimuli (Matson & DiLorenzo, 1984). Initially, aversive conditioning referred to a classical or respondent conditioning process in which a previously neutral stimulus, when paired with an aversive stimulus, comes to elicit an aversive reaction. The more common definition of the term, however, refers to an operant process in which a stimulus assumed to cause distress (discomfort, physical pain or anxiety) is administered contingent upon a preselected response. In essence, *aversive conditioning* refers to a punishment procedure, defined in operant terms as the reduction of the future probability of a response contingent upon the presentation of a stimulus.

The operant definition of punishment, of course, does not address whether the stimulus will be judged as aversive, unpleasant, undesirable, or distressful by the organism receiving it. Rather, the definition of whether a stimulus is a punishing stimulus or the process is punishment is based on the nature of the behavior change. It is certainly possible to think of a stimulus serving as a punishing stimulus in one situation and a reinforcing stimulus (i.e., a stimulus that results in the increased probability of a response) in another situation (cf. Mulick, 1988). For example, a father tickling his son in a playful situation may result in the son approaching the father more frequently and receiving increased tickling, whereas tickling by an older brother when the child does not wish to bothered may be very aversive and may lead to a change in the child's behavior (avoiding the older brother) in the future.

It appears to be the general consensus that the terms *aversive conditioning* and *aversive procedures* refer to treatment programming involving the use of the brief administration of stimuli that, in the perception of the observer, results in pain, discomfort, and distress. For the purpose of this chapter, I will review and describe procedures in which stimuli thought to cause pain, discomfort, or distress are presented for brief periods contingent upon the occurrence of the target behavior.

Interestingly, even those who have been at the forefront of a purely nonaversive approach discuss the appropriate use of mild punishers such as social time-out, verbal reprimand, and brief physical restraint. For example, Meyer and Evans (1989) justify the inclusion of specific punishment techniques in their treatment manual because they are described as mild and are intended to help the client pay attention to the learning environment. Determination of what makes one punisher mild and another aversive is subjective, and unless a client has the opportunity to choose which punisher he or she would rather experience, we have no way of knowing the subjective aversiveness of a punisher to the client other than by our own biases. It should also be kept in mind that distress is not engendered only by procedures involving so-called aversive stimuli. With any positively reinforced behavior on an intermittent schedule, there are times when the behavior occurs without being followed by positive reinforcement. It is certainly not uncommon for individuals to express distress when positive reinforcement is not forthcoming but is expected—Witness the gambler on a losing streak. Additionally, animal research has shown that aggression toward other animals can occur on certain schedules when behavior is maintained by positive reinforcement alone (Gentry, 1968). Additionally, Balsam and Bondy (1983) discuss in detail the negative side effects of positive reinforcement in humans.

In reality, this chapter defines aversive conditioning procedures by the punishing stimuli selected for review here. It is doubtful that there will ever be a universally agreed-upon definition of aversive conditioning or aversive procedures. For that reason, only techniques utilizing stimuli that the general public may perceive as being painful, disconcerting, or distress-inducing are included.

## Procedural Considerations

It must be emphasized from the outset that the procedures described in this chapter were never intended to be used in isolation but rather as a part of an overall program designed to teach appropriate and functional skills. They should be used both after reasonable attempts have been made to eliminate the severe behavioral difficulties by nonaversive means and for individuals whose ongoing behavior difficulties are interfering with their ability to profit from other therapeutic techniques. In addition, the use of these procedures should be considered for individuals whose behaviors are directly responsible for their continued placement in a more restrictive environment.

Aversive techniques should be evaluated on a number of parameters. First, procedures should be selected on the reasonable belief that they will be dramatically effective—That is, the procedure should result in a near-complete suppression of the target behavior very rapidly. When this occurs, only a very small number of the aversive stimuli are experienced by the individual, as the stimulus is not administered unless the behavior occurs. The goal when using an aversive conditioning procedure is not to decrease the rate by 50% or less, but to seek complete or near-complete suppression.

Second, can the procedure be realistically administered in all settings and environments? A procedure that requires extensive personnel, equipment, or supervision may not be practical. The goal with any client with mental retardation or developmental disabilities, of course, is to integrate that client into the normal community as much as possible. A procedure that prevents this should be seen as an undesirable procedure even though its effectiveness may be complete. Third, the punishment program using aversive stimuli should not interfere with or preempt an ongoing positively oriented training program.

In summary, an aversive program should be utilized only when individuals are engaging in behaviors dangerous to themselves or others and when reasonable attempts at nonaversive programming have failed to eliminate the problem; aversive procedures should be selected for use only if they have a substantial research basis to indicate that they will be effective in quickly eliminating or reducing the behavior to manageable levels. The technique should not interfere with or preempt ongoing positive programming and should be technically usable in all settings (e.g., school, community, home). Additionally, the nature of the punishing stimulus should have the properties that make for an effective punisher, as described in the following section.

## Punishment

Punishment in behavioral terms is quite different from the term *punishment* used in everyday language. The behavioral definition of punishment is based on behavior rate probabilities and says nothing regarding the therapeutic or corrective intent of a procedure. The term *punishment* was selected to describe a process in which the future probability of a response decreases based on the contingent presentation of the punishing stimulus.

A great deal of research on punishment has occurred over the past 40 years. This research has focused on the basic parameters of punishing stimuli, the interaction between positive reinforcement and punishment schedules and the effects of punishment on ongoing behavior maintained by positive reinforcement. In a landmark chapter, Azrin and Holz (1966) reviewed and summarized the research on punishment to that date. From their review and research, they examined the characteristics of the ideal punishing stimulus and described how punishment should be arranged in a treatment program in order to guarantee the maximum effectiveness. To set the stage for evaluating the punishment techniques and aversive stimuli reviewed in this chapter, the suggestions of Azrin and Holz are briefly reviewed here.

The ideal punishing stimulus should have several features or characteristics. First, the stimulus itself should be able to be measured in precise physical specifications. That is, dimensions of the stimulus, such as intensity and duration should be measurable in physical units of some kind. Second, a stimulus should be one that allows for consistency of the stimulus in its actual contact with subject. For example, in the case of a water-mist spray procedure (described later), one may be able to measure the amount of water leaving the squirt bottle nozzle in precise units; however, the amount of water actually making contact with subject's skin may be quite different, based on a number of factors, such as the distance of the subject from the spray bottle or the pattern of the spray (wide versus narrow).

A third characteristic of the punishing stimulus that can reduce its effectiveness relates to the subject's ability to either escape, avoid, or reduce the intensity of the aversive stimulus, based on the subject's behavior. The classic example of this is the observation that rats quickly learn to lie on their backs when receiving electric stimulation through floor grids in a operant chamber. This behavior, of course, introduces their fur as a insulating factor between the shock and their skin and reduces the actual intensity of the electrical stimulation that is received. To the extent that a subject can reduce, escape, or avoid the punishing stimulus, the effectiveness of the punishing procedure, of course, will be reduced in some proportional degree.

The absence of major or minor skeletal responses to the punishing stimulus is a fourth characteristic that is desirable. This is particularly true when using punishment with humans, as the intent is not to create such a strong physical response to the stimulus that more appropriate behaviors become impossible. The fifth characteristic of an ideal punishing stimulus as described by Azrin and Holz is its ability to be varied over a wide range of intensity. A stimulus that is not adjustable in intensity does not allow for determination of maximal effectiveness with minimal distress or aversiveness to the subject.

The preceding factors relate specifically to the characteristics of the stimulus itself. Once a stimulus has been selected based on the best characteristics, other factors should be considered in arranging for maximum effectiveness of the punishment procedure. Azrin and Holz described 14 components of a punishment program, which should be considered in maximizing the effectiveness of the punisher. First, the punishment stimulus should be arranged for delivery in a way that does not allow for any escape behavior. While Azrin and Holz suggested that the punishing stimulus should be as intense as possible, they did not mean that the punishing stimulus should be the maximal intensity possible for that stimulus but rather that the maximum intensity necessary to be effective should be utilized. Relatedly, the punishing stimulus should be introduced at that intensity rather than introduced at a low intensity with gradual increases to the final intensity level. Punishment should be delivered on a continuous schedule—that is, one administration of the punishing stimulus for each occurrence of the behavior. The punishing stimulus should also be delivered immediately following (or during) the response, with even slight delays resulting in decreased effectiveness. Extended periods of punishment, especially if the punishing stimulus is of a low intensity, may lead to adaptation and recovery of the punished behavior and should be avoided.

Azrin and Holz suggest strongly that it is crucial to prevent the delivery of punishment from being associated with the delivery of reinforcement, a situation in which a punishing stimulus could become a conditioned reinforcer (Hake & Azrin, 1965). Delivery of the punishing stimulus should also signal to the subject that a period of nonreinforcement or extinction is in effect for the behavior being punished. It is important when planning punishment procedures to eliminate, if possible, the source of reinforcement for the punished response. If this can be accomplished, the elimination of the behavior will be more rapid. The degree of motivation to omit the punished response should also be reduced to the extent possible. Reinforcements should be delivered for an alternative response, which is either trained or already in the subject's repertoire. If it is not possible to provide punishment on a continuous schedule—that is, one administration of the punishing stimulus for each behavior—then a conditioned punisher should be used. Interestingly, Azrin and Holz recommend the use of punishment through reduction of positive reinforcement (time-out procedures) as a seemingly less desirable alternative when the use of physical punishment is not possible for practical, legal, or moral reasons. For this to be effective, of course, the individual must be in a time-in or a high-density reinforcement situation.

Given that aversive conditioning procedures should be used rarely and for the purpose for treating behaviors that pose a severe danger to the client or others in the environment, such procedures should be selected for their probability of success. In other words, these procedures should not be utilized unless there is a near guarantee of success. Therefore, the punishing stimulus should meet all of the criteria proposed by Azrin and Holz and should be able to be incorporated practically into an ongoing positive program for maximum effectiveness. In reviewing the aversive conditioning procedures in the remainder of this chapter, the characteristics of the stimulus itself and the compatibility of the procedure with the preceding considerations are addressed.

# Aversive Conditioning Procedures

In the following section, punishment procedures that utilize stimuli thought of as physically painful or distressing are reviewed. Not all such stimuli are reviewed, as some have received little research attention or are not widely used, such as tickling (Greene & Hoats, 1971) and forced running (Borreson, 1980). One or two studies that are exemplary of each treatment technique are reviewed as examples. Also, studies that address behaviors other than self-injury (e.g., aggression) are included, to highlight relevant procedural concerns. Reported side effects are noted, and a comparison of the properties of the stimulus with the characteristics of an effective punisher, as described previously, are made. In addition, the appropriateness of the procedure for use within the community is addressed.

## *Water Mist*

In the first published demonstration of the use of water mist as a punishing stimulus, Dorsey, Iwata, Ong, and McSween (1980) treated the self-injurious behavior of institutionalized individuals with mental retardation. The procedure consisted of the use of a standard plastic plant sprayer to administer a spray of fine water mist to the face of the clients contingent upon the occurrence of a predefined self-injurious behavior. The water was administered at room temperature, and the sprayer was adjusted to provide a misting effect rather than a direct stream. The experimenters held the sprayer no closer than 0.3 meters from the client's face and estimated that approximately 0.6 cc of water were dispensed with each spray. Clients in Experiment 1 were seven different individuals, all functioning in the severely to profoundly mentally retarded range and all were nonambulatory. One client was treated in her bed, and the remaining clients were treated while seated in their wheelchairs. In Experiment 1 data were collected in an A-B-A-B reversal design format for six of the clients. The seventh client was evaluated using a simple A-B design.

In all cases, the contingent administration of the water mist reduced the rate of the various self-injurious behaviors quickly, and reinstitution of baseline conditions resulted in increases in the targeted self-injurious behaviors to pretreatment levels. Reintroduction of the water-mist treatment procedures again resulted in near-complete suppression of the behavior. In Experiment 2, the combination of a mild verbal reprimand (the word "No") and the utilization of a differential reinforcement of other behavior procedure (DRO) was investigated in two clients and in two separate settings for each client. Hand-biting was the target self-injurious behavior for both clients. Results suggested that the use of the word "No" as a punishing stimulus prior to its being paired with water mist was ineffective in altering the clients' rate of self-injurious behavior. Once "No" was paired with the water mist however, in a treatment that also included a DRO procedure, the word "No" plus the DRO was effective in maintaining response suppression even after the water mist was discontinued. DRO introduced by itself in a second setting was ineffective in altering the rate of self-injurious behavior. Interestingly, it was demonstrated that the word "No" when added to an ineffective DRO procedure in a setting in which "No" had never been paired with the water-mist spray did produce a dramatic decrease in the behavior, suggesting a generalization of the conditioned punisher, "No."

Bailey, Pokrzywinski, and Bryant (1983) report the successful treatment of a 7-year old boy's hand-mouthing and biting, using contingent water-mist spray. Previous attempts to treat the behavior with both positive reinforcement and punishment procedures had not been successful. The authors justified the selection of the water-mist procedure over other procedures on several grounds. First, the procedure could be done quickly, with little disruption of ongoing educational programming or increased attention to the child, as would be the case with a procedure such as overcorrection. Second, unlike a mechanical restraint (e.g., gloves), the procedure did not interfere physically with the child's normal activity. Third, the procedure did not allow for the increased probability of the child engaging in the target behavior, which may have been possible in a time-out procedure. Also, the water-mist technique was deemed subjectively (to the experimenters) less aversive than alternatives such as lemon juice squirted in the mouth or slaps.

The effectiveness of the treatment was evaluated over an 18-week period using an A-B-A-B design. Initial treatment resulted in an 89% reduction in the mouthing behavior from baseline levels. Withdrawal of treatment produced a return of the behavior to near-baseline levels and reinstitution of the procedure again resulted in a dramatic reduction (93%), compared to the initial baseline rate. Interestingly, the authors report approximately a 50% reduction in the target behavior in control or nonexperimental sessions. The child's response to receiving the water spray was one of surprise and mild displeasure, as described by the authors. No negative physical side effects such as chapped skin or increased colds were noted.

Unlike the subjects in the Dorsey et al. (1980) study, the subject in the Bailey et al. (1983) report was ambulatory and was treated in a public-school environment, as opposed to an institution, suggesting that the technique can be used in more normalized settings. Gross, Berler, and

Drabman (1982) also found acceptance of the procedure by teachers in their treatment of aggressive behaviors in a 4-year-old boy with mental retardation. Generalization from the classroom where treatment was conducted to the playground where no treatment occurred was also described. A differential reinforcement procedure for nonaggressive responding and a time-out program had been unsuccessful previously.

While there is evidence for the effectiveness of contingent water mist in reducing self-injurious behaviors, the intensity of the self-injury and aggression has been mild or the subjects young. Indeed, Singh, Watson and Winton (1986) found water-mist spray to be less effective than other procedures (facial screening and forced arm exercise) in two of three clients who had long histories of serious self-injurious behaviors.

Water-mist spray itself has several drawbacks when compared to the ideal punishing stimulus, as described by Azrin and Holz (1966). First, there may be a delay in the administration of the spray due to the requirement that a teacher (or therapist), unless holding the spray bottle at all times, must reach for the bottle and position it correctly before administering the spray. Second, while not described in the studies reviewed, clinical experience and observation in applied settings suggests that some clients learn to turn their head away from the mist or put their hands in front of their faces, thus reducing the intensity of the punisher or avoiding it altogether. Third, the presence of the spray bottle in the client's environment is a clear discriminative stimulus that the procedure is in effect and allows the client to easily determine whether responses will be consequated. Additionally, because the punisher must be administered by a person, no treatment of the behavior is possible when the client is alone.

## *Aromatic Ammonia*

By the mid-1970s, it had been very clearly established that punishment procedures could rapidly and effectively reduce self-injurious behavior (Corte, Wolfe, & Locke, 1971: Lovaas, Schaeffer, & Simmons, 1965). While contingent electrical stimulation had been shown to be most effective, there were problems related to the mechanics of delivering the treatment itself and concerns regarding generalization. Tanner and Zeiler (1975) attempted to find an effective punisher that could be used easily in everyday settings for the treatment of self-injurious behavior. They correctly pointed out that all staff could not be supplied with electrical stimulators so that contingent electrical stimulation programs could be conducted in all settings and at all times of the day. In addition, the devices used to deliver electrical stimulation were physically difficult to hide from the client, allowing the client to correctly discriminate when the treatment was in effect. Other aversive stimuli, such as loud noise or blasts of air to the face had similar drawbacks.

Aromatic ammonia was selected by Tanner and Zeiler (1975) as a punishing stimulus because of its aversive odor, which is physically safe if presented for brief periods in a diluted form. The ammonia is packaged in small, glass, pellet-shaped containers, which are crushed between the fingers when needed. As such, they are very portable, and their small size makes it possible for individuals in the client's environment to carry several in their pockets so that the treatment can be administered almost immediately upon the occurrence of the response. In addition, because the capsules are concealed, the client cannot discriminate when the treatment is in effect.

Tanner and Zeiler (1975) treated the self-injurious face-slapping behavior of a 20-year-old woman with autism by placing a capsule of aromatic ammonia under her nose contingent upon the occurrence of face-slapping and removing it when she ceased the slapping. By this procedure, the authors were punishing the initiation of face-slapping and negatively reinforcing its termination by removal of the aversive stimulus, a behavioral double-whammy.

Treatment was evaluated, using an A-B-A-B design in short experimental sessions. The initial baseline revealed rates of face-slapping ranging from 20 to 60 per minute. Treatment with the contingent aromatic ammonia reduced the rate to fewer than 5 in the first treatment session and to 0 by Session 4. Initial baseline rates were recovered during the second baseline, with an immediate return to a 0 rate when treatment was reinstated. Data recorded throughout the day for the 23 days following the initial evaluation showed that the procedure was capable of suppressing the face-slapping (range 0–3 per day) in the client's normal environment. Interestingly, this woman had been successfully treated using contingent electrical stimulation, but that treatment had been stopped 1 year previous to the present study, with the face-slapping slowly returning during the year. No reason was given for the termination of the electrical-stimulation program.

Subsequently, Singh, Dawson, and Gregory (1980) demonstrated the effectiveness of using aromatic ammonia as a punishing stimulus in the treatment of chronic hyperventilation in a 17-year-old woman with profound mental retardation. The treatment was evaluated using a multiple baseline design across settings (ward-wide, dining room, bathroom, and dayroom). In addition, a reversal was programmed in each setting, to further demonstrate experimentally the control of the behavior by the treatment.

Baseline condition mean rates of hyperventilation ranged from 6.75 to 10.82 per minute across the four settings. Initiation of treatment resulted in a 96% or greater reduction in all settings. Interestingly, and characteristic of treatment results obtained when using effective punishers, dramatic treatment effects were obtained in the first treatment session. Indeed, it is this immediate and extensive reduction in self-injurious behavior upon the initiation of punishment treatments that argues for their use in cases where the continuation of the behavior poses a serious health threat to the individual.

Doke, Wolery, and Sumberg (1983) used contingent aromatic ammonia to treat aggressive behavior in a child with mental retardation. They documented the success of the treatment and also documented two positive side effects of treatment—decreased inappropriate vocalizations and increased participation in activities—both of which were not treated directly. While the extent of these changes slowly decreased over time, after 14 months, the behaviors were still substantially better than prior to treatment.

Despite the strong evidence for the effectiveness of aromatic ammonia, there are a few considerations that question its use (cf. Jones & Anderson, 1981). First, while its portability and hideability serve to reduce problems of generalization, the treatment must be administered by an individual, and therefore the client must be under constant observation by someone who is capable of immediately administering the ammonia capsule. Second, because the ammonia is an irritant, there are risks to the client's health. Tanner and Zeiler (1975) describe the appearance of a scab on their client's nose which may have been caused by the direct touching of the ammonia to the nose during an administration. Doke et al. (1983) did not use the ammonia while their client had a cold, and Baumeister and Baumeister (1978) warn against the use of ammonia without medical supervision. Additionally, while noted only in passing in published reports, it has been my observation that clients quickly learn to turn away from the ammonia capsule or to hold their breath, both actions serving to reduce the intensity of the punisher.

The portability of the ammonia capsule would suggest that they could be used easily in community settings; however, if a client were to struggle with the person administering the ammonia or to show a violent reaction to the smell, it may attract the attention of others. The odor of the ammonia, once the capsule has been crushed, can also quickly permeate a small room, and for this reason, it may not be appropriate for use in public places, especially restaurants or theaters.

## *Aversive Tastes*

Punishment of self-injurious behavior by the contingent introduction into the client's mouth of aversive-tasting substances has been shown to be effective. Several substances have been used, including lemon juice (e.g., Becker, Turner, & Sajwaj, 1978; Sajwaj, Libet & Agras, 1974), Tabasco or pepper sauces (e.g., Altmeyer, Williams, & Sams, 1985; Murray, Keele, & McCarver, 1977), shaving cream (Conway & Bucher, 1974), and oral antiseptic, often used as part of an overcorrection program (cf. Foxx, Snyder, & Schroeder, 1979).

Aversive tastes have been used primarily to treat rumination in infants and individuals with mental retardation. Sajwaj, Libet, and Agras (1974) were the first to report the use of lemon juice squirted into a normal infant's mouth as a treatment for rumination. Becker, Turner, and Sajwaj (1978) successfully treated chronic rumination in a 36-month-old girl with profound mental retardation using the procedure described by Sajwaj et al. (1974). A brief reversal demonstrated the effectiveness of the contingent lemon-juice administrations, and the child was able to gain weight quickly. The authors were careful to document changes in other behaviors that occurred when rumination was being treated. The child cried less, interacted more with her environment, smiled more frequently, and babbled significantly more once the treatment was initiated. A slight increase in several stereotyped movements were observed early in treatment, but nearly all had disappeared by follow-up.

Favell, McGimsey, and Jones (1978) used contingent lemon-juice administration in the treatment of self-injurious behavior in a 15-year-old girl diagnosed with profound mental retardation. Use of the lemon juice as the only consequence for the self-injurious behavior produced a reduction in the behavior, from 75 to 85%, compared to baseline levels. The addition of both differential reinforcement (via contingent restraint) for periods of not engaging in self-injurious behavior and distraction reduced the self-injury to near-zero rates.

Altmeyer, Williams, and Sams (1985) used the contingent administration of Tabasco sauce in combination with time-out and DRO procedures to successfully treat the aggressive behavior of a 16-year-old girl with severe mental retardation. Unfortunately, it was not possible to isolate the effects of the aversive-tasting substance itself because all treatments were introduced simultaneously; however, the authors maintain that the Tabasco sauce was the significant component in the treatment.

While aversive-tasting substances appear to be an effective punishing stimuli, published studies have mostly covered its use in treatment of rumination or have used aversive tastes in combination with other procedures. There are also limited health risks with the aversive tastes, as they are generally irritants if presented in large quantities. For example, in the Altmeyer et al. (1985) study, the number of administrations of Tabasco sauce was limited to five per day in order to ensure that the client would not suffer oral tissue irritation.

As is the case with aromatic ammonia, the behavior of a client can serve to decrease the amount of the aversive tasting liquid received or to delay the administration of the punisher, thereby decreasing its effectiveness. The need to have the punisher dispensed by an individual again requires the close physical proximity of the therapist at all times so that each occurrence of the behavior can be treated as quickly as possible. Clients may be able to discriminate when treatment is in effect by the presence of the person administering the treatment or by the presence of the container of the aversive-tasting substance or equipment needed to administer it (e.g., a needleless syringe).

## *Electrical Stimulation*

The term "electrical stimulation" versus the more common term "electric shock" is used intentionally in order to decrease confusion regarding the procedure and to remove any subjective prejudices which may be attached to the word "shock". As Matson and DiLorenzo (1984) point out, the contingent administration of brief electrical stimulation for the purpose of behavior reduction is often confused with electroconvulsive shock therapy (ECT), used for the treatment of serious mental disorders such as depression. As such, it is not a behavior modification technique, as it is not applied contingently upon a specific behavior or set of behaviors. With ECT, the electrical charge is extremely intense, is directed to pass through the brain, and is designed to disrupt ongoing brain activity. In contrast, electrical stimulation used in behavior reductive procedures is mild by comparison, is generally administered to the extremities, and is not intended to interrupt current electrical activity of the brain. Additionally, the term *electric shock* conjures up images of capital punishment by electrocution and of injuries and even death from accidental contact with high voltage power lines.

Electrical stimulation can be varied over an extremely broad range from imperceptible to life-terminating. The level of stimulation used in behavior-reduction studies is on the extreme low end of this range and generally is not capable of producing any permanent or temporary physical damage to organ systems, skin tissue, or the nervous system. The intensity of stimulation required to produce behavior suppression is discussed in more detail later.

In 1982, the Association for the Advancement of Behavior Therapy issued a task force report on the treatment of self-injurious behavior (Favell et al., 1982). The report described aversive electrical stimulation as "physically harmless but subjectively noxious" (p. 540) and concluded,

> Aversive electrical stimulation (informally termed shock) is the most widely researched and, within the parameters of shock employed in the research literature, the most generally effective method of initially suppressing self-injury. (p. 540)

The quote is followed by 20 references to published research studies and goes on to warn that treatment with contingent electrical stimulation tends to be effective only in the specific situations where it is used (i.e., it does not generalize) and that periodic reapplications may be necessary. In addition, the procedure requires supervision by a qualified professional in settings where adequate informed consent, peer review, and procedural safeguards are in place.

One of the earliest and most well-known studies of the treatment of self-injurious behavior by contingent electrical stimulation was conducted by Lovaas and Simmons (1969). The authors treated the long-standing and severe self-injurious behavior of three children ages 8 to 11 years with contingent electrical stimulation, delivered via a device called a "Hot-Shot." Powered by five 1.5-volt flashlight batteries, this inductorium was used to deliver an electric shock for 1 second (volts = 1400 at 50,000-ohm resistance) to the child's leg. Upon introduction of the treatment procedure, in all three cases, the rate of self-injurious behavior dropped almost immediately to zero or near-zero. In two cases, the administration of the electrical stimulation was successfully ended without a return of the target behaviors after several sessions of treatment. In the third case, suppression of the behavior occurred only when the punishment program was in effect, with immediate returns of the target behavior to baseline levels when shock was not programmed. For one subject, the word "No" was paired with the administration of the electrical stimulation and when used alone in another experimental location with the same child produced the dramatic suppressive effects seen in the original test of the contingent electrical stimulation. In other words, "No," once paired with the contingent electrical stimulation became a conditioned punisher capable of suppressing the self-injurious behavior itself.

While the authors found that the suppressive effects of the procedure were generally confined to the physical situation in which the children received the contingent electrical stimulation, suppression of the target behavior could be accomplished in other settings using only a very few administrations of the electrical stimulation.

Problems in generalization have been noted by several authors (Birnbrauer, 1968; Corte, Wolfe, & Wolfe, 1971). Carr and Lovaas (1983) suggest that problems in generalization can be overcome by careful planning during the initial treatment procedures. Cunningham and Linscheid (1976) treated chronic rumination in an infant with contingent electrical stimulation and found that treating the infant in a variety of settings (e.g., a simulated living room) within the hospital resulted in the infant returning to his home without a single recurrence of the rumination.

One obvious reason for the difficulties in generalization of the suppressive effects of treatment with contingent electrical stimulation is the necessity for the treatment to be administered by an individual using a device not normally found in the subject's environment. For example, many studies have utilized a cattle prod as a means of administering the electrical stimulation, requiring that the therapist have the device with him or her at all times, and upon the occurrence of the target behavior, place the end of the prod against the subject's skin to administer the electrical stimulation. Individuals receiving the contingent electrical stimulation quickly discriminate the present or absence of the device and can easily come to learn that the absence of the therapist or the device in their environment signals the absence of the punishment contingencies.

It should not be surprising that clients treated with contingent electrical stimulation revert to their original behavior when they can discriminate that the treatment is no longer in effect. Punishment procedures suppress behavior and do not necessarily remove the original reason for the behavior's occurrence. Therefore, when the individual is able to discriminate that the treatment is no longer in effect, the target behavior would be expected to reappear unless specific training strategies or other efforts have been made to address the original reason for the self-injurious behavior or other target behavior.

In order to address the problem of readily discriminable cues indicating that the treatment is in effect, several different methods for the administration of the electrical stimulus have been developed, including devices that administer electrical stimulation to the client but are activated by a wireless remote control unit (Tri-tronics model AL-70, Whistle Stop, Farrell Instruments). These devices allow the delivery of the stimulation without requiring the immediate physical presence of the therapist. Of course, the physical presence of the stimulation device on the subject can serve as a discriminative stimulus that the program is in effect. Remote-control devices require that an attendant be in constant visual contact with the client and immediately activate the device upon the occurrence of the target behavior.

Devices have been also been developed, which are capable of detecting blows to the head and automatically delivering the electrical stimulation (Friauf, 1973; Yeakel, Salisbury, Greer, Marcus, 1970). Ball, Sibbach, Jones, Steele, and Frazier (1975) developed and used an automatic device to provide contingent electrical stimulation based on blows to the head. The device was fitted into a jacket, which each client could wear, and which did not restrict the client's free movement. A portable, battery-operated device generated an electrical stimulation and administered it to the client each time a blow to the head was detected by the accelerometer-activated switch. This device was used on five clients who had long histories of self-injurious and aggressive behavior. While results were somewhat variable across clients, all responded with rapid and near-total suppression of their targeted behaviors. One client exhibited self-injurious striking of his throat with his hand and additionally engaged in a stereotypical tapping of his mouth, tongue, and lips with his fingers. During baseline, rates of throat-hitting occurred between 110 and 400 times per day, and the tapping response occurred between 3800 and 7300 times per day. Initial treatment with the device resulted in total suppression of the throat hitting and a 99% reduction in the stereotypic tapping despite no consequences for the tapping behavior. This child was able to leave the treatment program after 20 days and showed only 4 occurrences of throat hitting in a $3\frac{1}{2}$-month period following the initial treatment. One year after initiation of treatment, he remained essentially free of self-injury, and it was possible to fade wearing of the jacket. The other four subjects showed varying degrees of success. Some of variability was attributed to reliability problems with the device.

Recently, Linscheid, Iwata, Ricketts, Williams, and Griffin (1990) published the results of the treatment of self-injurious behavior in five individuals with a device conceptually similar to that described by Ball et al. (1975) but technologically much more sophisticated. This device, called "SIBIS" (self-injurious behavior inhibiting system), was developed by the Applied Physics Laboratory at Johns Hopkins University and consists of two major components. The first, a sensor module, is worn on the client's head (within a cloth headband, concealed by a cap or a hat) and is capable of detecting blows to the head and of generating a radio signal, which is then sent to the second component, or the stimulus module. The stimulus module, generally worn on the client's leg, receives the coded radio signal and delivers an electrical stimulus with a maximum intensity of 3.5 milliamps at 85 volts.

The intensity of the stimulation delivered by SIBIS is in a safe range, as defined by Butterfield (1975). In fact, it is substantially lower than the intensity of electrical stimulation used in almost all previous reports in the literature. Electrical stimulation is delivered via two electrodes configured in a concentric circle, measuring approximately one inch in diameter. This configuration ensures that the electrical stimulation is localized to the site of the electrode and does not pass through any organ systems. The device is registered with the Food and Drug Administration as a Class II Medical Device and contains numerous safety features. Powered by two 9-volt batteries, SIBIS also provides for automated data collection via an internal counter, which records the number of electrical stimulations administered. This independent data collection system can be used as a check against staff abuse and inaccurate reporting of behavior rates. Foxx and his colleagues (Foxx, McMorrow, Rendleman, & Bittle, 1986) stressed this need for independent assessment of staff compliance with programs using aversive stimulation and described the simple modification of a digital wristwatch to independently record the time of administration of the electrical stimulus.

Linscheid et al. (1990) used single-subject reversal designs to evaluate the effectiveness of SIBIS. Two control conditions were used within these designs. For clients who routinely wore protective headgear, baseline data were taken with the headgear on (helmet condition). All clients were also observed in sessions in which SIBIS was worn but the electrical stimulation was not delivered (SIBIS-inactive condition). In order to be judged effective, the rate of self-injurious behavior needed to be significantly lower during the SIBIS treatment than during a pure baseline (no helmet, no SIBIS), the helmet condition, or the SIBIS-inactive con-

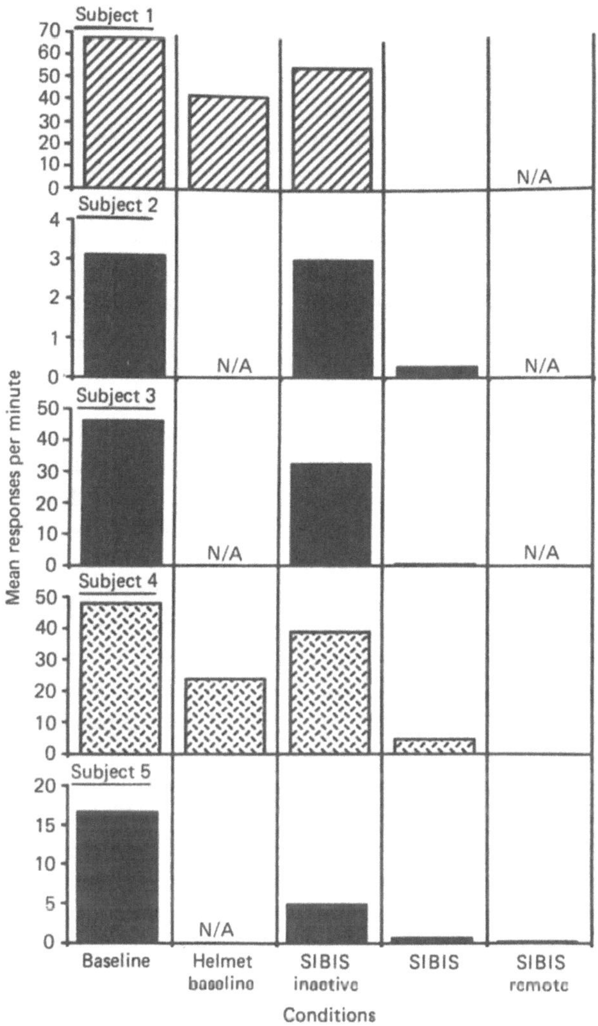


FIGURE 10.1. Mean number of self-injurious responses per minute across subjects and experimental conditions. (From Iwata, 1988, reprinted by permission of the Society for the Advancement of Behavior Analysis).

dition. In all five cases, contingent electrical stimulation delivered by SIBIS produced rapid and near-complete suppression of the severe and previously unsuccessfully treated self-injurious behavior (Figure 10.1).

In one client, the authors documented decreases in other undesirable and self-injurious behaviors, which were not directly treated by the contingent electrical stimulation. Improvements in general affect, interpersonal interaction, and interest in their environments were noted for all clients. In one case, the authors documented increases in behavior indicative of relaxation once treatment began. In other words, this client became less distressed during treatment with electrical stimulation than he had been during baseline sessions.

The positive side effects noted by Linscheid et al. (1990) are consistent with findings from reviews of other studies using electrical stimulation. Carr and Lovaas (1983) report positive side effects occurring at a rate of about five-to-one over negative side effects, and Lichstein and Schreibman (1976) found an even higher predominance of positive side effects in their review of the use of contingent electrical stimulation with individuals diagnosed with autism. Unfortunately, many of the reports of side effects, both positive and negative, are anecdotal and therefore should be considered with caution.

SIBIS, as an automated and technologically sophisticated device, has the advantage of maximizing the parameters of a contingently presented punishing stimulus. The automatic detection of the target behavior and the administration of the stimulus by the device itself, assures that all occurrences of the self-injurious behavior will be immediately consequated. The consistency and immediacy are probably the reasons that the device has proven to be effective despite using significantly lower intensities of electrical stimulation than reported in previous studies.

In addition, electrical stimulation, as delivered by SIBIS, does not result in any major skeletal response, is not necessarily associated with the presence or absence of individuals in the client's environment, and is not contingently tied to the delivery of reinforcement. Comparing these factors with the recommendations regarding effective punishment procedures made by Azrin and Holz (1966), it is clear that SIBIS operates in concert with scientifically validated operant principles.

To emphasize the low level of electrical stimulation needed to produce a therapeutic effect with SIBIS, I conducted a small experiment to determine whether individuals observing the client could tell when electrical stimulation was administered. Choosing one of the clients from the Linscheid et al. study, ten 5-second videotaped excerpts of the client's behavior beginning concurrent with the cessation of the electrical stimulus were edited onto a videotape for review. To reduce the influence of adaptation to the electrical stimulation, the 10 episodes were taken from the first 10 electrical stimulations received by the client. Twenty-three professionals who routinely work with individuals with developmental disabilities and who were in attendance at a conference served as subjects. They were told that they would be seeing several episodes of a client's behavior and were asked to indicate for each episode whether they thought the client had received an electrical stimulation. As shown in Figure 10.2, observers showed little agreement on when stimulation

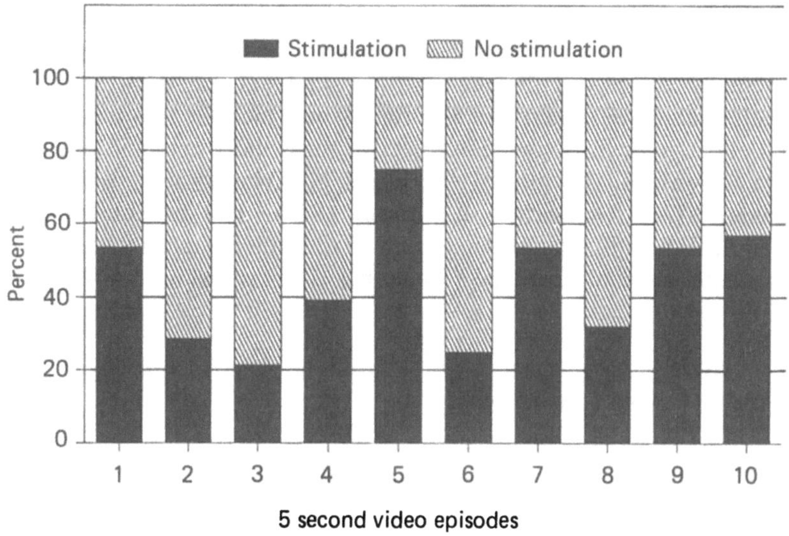


FIGURE 10.2. Percentage of subjects indicating whether an electrical stimulation had been received for 10 behavioral episodes.

occurred, and in no case did they all agree that an electrical stimulation had been delivered. Overall, they scored no better than chance. These data support the authors' observation that a client's response to the actual electrical stimulation is mild or in some cases nonexistent and call into question whether the effectiveness of the treatment is based on intensity alone.

The clients' response to the administration of electrical stimulation is extremely important in considering whether these techniques can be used in community settings. If it were true that clients screamed loudly, fell to the ground, and began to writhe in agony upon the administration of the electrical stimulation as delivered by SIBIS, obviously this technique would not be acceptable in the community, or for that matter in any setting. However, this in not the case, and it is clear that the response of the client to the administration of the electrical stimulation is minimal and not reliably detectable even by a panel of professionals in the field. Therefore, treatment with a device such as SIBIS in a community shopping center or a fast-food restaurant has very little potential for either stigmatizing a client or preventing the client from active participation in community-based activities. The stimulus module worn on the client's head can be easily hidden with a cap or hat, further decreasing the chance that treatment with the device will lead to stigmatization, especially when compared to the frequent need for individuals who engaged in self-injurious behavior to wear protective equipment such as helmets and arm restraints.

While there are more than 20 studies in the literature reporting effective treatment of self-injurious behavior in both normal and developmentally disabled individuals with contingent electrical stimulation (Favell et al., 1982), there are also reports in which the treatment has not been effective or has only been effective for a short time and one report of an increase in the rate of the target behavior (Jones, Simmons, & Frankel, 1974; Romanczyk & Goren, 1975). The use of contingent electrical stimulation has also been shown to be ineffective with individuals with Lesch–Nyhan syndrome (Anderson, Dancis, Alpert, & Hermann, 1977).

## Summary and Conclusions

The use of operant punishment procedures for the treatment of self-injury has been reviewed in the chapter. In general, results suggest that these procedures can be successful in rapidly reducing the rates of self-injurious behavior in individuals with developmental disabilities, as well as with individuals who are developmentally normal. Purposely, only aversive stimuli that may be thought of as physically painful or physically uncomfortable were reviewed herein. Obviously, many procedures, both reinforcing and punishing (in the operant sense), may instill emotional distress. For example, the failure to receive expected reinforcement if a target behavior occurs near the end of a DRO interval or the placing of an individual in a social time-out situation may both lead to distress.

Iwata (1988), in his presidential address to the Association for Behavior Analysis discussed the issue of advocating aversive interventions and the role of the behavioral scientist. Correctly, he concluded that the responsible behaviorist leaves decision making regarding the use of these procedures to the appropriate individuals—that is, parents or guardians, human rights and peer review committees, and adequately trained clinicians. However, until it is scientifically shown that self-injury (and other severe behavior disorders) can be successfully and safely treated without the need for aversive procedures, the development of these techniques and the documentation of their effectiveness is warranted and appropriate.

It is my conviction that clients have a right to have their severe behavior disorders treated rapidly and effectively, especially when the behaviors pose a threat to the individual's physical well-being or are responsible for preventing the individual from achieving his or her maximum development and integration into the community. Therefore, once it has been determined that the behaviors do indeed meet the preceding criteria, the individual has a right (Gardner, 1989; Van Houton et al., 1988) to be treated with the technique that is shown to have the greatest documented effectiveness with the specific behavior problem in question and that allows for the greatest degree of integration of the client into the community, even during the treatment itself. Given these considerations and despite emotional responses to the contrary, the use of contingent electrical stimulation should be given a high priority in treatment selection once it has been decided that an aversive procedure is necessary. This technique is the most widely researched, comes closest to the Azrin and Holz (1966) parameters of effective punishers, and—with recent advances in technology—is the safest of the procedures reviewed in this chapter. If selected for use, the excellent guidelines for programs using contingent electrical stimulation outlined by Foxx, Plaska, and Bittle (1986) should be followed.

## References

Altman, K., Haavik, S., & Cook, J. (1978). Punishment of self-injurious behavior in natural settings using contingent aromatic ammonia. *Behavior Research and Therapy*, *16*, 85–96.

Altmeyer, B. K., Williams, D. E., & Sams, V. (1985). Treatment of severe self-injurious and aggressive biting. *Journal of Behavior Therapy and Experimental Psychiatry*, *16*, 169–172.

Anderson, L. T., Dancis, J., Alpert, M., & Hermann, L. (1977). Punishment learning and self-multilation in Lesch–Nyhan disease. *Nature*, *265*, 461.

Azrin, N. H., & Holz, W. C. (1966). Punishment. In W. K. Honig (Ed.), *Operant behavior: Areas of research and application*, New York: Appleton-Century-Crofts, 380–447.

Bailey, S. L., Pokrzywinski, J., & Bryant, L. E. (1983). Using water mist to reduce self-injurious and stereotypic behavior. *Applied Research in Mental Retardation*, *4*, 229–241.

Ball, T. S., Sibbach, L., Jones, R., Steele, B., & Frazier, L. (1975). An accelerometer-activated device to control assaultive and self-destructive behaviors in retardates. *Journal of Behavior Therapy and Experimental Psychiatry*, *6*, 223–228.

Balsam, P. D., & Bondy, A. S. (1983). The negative side effects of reward. *Journal of Applied Behavior Analysis*, *16*, 283–296.

Baumeister, A. A., & Baumeister, A. A. (1978). Suppression of repetitive self-injurious behavior by contingent inhalation of aromatic ammonia. *Journal of Autism and Childhood Schizophrenia*, *8*, 71–77.

Becker, J. V., Turner, S. M., & Sajwaj, T. E. (1978). Multiple behavior effects of the use of lemon juice with a ruminating toddler-age child. *Behavior Modificiation*, *2*, 267–278.

Birnbrauer, J. S. (1968). Generalization of punishment effects—A case study. *Journal of Applied Behavior Analysis*, *1*, 201–211.

Borreson, P. M. (1980). The elimination of a self-injurious avoidance response through a forced running consequence. *Mental Retardation*, *18*, 73–77.

Butterfield, W. H. (1975). Instruments and technology: Electric shock—Safety factors when used for the aversive conditioning of humans. *Behavior Therapy*, *6*, 98–110.

Carr, E. G., & Lovaas, O. I. (1983). Contingent electric shock as a treatment for severe behavior problems. In S. Axelrod and J. Apsche (Eds.), *Punishment: Its effects on human behavior* (pp. 219–246). New York: Academic Press.

Conway, J. B., & Bucher, B. D. (1974). "Soap in the mouth" as an aversive consequence. *Behavior Therapy*, *5*, 154–156.

Corte, H. E., Wolf, M. M., & Locke, B. J. (1971). A comparison of procedure for eliminating self-injurious behavior of retarded adolescents. *Journal of Applied Behavior Analysis*, *4*, 201–213.

Cunningham, C. E., & Linscheid, T. R. (1976). Elimination of chronic infant ruminating by electric shock. *Behavior Therapy*, *7*, 231–234.

Doke, L., Wolery, M., & Sumberg, C. (1983). Treating chronic aggression: Effects and side effects of response-contingent ammonia spirits. *Behavior Modification*, *7*(4), 531–556.

Dorsey, M. F., Iwata, B. A., Ong, P., & McSween T. E. (1980). Treatment of self-injurious behavior using a water mist: Initial response suppression and generalization. *Journal of Applied Behavior Analysis*, *13*, 343–353.

Favell, J. E., Azrin, N. H., Baumeister, A. A., Carr, E. G., Dorsey, M. F., Forehand, R., Foxx, R. M., Lovaas, O. I., Rincover, A., Risley, T. R., Romanczyk, R. G., Russo, D. C., Schroeder, S. R., & Solnick, J. V. (1982). The treatment of self-injurious behavior. *Behavior Therapy*, *13*, 529–554.

Favell, J. E., McGimsey, J. F., & Jones, M. L. (1978). The use of physical restraint in the treatment of self-injury and as positive reinforcement. *Journal of Applied Behavior Analysis*, *11*, 225–242.

Foxx, R. M., McMorrow, J. J., Rendleman, L., & Bittle, R. G. (1986). Increasing staff accountability in shock programs: Simple and inexpensive shock device modifications [Letter to the editor]. *Behavior Therapy*, *17*, 187–189.

Foxx, R. M., Plaska, T. G., & Bittle, R. G. (1986). Guidelines for the use of contingent electric shock to treat abberrant behavior. In M. Herson, A. Bellack, & P. Miller (Eds.), *Progress in behavior modification* (Vol. 20, pp. 1–34). New York: Academic Press.

Foxx, R. M., Snyder, M., & Schroeder, F. A. (1979). A food satiation and oral hygiene punishment program to supress chronic rumination by retarded persons. *Journal of Autism and Developmental Disabilities*, *9*, 399–412.

Friauf, W. S. (1973). An aversive stimulator for autistic children. *Medical and Biological Engineering*, Sept., 609–612.

Gardner, W. I. (1989). But in the meantime: A client perspective of the debate over the use of aversive/intrusive therapy procedures. *The Behavior Therapist*, *12*, 179–181.

Gentry, W. D. (1968). Fixed-ratio schedule induced aggression. *Journal of the Experimental Analysis of Behavior*, *11*, 813–817.

Greene, R. J., & Hoats, D. L. (1971). Aversive tickling: A simple conditioning technique. *Behavior Therapy*, *2*, 389–393.

Gross, A. M., Berler, E. S., & Drabman, R. S. (1982). Reduction of aggression in a retarded boy using a water squirt. *Journal of Behavior Therapy and Experimental Psychiatry*, *13*(1), 95–98.

Guess, D., Helmstetter, E., Turnbull, H. R., & Knowlton, S. (1987). *Use of aversive procedures with persons with persons who are disabled: A historical review and critical analysis*. Seatle, WA: The Association for Persons with Severe Handicaps.

Hake, D. F., & Azrin, N. H. (1965). Conditioned punishment. *Journal of the Experimental Analysis of Behavior*, *8*, 279–293.
Iwata, B. A. (1988). The development and adoption of controversial default technologies. *The Behavior Analyst*, *11*, 149–157.
Jones, F. H., Simmons, J. Q., & Frankel, F. (1974). An extinction procedure for eliminating self-destructive behavior in a 9-year-old autistic girl. *Journal of Autism and Childhood Schizophrenia*, *4*, 241–250.
Jones, M., & Anderson, M. (1981). Problems involved in the use of ammonia in the treatment of self-injurious behavior. *Australian Journal of Developmental Disabilities*, *7*, 27–31.
LaVigna, G. W., & Donnellan, A. M. (1986). *Alternatives to punishment: Solving behavior problems with non-aversive strategies*. New York: Irvington Publishers Inc.
Lichstein, K. L., & Schreibman, L. (1976). Employing electric shock with autistic children: A review of the side effects. *Journal of Autism and Childhood Schizophrenia*, *6*, 163–173.
Linscheid, T. R., Iwata, B. A., Ricketts, R. W., Williams, D. E., & Griffin, J. C. (1990). Clinical evaluation of the self-injurious behavior inhibiting system (SIBIS). *Journal of Applied Behavior Analysis*, *23*, 53–78.
Lovaas, O. I., Schaeffer, B., & Simmons, J. (1965). Experimental studies in childhood schizophrenia: Building social behavior in autistic children by use of electric shock. *Journal of Experimental Research in Personalilty*, *1*, 99–109.
Lovaas, O. I., & Simmons, J. Q. (1969). Manipulation of self-destruction in three retarded children. *Journal of Applied Behavior Analysis*, *2*, 143–157.
Matson, J. L., & DiLorenzo, T. M. (1984). *Punishment and its alternatives: A new perspective for behavior modification*. New York: Springer-verlag.
Meyer, L. H., & Evans, I. M. (1989). *Non-aversive interventions for behavior problems: A manual for home and community* (p. 208). Baltimore: Paul Brooks Publishing.
Mulick, J. A. (1988, June). *Aversive in behavior therapy: When science and public policy clash*. Paper presented at the 112th meeting of the American Association on Mental Retardation, Washington, DC.
Murray, M. E., Keele, D. K., & McCarver, J. W. (1977). Treatment of ruminations with behavioral techniques: A case report. *Behavior Therapy*, *8*, 999–1003.
National Institutes of Health Consensus Development Conference Statement (1989). *Treatment of destructive behaviors in persons with developmental disabilities* (p. 23), Vol 7(9) Bethesda, MD: NICHD.
Romanczyk, R. G., & Goren, E. R. (1975). Severe self-injurious behavior: The problem of clinical control. *Journal of Consulting & Clinical Psychology*, *43*, 730–739.
Sajwaj, T., Libet, J., & Agras, S. (1974). Lemon-juice therapy: The control of life-threatening rumination in a six-month old infant. *Journal of Applied Behavior Analysis*, *1*(3), 557–563.
Singh, N. N., Dawson, M. J., & Gregory, P. R. (1980). Suppression of chronic hyperventilation using response-contingent aromatic ammonia. *Behavior Therapy*, *11*, 561–566.
Singh, N. N., Watson, J. E., & Winton, A. S. W. (1986). Treating self-injury:

Water mist spray versus facial screening or forced arm exercise. *Journal of Applied Behavior Analysis*, *19*, 403–410.
Tanner, B., & Zeiler, M. (1975). Punishment of self-injurious behavior using aromatic ammonia as the aversive stimulus. *Journal of Applied Behavior Analysis*, *8*, 53–57.
Van Houton, R., Axlerod, S., Bailey, J. S., Favell, J. E., Foxx, R. M., Iwata, B. A., & Lovaas, O. I. (1988). The right to effective behavioral treatment. *Journal of Applied Behavior Analysis*, *21*, 381–384.
Yeakel, M. H., Salisbury, L. L., Greer, S. L., & Marcus, L. F. (1970). An appliance for auto-induced adverse control of self-injurious behavior. *Journal of Experimental Child Psychology*, *10*, 159–169.

# 11
# Self-restraint

STEPHEN R. SCHROEDER and JAMES K. LUISELLI

In common parlance, the term *self-restraint* refers to one's ability to control one's own impulses, emotions, or desires. It is functionally equivalent to the dictionary definition of *self-control*. The clinical sense of the term is more restricted (i.e., self-control of undesirable or socially unacceptable behaviors). Usage of the term in conjunction with self-injurious behavior (SIB) is even narrower than usage in the general clinical sense. Here, *self-restraint* refers to the habit of some self-injurers to seek physical restraint devices, to entangle their arms and legs in clothing or furniture, or to sit or lie on their arms or legs, as a means of restraining themselves from self-injury.

In some cases, self-restraint can be very dramatic. The authors have observed clients who, when released from four-point restraints in bed, would scream, cry, and head-bang. Then they would put the ankle and wrist cuffs back on and tie themselves down to the bed again. One client used contorted wrist movements to execute triple slipknots on the homolateral wrist. The tendency in this client was so strong that even after having been free of bed restraints for more than 2 years, he still would tie himself down, if permitted. In fact, if he happened to be walking across the campus of the facility and viewed the building in which he was originally restrained, he would go directly to the building, crawl into bed, tie himself down, and smile.

The explanation of this bizarre behavior has eluded researchers for the past 20 years. Few of the clients who self-restrain can communicate expressively in order to relate the possible reasons. One exception to this rule might be those people who are emotionally disturbed and functioning at a high level or people with Lesch–Nyhan syndrome who may not have severe mental retardation, but who also self-restrain. Lesch–Nyhan syndrome is a sex-linked genetic disorder of purine metabolism, in which one of its many symptoms is ferocious self-biting of the lips, oral cavity, and hands, to the point of amputation (Lesch & Nyhan, 1964). Nyhan (1976) gives a graphic description of how these clients scream and show distress when released from physical restraints, and how they literally beg for restraints if they are verbal. The senior author has worked with three high-functioning self-restrainers. They have been acquaintances for a number of years and for a duration long enough to make it possible to ask them why they do it and how it feels. None could explain it. One of them, a man with Lesch–Nyhan syndrome and normal intelligence, related that "The captain makes me do it." Normally, during the day, he is not restrained. He is only tied down when he requests restraint. Various attempts at cognitive behavior modification or counseling treatments based on the treatment of multiple personality disorder have been unsuccessful with him. It does not seem likely, at least with our present technology, that the cognitive behavioral or psychotherapeutic approach would be successful with the most self-injurious self-restrainers. A functional approach to analysis and intervention is the only one that has show any success in treating self-restraint.

## Definition

Some confusion may remain as to the response classes that fall into the category of *self-restraint*. The most obvious behaviors involve hooking one's arms under the rungs of a chair, wrapping one's arms in another person's arms or in one's clothes, sitting on one's hands, tying one's self down with or towing physical objects, and so forth. Other more subtle self-restraining behaviors involve the use of symbolic behaviors, such as crossing one's limbs or wearing a hat or a pair of glasses (Foxx & Dufrense, 1984), or adaptive clothing (Rojahn, Mulick, McCoy, & Schroeder, 1978), or a wristband (Pace, Iwata, Edwards, & McCosh, 1986). In such cases, stimulus-fading techniques were used to transfer self-restraint to discriminative stimuli that publicly were more acceptable. A functional analysis of the behavior was required to identify them. Another functional kind of self-restraint occurs when a client, upon release from physical restraints with devices such as rigid arm splints, helmets, camisoles, beds, or chairs, engages in such dangerous behaviors that he or she must be restrained again for health and safety reasons. Sometimes, the physical devices used in this context are termed *self-protective devices* (see Luiselli, Chapter 9, this volume). It should be noted that this classification is a functional one, based upon its consequences. It may or may not be self-restraint because it may be used contingently or noncontingently and has consequences for the caregiver, as well as for the client (Rojahn, Schroeder, & Mulick, 1980).

Under some limited circumstances, self-restraint might be considered a form of self-control. If this is the case, then several implications would be presented for interpretation and analysis. Self-control is a broad concept in behavior theory, for which there is a variety of explanations. With regard to a severe behavioral pathology such as self-injury, it might be reasoned that the client's ability to self-restrain would be desirable because it would provide protection from physical harm. However, clients who self-restrain generally engage in the behavior continuously if allowed to do so rather than on a periodic basis that follows an urge to injure themselves. Also, as described previously, the typography of restraint usually is cumbersome and highly restrictive, to the extent that meaningful interactions with others is precluded.

## Prevalence

There are currently no prevalence estimates for self-restraint in people with mental retardation and developmental disabilities. Recently Fovel, Lash, Barron, and Roberts (1989) conducted a survey of self-restraint, self-injury, and other maladaptive behaviors in a 789-bed public residential facility. This was a well-conducted survey, which was performed in 1985 and repeated in 1988, and involved the caseloads of 40 psychologists. The behaviors surveyed were SIB, aggression, property destruction, tantrums, stripping, smearing feces, and oral behaviors, such as pica, mouthing, spitting, and vomiting.

Results were that 20 clients (2.5% of the total population of the facility) were identified as self-restrainers. For these 20 cases, prevalence of maladaptive behaviors was SIB—90%; aggression—50%; property destruction—60%; tantrums—45%; oral behaviors—35%; stripping—30%; and smearing feces—15%. Prevalence in the general population of the facility for these behaviors was 28%, 43%, 24%, 38%, 21%, 14%, and 8%, respectively. Only two self-restrainers with SIB problems did not engage in SIB. One was a severe SIB case involving a client whose behavior was under control through the use of behavior management techniques. The other self-restrainer buried her limbs in furniture cushions and would call for staff to rescue her, thereby precluding SIB taking place. Thus, it appears that the presence of self-restraint is almost perfectly correlated with the presence of SIB. This is a potentially important finding that needs replication in other populations and settings because it also may give clues to the causes and persistence of SIB. Furthermore, reducing SIB also should reduce self-restraint. Likewise, allowing some amount of self-restraint may be an important temporary alternative in a program to decrease SIB. This result is consistent with the interpretation that SIB is a negative reinforcing stimulus for self-restraint (Silverman, Watanabe, Marshall, & Baer, 1984). Finally, it suggests that the risk factors for self-restraint (Fovel et al., 1989) are the same as those for severe SIB (i.e., IQ, age of onset, organicity, chronicity, and communication handicaps; Schroeder, Schroeder, Smith, & Dalldorf, 1978).

## Etiological Theories of Self-restraint

The literature on the treatment of SIB contains several anecdotal references to the effect that *self-restraint appears to be operantly reinforcing* to the subjects, and that they only relax and calm down after being restrained (Duker, 1975; Jones, Simmons, & Frankel, 1974; Lovaas & Simmons, 1969; Myers & Diebert, 1971; Tate, 1972; Tate & Baroff, 1966). In a study by Favell, McGimsey, and Jones (1978), the positive reinforcing function of physical restraint (rigid arm splints) was demonstrated. Rapid and complete reduction of SIB was achieved when the subjects physically were restrained, contingent on increasing periods without self-injury and on providing them with toys and attention during intervals between the wearing of the restraints. Subjects also performed alternative tasks for the opportunity of restraint. When physical restraint was applied, contingent on toy play, the toy-play response increased. Favell, McGimsey, Jones, and Cannon (1981) replicated these findings. Three hypotheses were offered to explain the results. It was argued that (a) stimulus change components of restraint might constitute positive reinforcement in nonstimulating environments; or that (b) restraint may be paired with a reduction in aversive stimuli, such as staff-imposed demands, and that self-injury in some individuals may function as an escape *into* restraint conditions (negative-reinforcement hypothesis); or (c) restraint also could be paired with adult attention and, therefore, may be a conditional reinforcing response. The points raised for the explanation of these somewhat paradoxical properties of restraint are well-taken. Further research is needed to isolate and compare these explanations.

Favell et al. (1981) point out that the above reinforcement hypotheses for self-restraint may help to explain the persistence and maintenance of SIB in the face of competing reinforcement contingencies that might reduce SIB.

Using an ecobehavioral approach, Rojahn, Schroeder, and Mulick (1980) investigated the effects of restraints (a camisole and a fencing mask) on three mentally retarded persons with pica. Twenty-two client behaviors and six staff behaviors were observed simultaneously in a descriptive observational study. The study attempted an analysis of social dynamics in a special unit for profoundly mentally retarded clients with SIB (for the data collection system, see Schroeder, Schroeder et al., 1978). Although this was not an attempt to replicate the study by Favell et al. (1978), the results lend support for their second explanation: the self-protective devices tended to decrease social interactions between the restrained subjects and their caregivers. Staff behaviors, such as non-programmatic positive attention, instructions, and reinforcement in the form of verbal praise for specific tasks, decreased for all three subjects during the time they were wearing restraints, as compared to restraint-free periods. This pattern of responsiveness by the staff could reflect an increased demand situation for these clients when they were released from restraints. However, there was no indication with these three clients that the restraints had any reinforcing properties by themselves or provided an escape function of SIB (which consisted of pica). How much self-protective devices and their situational consequences actually contribute to the development and maintenance of problem behaviors such as SIB beyond their preventive function is an important question for ecobehavioral research.

A fourth hypothesis, raised by Silverman et al. (1984), is that self-restraint is behaviorally chained to self-injury and is maintained by escape and avoidance of demands. This seems like a plausible hypothesis that could be tested empirically by experiments on response chaining. This type of research has not been published as yet.

A fifth hypothesis is that restraint devices may provide tactile sensations (warmth and pressure) that are very reinforcing. This speculation was put forward by Temple Grandin in her remarkable autobiography (Grandin & Scariano, 1986). Grandin is a person with autism who has a doctorate in animal behavior science and who is recognized as a world expert in the constructing and handling of livestock facilities. As a young girl, she manifested extreme tactile defensiveness. One summer, while working on a relative's ranch, and cattle were being branded, she became struck with her observation that the cattle became completely calm when restrained in stanchions. She began reading the literature on animal taming and infant swaddling and became convinced that such restraints were comforting. She even tried them on herself and found them very pleasurable. She then developed her own "squeeze machine," where she could regulate the temperature and pressure. She used this device regularly to calm herself down. Her own words are eloquent:

> I remember when I was young, I sort of liked stimulation that was painful. So it might be with kids who mutilate themselves. Perhaps they could be directed into a more positive, less destructive form of self-stimulation. And possibly my "machine" could help these youngsters. Maybe if the child learned to like the stimulation from the squeeze machine, he would not bite his fingers. Recent research on animals indicates that self-stimulation and stereotyped behavior will reduce arousal in frustrated animals. The stereotyped behavior lowered cortisol (stress hormone) levels. Autistic children have an overactive nervous system. People and animals that are sensorily deprived have an overly sensitized nervous system resulting in lower thresholds to sensory stimuli.
>
> Perhaps if a child used the squeeze machine, he could apply intense yet pleasant stimulation to himself. Since the chute is designed to feel very much like being held by a person, it might help the child learn to like being held or touched by a person. Once the child can operate the chute and likes it, the next step would be human affection. The chute is an important step because the child controls it.
>
> Obviously, if a child is mutilating his body, he has to be stopped. But other types of fixations should not always be discouraged. They can be the means of

communicating, as in Jake's case. Turning a negative act into a positive one is possible. Also, I believe that Jake would have been helped immeasurably by my squeeze machine. I have been corresponding with an adult autistic woman. She has difficulty controlling her temper. In her letters her craving for tactile stimulation is apparent. She uses tactile words to describe things—words like fluffy and soft. She likes the idea of the squeeze machine. Perhaps the squeeze machine would help her. (p. 110)

This remarkably introspective account by a person who also is a highly trained professional observer should be researched more extensively. It is a very different perspective on the nature of self-restraint and the general restrictiveness of restraint devices as perceived by the public and reflected in current regulations for residential facilities.

The only quantitative data possibly having a bearing on this issue of the sensory reinforcing nature of self-restraint with which we are familiar come from an ecobehavioral analysis of developmental day care for chronic SIB clients conducted by Schroeder, Kanoy, Thios, Mulick, Rojahn, Stevens, and Hawk (1982), in which self-restraint routinely was recorded on all clients in the program. Self-restraint was not affected by the time of day, staff–client ratio, or presence of toys. It was affected by the presence of a self-protective device, in that clients found some other way to restrain themselves if their self-protective device was removed. In addition, people who had severe sensory impairments, especially visual impairments, tended to self-restrain much more than people without severe sensory impairments.

## Treatment

When confronted with a self-injurious client who displays self-restraining behavior, the clinician has several treatment options. One approach is to make pleasurable stimuli available for the absence of SIB/self-restraint (differential reinforcement of other behaviors—DRO) or the occurrence of alternative behaviors (DRA). A variation of this strategy is to incorporate the reinforcing properties of restraining, whereby access to restraint becomes the reinforcing consequence. A second method is to transfer gradually the control exerted by self-restraint to a functionally equivalent stimulus that does not restrict the hands or body. Finally, procedures can be employed to shape acceptable forms of restraint. It should be noted that treatment programs often include a combination of treatment methods.

In what follows, treatment programs that address the issue of SIB and self-restraint are discussed. However, in comparison to other topics presented in this volume, there is very little in the way of systematic research. Additionally, very few papers quantitatively recorded self-restraint and/or the use of protective devices as covariates of SIB. In hindsight, this seems to be a serious oversight in the analysis of interventions for SIB.

## *Positive Reinforcement*

To our knowledge, the first experimental study investigating self-restraint and SIB was by Peterson and Peterson (1968). The subject was an 8-year-old boy, living in a state institution, who spent most of his day rocking or lying in his bed, wrapped in a small quilt. Whenever the quilt was removed, he engaged in high-rate head-banging until it was returned to him.

A major breakthrough in the conceptualization of self-restraint as *positive reinforcement* was a paper presented by Favell and McGimsey (1976) and subsequently replicated and extended by this group and by others (Favell, McGimsey, & Jones, 1978; Favell, McGimsey, Jones, & Cannon, 1981; Hamad, Isley, & Lowry, 1983). In all of these studies, treatment basically consisted of three procedures: (1) applying physical restraint as a consequence for absence of SIB for a certain period of time, (2) distracting subjects during periods of nonrestraint, and (3) delaying the restraint consequence, contingent upon episodes of SIB. Distractions consisted of walking, toy play, entertainment of the client—anything to prevent self-injury. Over a number of sessions, the amount of physical restraint imposed by distractors was reduced, and longer periods of non-SIB were required for the client's opportunity to have shorter and shorter periods of restraint. The Favell et al. (1978) experiment also combined this treatment with lemon juice for severe eye-poking and scratching for one subject. All of these combinations were effective in reducing the rate of SIB. Generalization data were not reported, but maintenance was still good 5 months later. This set of papers has been very influential in the SIB literature, encouraging interventions for SIB, based on positive reinforcement techniques.

Foxx and Dufrense (1984) described the use of contingent restraint for periods of non-SIB, coupled with stimulus fading, in the treatment of multiple self-injury in a 22-year-old man diagnosed as severely mentally retarded and psychotic. This project also was the basis for the film, *Harry*, which has been widely distributed as an exemplary model of behavioral treatment for SIB. The client had a long-standing history of self-restraint and, at the time of the study, was wearing arm splints continuously during the day. He routinely asked for the splints, was relaxed when they were on, and became agitated and self-injurious if they were removed. During treatment sessions, the restraints were removed, and he was informed that he could "earn them back" if he did not injure himself. The duration of required non-SIB was advanced slowly during sessions, based upon the judgment of the therapist. Each time the client received his restraints, he wore them for 5 minutes. When SIB was displayed, the therapist left the room for a brief period as a form of time-out. This treatment produced substantial reductions in the rate of SIB and corresponding increases in the amount of time spent out of restraints. Subsequently, the restraints were faded to an alternative stimulus, the results of which are described in the following section.

## *Stimulus Control and Transfer*

A second phase of treatment in the Foxx and Dufrense (1984) study evaluated a naturally occurring condition of restraint fading. Following initial treatment, the client began to self-restrain by holding objects in his hands. His preferred method was to grasp a drinking glass in each hand, and so fading was instituted by systematically reducing the size of the glasses until eventually he was holding just the glass rims. Next, he was shaped to wear a wristwatch instead of holding the rims. When he requested to wear eyeglasses instead of the watch, this item acquired stimulus control and remained effective without attempts being made to secure previous forms of restraint.

The fading sequence described by Foxx and Dufrense (1984) was determined largely by the behavioral preferences of the client. For persons who are not as cognitively advanced, there would be few cues to dictate a fading prcedure. In such cases, the clinician must decide upon how restraint should be induced and then construct a *predetermined* sequence to transfer stimuli control. A study by Pace et al. (1986) involved treating two self-injurious, mentally retarded adolescents who engaged in self-restraint, one by grasping the bottom of rigid arm tubes that were worn continuously, and the second by placing his hands into his pockets or under his thighs (this client also wore elbow splints to prevent SIB). Fading for the first client was accomplished by cutting back the length of the arm tubes in successive steps. When they achieved a length of 5 cm, they were covered with fabric and subsequently changed to tennis wristbands. For the second client, the elbow splints were discarded and, in their place, restraint was induced via inflatable air splints. By gradually reducing the pressure of the splints, it was possible to deflate them as a means of stimulus fading. Low rates of SIB and an absence of self-restraint were achieved with both clients under fading and postfading conditions.

## *Establishing Acceptable Self-restraint*

This method attempts to shape alternative and more acceptable typographies of self-restraint. Unfortunately, only one study has evaluated this strategy empirically, and the results were equivocal. Rojahn et al. (1978) targeted SIB in two men with profound mental retardation. One man hit his head with his hands, hit his forehead with his knuckles, and banged his head against his shoulders. Rates of SIB were recorded in daily sessions, along with frequencies of inappropriate self-restraint (wrapping arms in clothing, placing hands under rests of chairs) and appropriate self-restraint (putting hands in pockets). Appropriate self-restraint was established, and face/head hitting was reduced when the client wore a jacket with large side pockets. Inappropriate restraint was encountered only when the jacket was not worn.

For the second client, levels of self-restraint were recorded when he wore either a T-shirt that permitted the wrapping up of his hands or a jumpsuit that prevented this behavior. Frequency of SIB was higher when the jumpsuit was worn, but it also occurred when he wore the T-shirt, even though self-restraint continued. Self-restraint in this case was not associated consistently with decreased SIB, and it competed with training sessions.

Based on the results of Rojahn et al. (1978), it may be concluded that attempting to train clients in alternative typographies of self-restraint is not a recommended treatment strategy until more extensive experimental analyses are conducted. One important contraindication is that although isolating is a more acceptable form of self-restraint, and may seem desirable (e.g., putting hands in pockets instead of placing them in the rungs of a chair), the outcome still may be a client who continues in restraint and resists efforts to discontinue the behavior. In a rejoinder to the Rojahn et al. (1978) study, Murphy (1978) emphasized that replacing SIB with self-restraining behavior was not a long-term solution, given the interference of self-restraint on habilitative care. One option would be to develop different typographies of self-restraint that are more acceptable by virtue of the fact that they can be faded more easily or shaped via stimulus-control procedures.

## *Protective Devices*

An interesting phenomenon that has been observed by the authors on several occasions is the finding that protective equipment can function as a form of self-restraint, even though it does not restrict movement or the ability to engage in SIB (also see Luiselli, Chapter 9, this volume). As an illustration, a child who displays self-injurious head-striking with his fists and corresponding self-restraint (e.g., wrapping fingers in belt loops, sitting on hands) may stop, or greatly reduce, self-restraining behavior when he is placed in a protective helmet. When the helmet is removed, self-restraint increases to previous levels. Persons who exhibit this pattern of behavior also demonstrate a strong preference for, and desire to wear, the equipment. For example, they will readily approach staff and request the device, seek it out, and become agitated when it is not available.

Silverman et al. (1984) provided an empirical demonstration of the association between self-injury, self-restraint and the wearing of protective equipment in a single-case study with a 13-year-old boy who was legally blind and profoundly mentally retarded. Various typographies of leg and arm SIB, plus leg and arm self-restraint, were recorded during daily experimental sessions that featured application of a helmet, a helmet and protective slipper, or no equipment. This investigation revealed decreases in arm SIB and restraint when the client wore the helmet, and a similar effect on leg SIB and restraint was obtained when he wore the protective slippers. In effect, as each body part was protected from SIB, the client engaged less frequently in self-restraint.

The fact that the wearing of protective devices apparently can acquire a self-restraint function suggests several interpretations of the covariation between self-injurious and self-restraining behaviors. As noted previously, a common theory is that the act of self-restraint is negatively reinforced, in that it prevents or avoids discomfort and pain that are the outcome from SIB. This interpretation is the one offered by Silverman et al. (1984) in explaining their results. They stated, "Self-restraint showed the selective characteristics that it should if its function were to escape, avoid, hinder, or delay self-injurious behaviors" (p. 55).

A second interpretation is that the wearing of a protective device provides a distinctive and conspicuous cue that signals the avoidance of social interactions and task demands. It is our experience that virtually all self-injurers who perform self-restraining behaviors do not show a preference for task engagement. The most obvious reason for such avoidance is that by interacting or working with an adult, the client will be required to stop self-restraint. At the same time, prolonged periods of self-restraint are preferred by many staff members because this condition avoids occurrences of SIB. Self-restraint, therefore, may function as a discriminative stimulus for the withholding of adult demends and, similarly, learning may be conditioned and enhanced by the wearing of protective equipment. Determining the variability between task engagement, SIB, and self-restraint with and without protective devices represents a fascinating research topic that would have meaningful clinical implications.

## Critical Issues

This review of self-restraint reveals several issues worthy of discussion. One interesting feature is that, although self-restraint is virtually always associated with SIB, the majority of self-injurers do not self-restrain. The institutional survey conducted by Fovel et al. (1989) found that, in contrast to the general residential population, the self-restraining clients were younger and all were classified as severely to profoundly mentally retarded. However, age and degree of mental retardation do not appear to be valid predictors of self-restraint. Therefore, we are left with an uncertain picture of how self-restraint is generated, what factors predispose development of the behavior, and whether interventions can be identified to prevent its occurrence.

The near perfect correlation between self-restraint and SIB underscores the question of why restraint is not encountered in clients who are behaviorally problematic (e.g., those who have tantrums or are aggressive), but do not engage in self-injury. The data from Fovel et al. (1989) revealed that aberrant behaviors, such as property destruction, aggression, tantrums, pica, stripping, and smearing of feces, occurred in the population of self-restrainers. However, because 90% of the clients who engaged in self-restraint displayed SIB, it appears that the other behaviors simply occurred concurrently, with self-injury as the dominant problem. That is, clients do not present with self-restraint and either aggression or destruction as the *only* targeted behavior. This observation supports the negative reinforcement hypothesis that was articulated previously, in that it is the avoidance and interruption of pain/discomfort that reinforces self-restraint. Behaviors that do not produce painful effects are unlikely to have self-restraint as a covariant.

Another important question is whether treatment should begin with efforts to reduce SIB, self-restraint, or both behaviors simultaneously. Conceptually, a program of differential reinforcement for the absence of SIB (DRO) or the display of alternative behaviors (DRA) should result in corresponding reductions in self-restraint. On a clinical level, however, this strategy can be problematic with a client who spends the majority of time in self-restraint, as most self-restrainers do. In this situation, the client may demonstrate low rates of SIB, but only because he or she is self-restraining continuously. This condition has prompted some authors to suggest that if self-restraint is occurring with regularity, it may be more efficacious to allow the behavior to be performed and to design interventions that focus on restraining versus SIB. Silverman et al. (1984), for example, warn that trying to eliminate self-restraint may leave the client defenseless against SIB. Fovel et al. (1989) stated that, "the modification of self-restraint should be conducted cautiously and monitored carefully for corresponding changes in SIB" (p. 381). The two most relevant procedures in this regard would be to reinforce gradually increasing durations without restraint/SIB or to transfer stimulus control via restraint fading.

Once self-restraint has been reduced significantly or eliminated, do the results persist over an extended period? There appear to be some promising findings, considering the few studies that have addressed this topic. Pace et al. (1986) reported reduced rates of SIB and an absence of self-restraint upon a 2-year follow-up for one client who had undergone restraint fading treatment. Recently, Foxx (1990) conducted a 10-year follow-up of "Harry," and found that this client's self-injury remained infrequent and that there had never been a need to resort to previous mechanical restraint devices. Interestingly, the client was demonstrating two types of self-restraint, which consisted of holding task materials in his hands or wearing a baseball cap. Foxx (1990) commented that, "Such restraint is viewed as a form of self-control that is quite appropriate so long as it does not interfere with the task for more than a brief period and will cease when Harry is requested to do so" (p. 74).

## Conclusion

Not a great deal is known about self-restraint among people with mental retardation. It appears to be highly correlated with self-injury and not with other forms of aberrant behavior. Whether it is positively or negatively related to SIB probably depends on a variety of cofactors, most notably the availability of preferred self-protective devices and the presence of sensory handicaps. It can be decreased by a variety of positive and negative reinforcement techniques without markedly increasing the risk of SIB if done in combination with stimulus control techniques involving fading and transfer to more adaptive forms of self-restraint. At present, the most plausible interpretation is that self-restraint develops and persists as an escape or avoidance of SIB.

*Acknowledgments.* The senior author wishes to acknowledge MCH Project #922 and ADD #24882 for support during the writing of this paper.

## *References*

Duker, P. (1975). Behavior control of self-biting in a Lesch–Nyhan patient. *Journal of Mental Deficiency Research*, *19*, 11–19.

Favell, J. E., & McGimsey, J. F. (1976, August). *The control of self-injury by a combination of procedures*. Paper presented at the 84th annual convention of the American Psychological Association, Washington, DC.

Favell, J. E., McGimsey, J. F., & Jones, M. L. (1978). The use of physical restraint in the treatment of self-injury and as a positive reinforcement. *Journal of Applied Behavior Analysis*, *11*, 225–241.

Favell, J. E., McGimsey, J. F., & Jones, M. L., & Cannon, P. R. (1981). Physical restraint as positive reinforcement. *American Journal of Mental Deficiency*, *85*, 425–432.

Fovel, J. T., Lash, P. S., Barron, D. A., & Roberts, M. S. (1989). A survey of self-restraint and other maladaptive behaviors in an institutionalized population. *Research in Developmental Disabilities*, *10*, 377–382.

Foxx, R. M. (1990). "Harry": A ten year follow-up of the successful treatment of a self-injurious man. *Research in Developmental Disabilities*, *11*, 67–76.

Foxx, R. M., & Dufrense, D. (1984). "Harry": The use of physical restraint as a reinforcer, timeout from restraint, and fading restraint in treating a self-injurious man. *Analysis and Intervention in Developmental Disabilities*, *4*, 1–13.

Grandin, T., & Scariano, M. M. (1986). *Emergence: Labelled autistic*. Novato, CA: Arena Press.

Hamad, C. D., Isley, E. M., & Lowry, M. (1983). The use of mechanical restraint and response incompatibility to modify self-injurious behavior: 4 Case studies. *Mental Retardation*, *21*, 213–218.

Jones, Simmons, & Frankel (1974). An extinction procedure for eliminating self-destructive behavior in a nine-year-old autistic girl. *Journal of Autism and Childhood Schizophrenia*, *4*, 241–250.

Lesch, M., & Nyhan, W. (1964). A familial disorder of uric acid metabolism and central nervous system function. *American Journal of Medicine*, *36*, 561–570.

Lovaas, O. I., & Simmons, J. Q. (1969). Manipulation of self-destruction in three retarded children. *Journal of Applied Behavior Analysis*, *2*, 143–157.

Murphy, G. H. (1978). Comment to J. Rojahn, J. A. Mulick, D. McCoy, and S. Schroeder. *Behavioral Analysis and Modification*, *2*, 197–199.

Myers, J. J., Jr., & Diebert, A. N. (1971). Reduction of self-abusive behavior in a blind child by using a feeding response. *Journal of Behavior Therapy and Experimental Psychiatry*, *2*, 141–144.

Nyhan, W. L. (1976). Behavior in the Lesch–Nyhan syndrome. *Journal of Autism and Childhood Schizophrenia*, *6*, 381–389.

Pace, G. M., Iwata, B. A., Edwards, G. L., & McCosh, K. L. (1986). Stimulus fading and transfer in the treatment of self-restraint and self-injurious behavior. *Journal of Applied Behavior Analysis*, *19*, 381–389.

Peterson, R. F., & Peterson, L. R. (1968). The positive reinforcement in the control of self-destructive behavior in a retarded boy. *Journal of Experimental Child Psychology*, *6*, 351–360.

Rojahn, J., Mulick, J. A., McCoy, D., & Schroeder, S. R. (1978). Head banging and self-restraint in two profoundly retarded adults. *Behavioural Analysis and Modification*, *2*, 185–196.

Rojahn, J., Schroeder, S., & Mulick, J. (1980). Ecological assessment of self-protective restraints for the chronically self-injurious. *Journal of Autism and Developmental Disorders*, *10*, 59–65.

Schroeder, S., Kanoy, R., Thios, S., Mulick, J., Rojahn, J., Stephens, M., & Hawk, B. (1982). Antecedent conditions affecting management and maintenance of programs for the chronically self-injurious. In J. Hollis & C. E. Myers (Eds.), *Life-threatening behavior: Analysis and intervention* AAMD Monograph Series No. 5, pp. 105–159. American Association of Mental Deficiency.

Schroeder, S. R., Rojahn, J., & Mulick, J. A. (1978). Ecobehavioral organization of developmental day care for the chronically self-injurious. *Journal of Pediatric Psychology*, *3*, 81–88.

Schroeder, S. R., Schroeder, C. S., Smith, B., & Dalldorf, J. (1978). Prevalence of self-injurious behaviors in a large state facility for the retarded: A three-year follow-up study. *Journal of Autism and Childhood Schizophrenia*, *8*, 261–269.

Silverman, K., Watanabe, L., Marshall, A. M., & Baer, D. M. (1984). Reducing self-injury and corresponding self-restraint through the strategic use of protective clothing. *Journal of Applied Behavior Analysis*, *17*, 545–552.

Tate, B. (1972). Case study: Control of chronic self-injurious behavior by conditioning procedures. *Behavior Therapy*, *3*, 72–83.
Tate, B. G., & Baroff, G. S. (1966). Aversive control of self-injurious behavior in a psychotic boy. *Behaviour Research and Therapy*, *4*, 281–287.

# 12 Psychopharmacology of Self-injury

NIRBHAY N. SINGH, YADHU N. SINGH, and CYNTHIA R. ELLIS

A long-held view of mental retardation is that it is primarily a problem of learning, and that the behavioral deficits and excesses exhibited by individuals with mental retardation can be treated through learning-based therapies. This view has led some professionals to question the need for using psychotropic medication to treat behavior problems in this population. Historically, this view may have been reinforced by the use of many ineffective and even toxic substances prior to the chlorpromazine era (Caldwell, 1978). The use of medication has been likened to a "chemical straitjacket" by some professionals who questioned whether individuals with mental retardation actually learned anything while on medication (see Aman, 1984). However, based on the "magic bullet" theory (Wolfensberger & Menolascino, 1968), others espoused the use of various drugs in the hope of reversing the intellectual deficits of individuals with mental retardation. Although the fallacy of this theory has always been very clear, individuals with mental retardation are still the single most medicated group of individuals in our society today (Singh & Winton, 1989).

When medication is used with this population primarily for its psychotropic effects, it is prescribed for the treatment of behavior problems. National incidence studies indicate that aggressive behavior, self-injury, agitation, property destruction, and stereotypy are the major classes of behavior that lead to medication of this population (Hill, Balow, & Bruininks, 1985). Drug prescription in this population is also affected by a number of other factors, including the age and level of retardation (Aman, Field, & Bridgman, 1985; Hill et al., 1985), type of residential facility (Aman et al., 1985; Martin & Agran, 1985), and presence of psychiatric disorders (Tu & Smith, 1983). Of course, even when medication is indicated as the treatment of choice, there is no guarantee that it will be prescribed appropriately. For example, Bates, Smeltzer, and Arnoczky (1986) examined the medication prescribed for the psychiatric problems of 242 residents and found that only 45% of the diagnosis–medication combinations were appropriate.

## Assessment Considerations

The treatment of choice for self-injury usually can be derived through an experimental (or functional) analysis of behavior, although other, less rigorous, methods also can be used to determine not only the motivation for the behavior but also whether the self-injury may have medical etiologies (see Repp & Singh, 1990). However, given that self-injury often has multiple and complex components, a multimodal or multidisciplinary assessment best facilitates valid analyses of its maintaining contingencies (see Singh, Parmelee, Sood, & Katz, in press; Singh, Sood, Sonenklar, & Ellis, 1991).

In an experimental analysis, antecedents and/or consequences of self-injury can be experimentally manipulated in either a clinical or an analogue setting, in order to identify the factors that produce systematic changes in the level of the behavior (see Chapter 5 of this volume). For example, such an analysis might indicate whether self-injury is maintained by positive, negative, or automatic reinforcement (Iwata, Vollmer, & Zarcone, 1990). Other, less rigorous, methods also can be used, but these have associated problems. For example, *ecobehavioral analysis*, or the direct observation of behavior without the manipulation of any variables, provides only correlational data on the probable cause of self-injury. Rating scales and interviews can be used to derive tentative hypotheses of factors that may maintain self-injury, although such methods heavily rely on the knowledge of significant others regarding the individual's behavior (O'Neil, Horner, Albin, Storey, & Sprague, 1990). Regardless of which instrument or assessment procedure is used, intervention should be based on the assumed causes of the problem behavior (Repp, Felce, & Barton, 1988).

In addition to a behavioral analysis of self-injury, it is important that a full medical evaluation, including comprehensive testing (e.g., metabolic, genetic), is concurrently undertaken. Thus, if the motivation for the behavior is unclear, it may well be that the genesis of the problem is medical and in need of medical intervention.

## Treatment Modalities

The mainstay of treatment for severe self-injury is behavioral intervention (National Institute of Mental Health [NIMH], 1989; Schroeder, Rojahn, Mulick, & Schroeder, 1990; Singh, 1981; Singh & Repp, 1988). Although sometimes it is difficult to determine the cause of self-injury in certain individuals, it is likely that the majority do not engage in self-injury for neurobiological reasons (see Chapter 3 of this volume). Despite this fact, there are a number of reasons why pharmacological intervention may be considered for use in some self-injurious individuals. Foremost among these is that good theoretical rationales are available for the use of some classes of drugs to treat self-injury (Deutsch, 1986; Goldstein, 1989; Goldstein, Anderson, Reuben, & Dancis, 1985; Konicki & Schulz, 1989; Richardson & Zaleski, 1983). In addition, a pharmacotherapeutic trial is often the only alternative to long-term physical restraint of some individuals who have proven intractable to all other forms of treatment.

In this chapter, we present what is currently known about psychopharmacological treatment of self-injury in individuals with mental retardation. We provide a brief overview of the prevalence of drug prescription for the treatment of problem behaviors in this population, followed by the scientific evidence attesting to the usefulness of various classes of drugs for treating self-injury. By design, the coverage will be comprehensive rather than exhaustive because several reviews are already available. For example, interested readers may consult Singh and Millichamp (1985) and Farber (1987) for brief reviews of drug effects on self-injury, and Aman and Singh (1988) as well as Gadow and Poling (1988) for more extensive reviews on the psychopharmacology of the developmental disabilities in general.

## Psychopharmacology of Self-injury

Some of the earliest published studies on the use of drugs with individuals who are mentally retarded were related to the treatment of self-injurious behavior. These studies were published when little was known about the effects of drugs on behavior, and psychotropic medication usage was based on the apparent similarity between the behavior of individuals with mental retardation and those with mental illness. Although there has been a resurgence in the use of drugs over the past 20 years, it has been based more on trial and error than on rational pharmacotherapy. In addition, most of the studies published before 1980 were methodologically flawed to the extent that a substantial number are scientifically uninterpretable. Some methodologically elegant studies have been published in the past few years, but, unfortunately, most of these have not involved individuals who engage in self-injury.

In the following sections, we review what is currently known about the effects of drugs on self-injury, based on an evaluation of the clinical and empirical literature. Typically, studies were reviewed only if they had self-injury as a separate variable, and studies that included self-injury within other categories (e.g., destructive behavior, aggressive behavior) were excluded. The review is organized by drug class rather than by response topography.

## *Antipsychotics*

Subsequent to Lipman's (1970) seminal study, a number of other prevalence studies showed that about 40% to 50% of institutionalized individuals with mental retardation received antipsychotic drugs. However, there has been a major emphasis in recent years on reducing drug prescriptions for behavior problems in this population (Briggs, 1989; Findholt & Emmett, 1990; Poindexter, 1989), resulting in a considerable decline in these figures. For example, in a more recent national study of prescribed drugs in residential facilities, Hill et al. (1985) reported that only 30% of individuals in institutions were on antipsychotics. In another recent statewide prevalence study, it was found that only 27% of California's institutionalized developmentally disabled population were treated with antipsychotics (Stone, Alvarez, Ellman, Hom, & White, 1989). Comparative prevalence figures for individuals in community residential facilities are typically lower, ranging from 11% (Aman et al., 1985) to 29% (Intagliata & Rinck, 1985).

### Mode of Drug Action

Antipsychotic drugs act primarily at several subcortical brain sites, including the limbic system, hypothalamus, and brainstem. The known effects of the drugs include both reduction of neuronal levels of the second messenger cyclic adenosine monophosphate in brain regions associated with emotion and behavior and decrease of cortical sensory input to the reticular formation (Malseed & Harrigan, 1989, p. 500).

All chemical compounds with antipsychotic efficacy are thought to exert their major effect as a result of their ability to block dopamine (DA) receptors. Studies in Snyder's laboratory, utilizing a technique of direct labeling of dopamine receptors, have identified two physically distinct dopamine receptors within the brain (Snyder, 1981). The first of these, known as "$D_1$," is linked to adenylate cyclase, the enzyme that catalyzes the formation of cyclic AMP. The $D_1$ receptor is blocked by phenothiazines such as chlorpromazine, thioridazine and mesoridazine, in rough proportion to their clinical efficacy. However, haloperidol and other nonphenothiazine drugs, which are among the most potent antipsychotic agents, act only as weak inhibitors of the cyclase enzyme. The other type of dopamine receptor, referred to as "$D_2$," is not associated with adenylate cyclase and is labeled by tritiated butyrophenones such as $^3$H-haloperidol (Snyder, 1981). The clinical potency of all antipsychotic agents that have been studied thus far correlates well with the extent of $D_2$ receptor binding (Creese, Burt, & Snyder, 1976; Snyder, 1981). Other biochemical actions of these drugs that may contribute to antipsychotic efficacy include increasing dopamine turnover, inhibition of neuronal uptake of norepinephrine and serotonin, and suppression of acetylcholine release.

## Therapeutic Effects on Self-injury

### *Chlorpromazine*

In one of the earliest double-blind, crossover studies, Adamson, Nellis, Runge, Cleland, and Killian (1958) compared the effects of chlorpromazine, reserpine, their combination, and placebo on the severe behavior problems of 40 individuals with mental retardation. Although the level of their retardation was not specified, they were categorized as being "low-grade." The dosages ranged from 300 mg to 500 mg per day for chlorpromazine, 3 mg to 5 mg per day for reserpine, and 1.25 mg to 2.5 mg of reserpine in combination with 150 mg to 250 mg per day of chlorpromazine. Results showed that chlorpromazine alone was the most effective in controlling the severe behavior problems of the residents, followed by reserpine, and the combination, with the least effective being placebo. Given that most of the subjects had severe behavior problems, including self-injury, it can be concluded that chlorpromazine may play some role in the suppression of self-injury. However, the data were not presented in a manner that enables us to isolate the effects of chlorpromazine specifically on self-injury.

In another double-blind crossover study, Vaisanen, Kainulainen, Paavilainen, and Viukari (1975) evaluated the effects of sulpiride (150 to 300 mg/day), chlorpromazine (75 to 150 mg/day) and placebo on 60 individuals with moderate to profound levels of retardation. Self-injury was rated on a 5-point scale by the ward personnel. The results showed that, overall, sulpiride was more effective than chlorpromazine in reducing a range of behavior problems, but there was virtually no difference between the two drugs in relation to their effects on self-injury. Both drugs, however, were superior to placebo in reducing the rate of self-injury.

In a drug withdrawal study, Marholin, Touchette, and Stewart (1979) observed the behaviors of five adults who were severely mentally retarded, while they were on and off chlorpromazine. All had been on the drug for 6 to 12 years and, with the exception of one subject who was on a dosage of 800 mg/day (14.18 mg/kg), all subjects were on 200 mg/day. The only subject who exhibited self-injury showed an increase in the rate of this behavior when he was on chlorpromazine (3.36 mg/kg) but did not engage in self-injury when on placebo. In his case, the drug functioned to increase rather than control his self-injury.

In a drug-reduction study with 11 individuals with mental retardation who exhibited self-injury and other maladaptive behaviors, Schroeder, Rojahn, Hawk, Kanoy, Thios, Mulick, and Stephens (1982) reported a single case in which chlorpromazine was reduced from 400 mg/day to 200 mg/day. The systematic reductions in medication resulted in a temporary increase in self-injury over the 2-week period, immediately following dosage reduction, with the subsequent disappearance of the effect. Overall, there was no change in the rate of self-injury at half the dose, although there was a concomitant increase in stereotypy with the reduction in drug dosage.

In a single-subject study, Singh and Winton (1984) carried out detailed observations of the self-injurious behavior of a 15-year-old boy who was profoundly mentally retarded. He was sequentially treated with chlorpromazine, thioridazine, and carbamazepine. His rate of self-injury increased with the introduction of chlorpromazine (75 mg/day), decreased slightly when the dosage was doubled (150 mg/day), and then increased again when the dosage was increased to 300 mg/day.

Millichamp and Singh (1987) conducted a double-blind, placebo-controlled study to assess the effects of a drug-reduction schedule on stereotypy and collateral behaviors of six adults who were profoundly mentally retarded. Two of the six subjects had been on chlorpromazine (2.2 mg/kg and 3.0 mg/kg) for 6 years prior to the study. The others had been on methotrimeprazine for 3 to 6 years. All subjects had their medication reduced gradually by almost half. While there was individual variation across behaviors and subjects, the main finding was that despite the marked reduction in medication, there were no general changes of clinical significance in any of the behaviors. Of the two subjects who were on chlorpromazine, neither showed a clinically significant change in their rate of self-injury. These results are in accord with those of Schroeder et al. (1982).

In summary, the two earliest studies reported that chlorpromazine was effective in reducing self-injury in this population. However, more recent studies using rigorous methodologies indicate that chlorpromazine either has no effect or may in fact increase self-injury. The data are limited, and further research is needed to establish the efficacy of this drug in controlling self-injury.

### *Thioridazine*

Abbott, Blake, and Vince (1965) evaluated the effects of three doses of thioridazine (75 mg/day, 150 mg/day, 300 mg/day) in an open trial on the problem behaviors of 141 individuals with mild to profound mental retardation. Problem behaviors included aggression, hyperactivity, temper tantrums, and property destruction, as well as self-injury. About 34% of the subjects showed a marked improvement on medication, particularly in their levels of self-injury, hyperactivity, and temper tantrums; 55% showed some improvement; and 11% showed no change in their problem behavior. In addition, there was a strong correlation with IQ, with greater improvement being evident in those with lower IQs.

Llorente (1969) evaluated the effects of thioridazine (150–300 mg/day) in a retrospective study of 65 individuals who had mental retardation that ranged from mild to profound, and were between ages 7 and 63 years. The results showed a statistically significant reduction in self-injury when behavioral ratings of the subjects taken before and after drug treatment were compared. These findings must be cautiously interpreted because the data were collected retrospectively from the subjects' medical case notes, and no experimental controls were used.

The comparative effects of thioridazine (1.3 mg/kg/day) and methylphenidate (0.44 mg/kg) were evaluated by Davis, Sprague, and Werry (1969) in a placebo-controlled, crossover study with nine individuals, diagnosed as profoundly mentally retarded. There was a clinically significant decrease in stereotypy—a class of behaviors that included several topographies of self-injury—with thioridazine but not with methylphenidate.

Vaisanen, Rimon, Raisanen and Viukari (1979) and Vaisanen, Viukari, Rimon, and Raisanen (1981) conducted a double-blind crossover study of the comparative effects of thioridazine (up to 600 mg/day) and haloperidol (up to 60 mg/day) with 30 individuals who were moderately and severely mentally retarded. Initiation of thioridazine following placebo increased the subjects' self-injury during the first 2 weeks, which then decreased slightly, but never below levels observed during the initial placebo condition. Although no statistical data were provided, a visual inspection of the data suggests that similar results were observed with haloperidol.

Singh and Aman (1981) compared the effects of two doses of thioridazine on the stereotypy and collateral behavior of 19 individuals with severe mental retardation in a double-blind, placebo-controlled crossover study. A low standardized dose (2.5 mg/kg/day) and the subjects' previous individualized doses (mean dose of 5.23 mg/kg/day) were compared against a placebo condition. Both active drug conditions caused a reduction in hyperactivity, bizarre behavior, and self-stimulation, but there were no significant therapeutic differences between the two doses. There was a small but statistically insignificant reduction in the subjects' rate of self-injury.

Heistad, Zimmerman, and Doebler (1982) conducted a double-blind, placebo-controlled crossover study of thiorizadine in 106 individuals, about half of whom were profoundly mentally retarded. The primary target symptoms were aggression, self-injury, yelling and screaming. Thioridazine caused a moderate suppression of inappropriate target behaviors, including self-injury, and a nonsignificant increase in prosocial behaviors. The most notable effect was an increase of about 18% in self-stimultion during the placebo condition.

Jakab (1984) evaluated the short-term effects of thioridazine tablets versus thioridazine in suspension on the behavior problems of 10 children who were diagnosed as emotionally disturbed, with mild to profound levels of mental retardation. This study was designed to compare the children's pre- and postmedication behavior on a daily basis, using a single-subject reversal design (Singh & Beale, 1986). The behaviors of interest were aggression, disruptive tantrumming, self-injury, stereotyped self-stimulation, and pica. There was no difference between the effects of thioridazine tablet and suspension. In the short term, both forms of thioridazine (mean dose of 3.44 mg/kg/day; range 2.14–5.71 mg/kg) were effective in reducing all target behavior problems, including self-injury. However, because this was not really an efficacy study employing placebo controls, no data on individual target behaviors were reported, although there was an overall average symptom reduction of 27.4% within 35 minutes following medication intake.

Schroeder and Gualtieri (1985) evaluated the effects of rapid or gradual withdrawal of drugs, primarily thioridazine, in a sample of 23 individuals with profound mental retardation. Direct behavioral observations showed a differential effect on the subjects' self-injury that depended on whether they were in school or in the dayroom. There was no consistent effect on the very low rate of self-injury that occurred in the dayroom, but a much higher rate was observed in the classroom after both abrupt and gradual drug withdrawal conditions. This study highlighted the need to assess the complex interactions that may occur between drugs and the environment.

In the final study, 11 individuals with moderate to profound mental retardation receiving long-term thioridazine treatment were studied while receiving their baseline dose (0.45 mg/kg–4.11 mg/kg/day), standardized low (1.25 mg/kg) and high doses (2.5 mg/kg/day), and placebo (Aman & White, 1988). The results showed that ratings of self-injury were significantly lower on the higher dose (2.5 mg/kg) when compared to the lower dose (1.25 mg/kg) of thioridazine. However, no significant drug effects were detected when all four experimental conditions were compared. Aman and White (1988) suggested that this might have been due to increased variability in one of the other conditions.

In summary, although the results are mixed, the better-controlled studies do suggest that thioridazine may be effective in controlling the self-injury of some individuals with mental retardation. In addition, there is some suggestion in the dose–response literature that a dose of 2.5 mg/kg/day may prove to be the most efficacious.

### *Haloperidol*

In a double-blind, placebo-controlled study, Burk and Menolascino (1968) evaluated the effects of haloperidol (0.2 mg to 7.8 mg/day) on the problem behaviors of 50 individuals with moderate mental retardation. Target problem behaviors included hyperactivity, aggression, impulsivity, and self-injury. The results showed haloperidol to be superior to placebo in controlling all target behaviors, including self-injury.

Similar results were obtained by Le Vann (1969) in an open trial of haloperidol (average dose of 3.1mg/day) on 100 institutionalized children and adolescents (54 with mental retardation, 46 with behavioral disorders) who exhibited hyperactivity, aggression, and self-injury. Although it was not reported how many subjects initially engaged in self-injury, 34 subjects decreased their self-injury while on haloperidol.

In another open trial, Grabowski (1973) reported an evaluation of haloperidol (final titrated dosage unspecified) on 148 individuals with mental retardation. Although the methodology used and the reporting of the data were very poor, the author reported major reductions in hyperactivity, and improvements in social behavior, concentration, and "emotion" while the subjects were on haloperidol. Two illustrative case presentations reported major reductions in self-injury as well.

In the previously described studies, Vaisenan et al. (1979, 1981) compared the effects of thioridazine and haloperidol and reported an increase in the rate of self-injury while the subjects were on haloperidol, probably due to the very high doses of the drug (60 mg/day). Similar results were reported for thioridazine.

Durand (1982) used a single-subject withdrawal design to evaluate the effects of haloperidol alone (4 mg/day) and in combination with a punishment procedure, and the punishment procedure alone in the control of self-injury in a 17-year-old man with profound mental retardation. Self-injury increased while the subject was on haloperidol or punishment alone but decreased when the two procedures were combined. Durand (1982) suggested that haloperidol may have acted as a "setting event" for the successful use of the punishment procedure. However, as noted by Schroeder (1988), these results are counterintuitive because neuroleptics tend to disrupt rather than facilitate conditioned avoidance learning and, in addition, have little effect on punished responding. Further, this study was not placebo controlled. These data must be treated with great caution.

Anderson, Campbell, Grega, Perry, Small, and Green (1984) carried out a double-blind, placebo-controlled study of haloperidol (0.019–0.217 mg/kg/day) in 40 children with autism. Target behaviors included a range of behavioral symptoms, clinical indices, and discrimination learning. The results showed a significant decrease in behavioral symptoms, general clinical improvement, and facilitation and reten tion of discrimination learning on haloperidol. Although only 6 of the 40 children engaged in self-injury when they were on placebo, suggesting that haloperidol had a suppressive effect on self-injury in these children, we do not know how many children initially engaged in self-injury, the topography of their self-injury, or the motivation(s) for their self-injury.

Luiselli, Evans, and Boyce (1986) successfully eliminated the use of haloperidol in an 11-year-old boy while concurrently instituting a behavioral treatment program for self-injury. Although the self-injurious behavior was unaffected by medication, haloperidol was reinstated at a low dose after the boy's communication skills had deteriorated when he was not on medication.

Mikkelsen (1986) reported on the effects of low-dose haloperidol (0.25 mg to 6 mg/day) on the self-injurious behavior of six adults with severe mental retardation. All subjects had received behavioral treatments, and four of the six also had been on various medications for their self-injury. Low-dose haloperidol eliminated self-injury in all four subjects with whom other drugs have proven ineffective, and it reduced self-injury to very low levels in the other two subjects. This was an uncontrolled study, and the data should be interpreted with appropriate caution.

Grossett and Williams (1988) investigated the effects of haloperidol (3 mg/day) alone and in combination with a differential reinforcement procedure (DRO) to control the self-injurious behavior of a woman diagnosed as profoundly mentally retarded with atypical psychoses. Haloperidol caused a major reduction of her self-injury, but only when the treatment was combined with a DRO procedure did she increase her participation in daily programs, activities, and on-task behaviors. Follow-up at 2 years showed that she remained free of self-injury.

Finally, in the most recent study, Aman, Teehan, White, Turbott, and Vaithianathan (1989) conducted a double-blind, placebo-controlled, crossover study of two doses of haloperidol (0.025 mg and 0.05 mg/kg/day) with 20 individuals who had moderate to severe mental retardation. Among other main effects, the results showed that self-injury decreased under both active medication conditions when compared to placebo, with greater reduction being evident at the lower dose of haloperidol. However, the effects were reversed for stereotypy, with greater reduction being evident at the higher dose. These are interesting dose-dependent findings that must await replication before general conclusions can be drawn.

In summary, there is some indication from these studies that haloperidol may have therapeutic effects on self-injury, particularly at low doses. In addition, if this finding is to be used clinically, clinicians may wish to monitor the rate of stereotypy in their clients because the Aman et al. (1989) data suggest that stereotypy and self-injury are controlled at different doses of haloperidol. Given that better controlled recent studies indicate that haloperidol may be effective in controlling self-injury, further research focused specifically on intractable cases of self-injury should be undertaken to provide the scientific basis for such treatment.

### Miscellaneous Antipsychotics

There are a number of studies, generally uncontrolled or anecdotal, that have investigated the effects of miscellaneous antipsychotics on the self-injurious behavior of individuals with mental retardation. These are briefly discussed in the hope that future research on these drugs may provide more definitive data on their usefulness.

*Mesoridazine*

The effects of mesoridazine on self-injurious and other behaviors were evaluated in two uncontrolled studies. In one, mesoridazine (75 mg to 300 mg/day) was given to a group of 49 individuals who had moderate mental retardation (Zaleski, 1970). An 8-week drug trial showed that all problem behaviors (e.g., aggression, tantrums, destruction), including self-injury, were significantly reduced. In the other, mesoridazine (75 mg to 300 mg/day) was administered to 45 young adults diagnosed as severely or profoundly mentally retarded (Lacny, 1973). The results were similar to those reported for the earlier study, including a statistically significant decrease in self-injury. Both studies suffered from major methodological problems, and these results should be taken as preliminary and only suggestive of the effects of this drug, pending more rigorous evaluation.

*Droperidol*

Burns (1980) reported a trial of droperidol (10–60 mg/day), a butyrophenone closely related to haloperidol, with 16 individuals with mental retardation who engaged in a variety of problem behaviors, including self-injury. Some of the patients who engaged in self-injury were reported to have improved on droperidol. However, this was an uncontrolled study.

*Pipamperon*

Haegeman and Duyck (1978) reported a trial of pipamperon (40–180 mg/day), a butyrophenone derivative, with 19 young adults diagnosed as severely mentally retarded. Some improvements were noted across most of the problem behaviors, including self-injury. Again, this was an uncontrolled trial of the drug, and the data must be interpreted with caution.

*Reserpine*

As discussed previously, the comparative effects of reserpine, chlorpromazine, and their combination were evaluated against a placebo in a study by Adamson et al. (1958). There were some global clinical changes in a number of problem behaviors, including self-injury, that could be attributed to reserpine.

*Loxapine Succinate*

Varga and Simpson (1971) evaluated the effects of loxapine, a dibenzoxazepine derivative, on the behavior of 16 individuals, half of whom were mentally retarded and the other half, schizophrenic. Subjects were on a wide range of doses, and it was found that subjects who were schizophrenic showed the greatest improvement. There was no reported change in the self-injury of any subject.

*Summary*

There is some literature on miscellaneous antipsychotics suggestive of their efficacy in treating self-injury, but the data are simply not strong enough to warrant recommendation for clinical use at this time.

## Side Effects of Antipsychotics

Although the antipsychotics include several compounds from different structural classes that are all very similar in their actions, the side effect profiles for each structural class and for the individual antipsychotics within these classes are somewhat different. The majority of the adverse effects, some of which are potentially life-threatening and irreversible, are directly related to the pharmacologic actions of the individual antipsychotic agents.

*Central Nervous System (CNS)*

There are several neuromuscular (extrapyramidal) syndromes that may result from antipsychotic use, especially the high-potency agents such as haloperidol. Acute dystonia (a Parkinsonian syndrome very similar to idiopathic Parkinsonism), malignant neuroleptic syndrome, and akathesia are extrapyramidal syndromes that usually appear concomitantly with the initiation of antipsychotic drugs. Tardive dyskinesia and perioral tremor (a rare extrapyramidal reaction) tend to appear after prolonged treatment. Autonomic nervous system (anticholinergic) effects, including blurred vison, dry mouth, priapism, ejaculatory disorders, and constipation, may also present as adverse effects. Sedation is another side effect common to antipsychotics and is highest with the lower potency agents, although transient drowsiness also can be seen after the initiation of treatment with the higher-potency antipsychotics. Cognitive blunting and fatigue unrelated to the sedative side effects of the medications are other common adverse effects. Psychotic symptoms, confusion, and excitement are rare side effects of antipsychotics.

*Cardiovascular*

EKG changes consisting of abnormal T-waves are frequently seen in individuals on antipsychotic drugs, especially thioridazine and mesoridazine. Orthostatic hypotension is a common side effect, which appears to be more pronounced with chlorpromazine.

*Endocrine*

Menstrual irregularities and galactorrhea in females, and gynecomastia, decreased libido, and impotence in males, and the syndrome of inappropriate ADH secretion in both are side effects of many of the antipsychotics. Weight gain is a common side effect that is, however, not a problem with loxapine.

*Other*

Skin photosensitivity, blood dyscrasias, impaired liver functions and/or jaundice, ocular complications, allergic reactions, and symptoms of gastrointestinal distress are other occasional complications of the various antipsychotics.

## *Stimulants*

The stimulants are not very widely used in individuals who are mentally retarded (Chandler, Gualtieri, & Fahs, 1988). Lipman (1970) reported that less than 3% of institutionalized individuals with mental retardation were prescribed stimulants. Recent surveys of institutions show even lower drug prescription rates for stimulants: 0% (Briggs, 1989; Poindexter, 1989), 0.4% (Hill et al., 1985), and 1.2% (Intagliata & Rinck, 1985). Similar figures have been reported from community surveys: 0.3% (Intagliata & Rinck, 1985) and 1.0% (Hill et al., 1985), although Gadow (1985) has reported 5.5% and 3.4% for students with mild and moderate mental retardation, respectively, who attended public schools in Illinois.

### Mode of Drug Action

Methylphenidate is a CNS stimulant that has a mechanism of action that is not fully understood. Its pharmacologic profile of action resembles that of amphetamine but has a more marked effect on mental rather than physical or motor activities at therapeutic doses. Thus, methylphenidate is assumed to both stimulate the release and inhibit the uptake of the catecholamines norepinephrine and dopamine at the nerve terminals. The net increase in these catecholamines induced by the drug, together with its direct stimulation of postsynaptic receptor sites, is thought to mediate its observed clinical effects (Tesar, 1982).

### Therapeutic Effects on Self-injury

The effects of stimulants on self-injury have been evaluated in two well-controlled studies. As discussed previously, Davis et al. (1969) reported a comparative study of the effects of methylphenidate (0.44 mg/kg), thioridazine (1.3 mg/kg), and placebo on nine males who were profoundly mentally retarded. There was no apparent effect on self-injury. In a dose–response study, Aman and Singh (1982) evaluated the effects of two doses of methylphenidate (0.3 mg/kg, 0.6 mg/kg) on the behavior of 28 adolescents and adults who were severely or profoundly mentally retarded. When compared to placebo, a small but statistically insignificant reduction in self-injury was observed under the high dose.

These two studies suggest that stimulants may not be indicated as a drug of choice for treating self-injury in individuals who are mentally retarded, particularly the severely or profoundly retarded.

### Side Effects

Given that the research on stimulants has focused only on methylphenidate, this section focuses on the side effects of this drug. The majority of the adverse effects associated with methylphenidate are short term and dose related.

#### *Gastrointestinal*

Anorexia with subsequent weight loss and abdominal pain are frequently reported, although these are usually transient effects. Nausea, vomiting, constipation and dryness of the mouth are other adverse gastrointestinal effects associated with both the central and peripheral actions of methylphenidate.

#### *Central Nervous System*

Irritability, nervousness, fatigue, dizziness, alteration of mood (including dysphoria), and insomnia have been frequently reported. Although uncommon, the precipitation of psychotic or psychoticlike symptoms, and the worsening of preexisting stereotyped or compulsive behaviors also has been noted. Methylphenidate usage appears to exacerbate and/or precipitate motor and phonic tics, as well as other dyskinesias, in a small percentage of patients.

#### *Cardiovascular*

Changes in baseline pulse rates and blood pressure are uncommon findings. Palpitations and arrhythmias also have been reported.

#### *Others*

A clinically insignificant slowing of height gain, probably due to an alteration in cartilage metabolism that is related to dose and duration of treatment, has been reported in some children treated with methylphenidate. A return to within 1% of projected height can be expected by adulthood or following withdrawal of long-term medication.

## *Anxiolytics*

In Lipman's (1970) survey, anxiolytics (chlordiazepoxide and diazepam) were prescribed for about 8% of institutionalized individuals with mental retardation. Prevalence studies from the mid-1980s reported a somewhat higher rate of 9.4% (Intagliata & Rinck, 1985) and 12.7% (Hill et al., 1985), but recent studies of institutional drug prescriptions have reported prevalence rates of only 6% (Poindexter, 1989) and 3% (Stone et al., 1989). The prevalence rates in community settings have varied between 2% and 12% (Aman et al., 1985; Fox & Westling, 1986; Hill et al., 1985; Intagliata & Rinck, 1985).

## Mode of Drug Action

The benzodiazepines, which include diazepam and chlordiazepoxide, potentiate the action of gamma-aminobutyric acid (GABA), the major inhibitory neurotransmitter in the CNS, by increasing neuronal membrane permeability to chloride ions (Insel, Ninan, Aloi, Jimerson, Skolnick, & Paul, 1984; Skolnick & Paul, 1983). The entry of chloride ions into the neurons leads to a greater membrane hyperpolarization (a less excitable state), diminished synaptic transmission and membrane stabilization. The benzodiazepines appear to act at several subcortical brain sites, most notably the limbic system and the reticular formation. Higher cortical function is largely unaffected by therapeutic doses of these drugs.

## Therapeutic Effects on Self-injury

As noted by Singh and Winton (1989), only a few studies have investigated the effects of anxiolytics on the behavior of individuals with mental retardation. In the only study that included self-injury as a variable, Galambos (1965) evaluated the effects of diazepam (2 mg to 105 mg/day) on a number of behaviors of 42 adults with moderate to profound mental retardation. Of the 7 residents who engaged in self-injury, all showed a marked improvement with the introduction of diazepam. Little can be concluded from this study, however, because it was totally uncontrolled and had other methodological problems (e.g., no standardized ratings or inferential statistics were used).

## Side Effects

The most commonly experienced side effects of diazepam are related to the CNS-depressant properties of the drug.

### *Central Nervous System*

Fatigue, drowsiness, and ataxia are the most commonly reported adverse effects. Blurred vision, diplopia, headaches, slurred speech, and tremor have also been noted. Paradoxical reactions of behavioral and central nervous system disinhibition featuring overexcitement, hyperactivity, increased aggression or rage outbursts, anxiety, hallucinations, increased muscle spasticity and sleep disturbances have been seen.

### *Gastrointestinal*

Infrequently occurring adverse effects include constipation, nausea, and changes in salivation.

### *Abuse*

There is a potential for the development of physical and psychological dependency with diazepam usage.

### *Other*

Hematologic abnormalities including leukopenia, thrombocytopenia, and agranulocytosis are rare but have been reported. Incontinence, urinary retention, dysarthria, skin rashes, impairment of sexual function, and weight gain are other uncommon adverse effects of diazepam.

## *Antimanics*

The antimanics, mainly lithium carbonate, have not been widely used in either residential or community settings, with most prevalence studies reporting rates less than 1% (Hill et al., 1985; Intagliata & Rinck, 1985). Two studies, however, have reported rather high prevalence rates. Martin and Agran (1985) reported a prevalence of 8% in one community setting, and Poindexter (1989) reported 13% in a residential facility.

### Mode of Drug Action

It is difficult to assign a specific mechanism of action to lithium because of its many and varied pharmacological properties. Currently, an effect of lithium on modulation of neurotransmitter function, the endocrine system, circadian rhythms, and cellular processes are though to be the likely explanations for its therapeutic action.

Lithium has been shown to interact with catecholamine (norepinephrine and dopamine) and serotonin systems as well as cholinergic transmission. In the CNS, it decreases release and increases neuronal reuptake of norepinephrine, the neurotransmitter thought to be most influential in the causation of primary affective disorders (Ortiz, Dabbagh, & Gershon, 1984). Furthermore, lithium's ability to block dopamine receptor sensitivity concurs with the view that the onset of mania may be associated with a supersensitivity of dopamine receptors. It is known that lithium blocks the release of thyroid hormones, which may potentiate beta-adrenergic activity. This has led to the suggestion that thyroid hormones may precipitate an episode of mania in susceptible individuals and that lithium's antimanic effect can be attributed to its antithyroid actions (Janicak & Vadis, 1987). Studies on biological rhythms have shown that changes in circadian rhythms of sleep, temperature, and hormones can be associated with bipolar disorders. From the available data, it has been postulated that lithium lengthens and resynchronizes the circadian rhythms.

Because of many physicochemical similarities, lithium is able to partially substitute for sodium and potassium, and to a lesser extent, calcium and magnesium in a number of physiological functions. Distribution of ions across cell membranes are disrupted during manic–depressive episodes (Naylor, Dick, Dick, & Moody, 1974), and lithium appears to produce its therapeutic effect in part by modulating cation movement and by restoring ionic gradients across cell membranes.

### Therapeutic Effects on Self-injury

In an early case report, Cooper and Fowlie (1973) treated a 27-year-old woman, diagnosed as severely mentally retarded, with lithium carbonate (serum level 0.9 mEq/l). She had a 9-year history of self-injury and hyperactivity. Informal clinical assessment showed that she became quiet, docile, and cooperative within 1 week of being on lithium. In addition, her self-injury ceased and her chronically ulcerated hands healed. Not self-injury was observed during a 5-year follow-up period.

Micev and Lynch (1974) evaluated the effects of lithium carbonate (0.6–1.4 mEq/l) on the self-injurious and aggressive behavior of 10 adults with severe mental retardation. Six of 8 subjects ceased their self-injurious behavior, 1 showed some improvement, and the other showed no change. However, all subjects became less irritable, more cooperative, and developed increased social tolerance.

Sovner and Hurley (1981) reported two case studies, one of which involved a 44-year-old woman who was severely mentally retarded and engaged in hyperactivity, sleeplessness, and self-injury. It was reported that her hyperactivity significantly decreased while on lithium carbonate (1.0 mEq/l), but no specific mention was made of its effects on her self-injury.

In a double-blind crossover study, Tyrer, Walsh, Edwards, Berney, and Stephens (1984) evaluated the effects of lithium carbonate (0.5–0.8 mEq/l) on 26 adults with mental retardation. Seventeen of the 26 subjects showed some improvement in their rate of self-injury when compared to placebo.

Amin and Yeragani (1987) reported a case study of a 48-year-old woman with mental retardation who engaged in a high rate of aggressive and self-injurious behaviors and had to be in physical restraints. After 3 weeks on lithium carbonate (0.9 to 1.2 mEq/l), her aggression and self-injury ceased, and she began responding socially. She no longer required physical restraint.

Finally, in a retrospective analysis of case records, Luchins and Dojka (1989) reported that of the 11 adults with mild to profound levels of mental retardation treated with lithium carbonate (0.6 to 0.95 mEq/l), 8 showed a decrease in their rate of self-injury. Of the 3 who showed no improvement, 2 were profoundly retarded, and 1 was severely retarded.

In summary, there are several case studies of the effects of lithium carbonate on the self-injurious behavior of individuals with mental retardation. While these results suggest that lithium carbonate may be useful, the lack of well-controlled studies is a major problem. In addition to efficacy studies, future research efforts should be directed at predictors of drug response in this population.

## Side Effects

Lithium toxicity is directly related to elevated serum lithium levels, although frequently there are other untoward effects of lithium within the therapeutic range. These side effects may appear at varying times after the initiation of lithium therapy.

### *Gastrointestinal*

Mild and transient nausea is commonly experienced within the first few days of beginning lithium therapy. Anorexia, vomiting, and diarrhea also are occasionally reported.

### *Neuromuscular*

A fine hand tremor may appear during the initial treatment phase, which can persist throughout the course of lithium therapy. Muscle hyperirritability, weakness, and ataxia also are less commonly seen.

### *Endocrine*

Reported thyroid abnormalities in patients treated with lithium include euthyroid goiter formation and, less commonly, hypothyroidism. Weight gain is frequently seen secondary to lithium usage, as is transient edema and sodium retention following the initiation of therapy.

### *Renal*

Early effects of lithium on the distal renal tubule and excessive free-water clearance frequently result in polyuria and polydipsia. A usually reversible diabetes insipidus of nephrogenic origin may also be seen. Up to one fourth of patients treated with long-term lithium therapy may develop a nephropathy characterized by a reduction in renal concentrating ability, with the degree of damage to the renal interstitium dependent on the duration of treatment and the serum lithium concentrations.

### *Central Nervous System*

Sedation, irritability, headache, subtle cogwheel rigidity, EEG abnormalities, psychomotor retardation, confusion, and slurred speech are all occasional untoward effects of lithium treatment. Although rare, pseudotumor cerebri also has been reported.

### *Other*

Orthostatic hypotension, EKG abnormalities, cardiac arrhythmias, allergic reactions including dermatitis and vasculitis, transient scotomata, and metallic taste are other less commonly seen adverse effects.

## *Antidepressants*

Up to 4% of institutionalized individuals with mental retardation have been prescribed antidepressants (Hill et al., 1985; Lipman, 1970), although recent studies indicate that this rate may be decreasing. For example, two recent studies reported prevalence rates of 2.6% (Stone et al., 1989) and 2%(Poindexter, 1989). The prevalence rates for community samples range from 1% to 6% (Aman et al., 1985; Hill et al., 1985; Intagliata & Rinck, 1985).

### Mode of Drug Action

Tricyclic antidepressants inhibit neuronal uptake of norepinephrine and serotonin into presynaptic nerve endings, thereby blocking a major mechanism of their inactivation and enhancing their pharmacological effects. They also exert a blocking effect on presynaptic alpha-adrenergic receptors, which results in increasd neurotransmitter release from nerve endings. The increased amount of available neurotransmitters results in a decrease in the number and sensitivity of the adrenergic and serotonergic receptor sites by the process of downregulation of receptors. The clinical efficacy of these agents is now thought to be primarily due to the reduced responsiveness of these receptors in the CNS (Malseed & Harrigan, 1989, p. 536).

### Therapeutic Effects on Self-injury

No empirical data on the effects of antidepressants in the treatment of self-injurious behavior of individuals with mental retardation are available in the published literature. However, Huessy and Ruoff (1984) have anecdotally reported the success of tricyclic antidepressants in controlling self-injury, as well as mood, unpredictable behavior, aggression, and problems in attention span, in this population.

### Side Effects

Tricyclic antidepressants are associted with a spectrum of adverse effects, the specific profiles of which vary among the individual tricyclics and their slightly different pharmacologic properties.

#### *Anticholinergic*

The most frequently reported side effects associated with all tricyclic antidepressants are related to the anticholinergic effects, including dry mouth, constipation, blurred vision, and occasional urinary retention. These symptoms are usually transient and improve with a reduction in the drug dosage. First-generation tricyclic antidepressants (e.g., imipramine) are more likely to produce these adverse anticholinergic effects than the newer products (e.g., trazodone).

*Cardiovascular*

Orthostatic hypotension, delayed cardiac conduction with mild increases in the P-R and Q-R-S intervals, arrhythmias, and heart block are potential untoward effects of tricyclic antidepressant usage. In addition, the autonomic effects of the compounds may cause tachycardia and an increase in diastolic blood pressure, especially in patients with preexisting hypertension.

*Central Nervous System*

A lowering of the seizure threshold may be seen with any antidepressant. A rare worsening of preexisting EEG abnormalities has been reported with imipramine. Mental confusion, sedation, anxiety and agitation, insomnia, and the precipitation of the psychosis, including mania (which may actually represent true psychopathology rather than a drug effect) also have been described.

*Dermatologic*

Skin rashes are occasionally associated with the use of tricyclic antidepressants. These rashes may represent actual allergic responses to the active antidepressant compounds themselves or to tartazine, the FD&C Yellow No. 5 dye frequently incorporated into some formulations.

*Endocrine*

Gynecomastia in males using tricyclic antidepressants, along with breast enlargement and galactorrhea in females are potential adverse effects.

*Other*

Nausea and vomiting, anorexia, liver function abnormalities, jaundice (simulating obstruction), peripheral neurologic symptoms and bone-marrow depression including agranulocytosis all have been reported in association with tricyclic antidepressant usage.

## Other Drugs

A number of other drugs have been used in the specific treatment of self-injurious behavior of individuals with mental retardation. Indeed, some of the best work in the psychopharmacology of self-injury has been undertaken with these drugs.

### Opiate Antagonists (Naloxone and Naltrexone)

No prevalence data on the use of opiate antagonists is available.

## Mode of Drug Action

Opiate antagonists were formerly thought to act through their ability both to combine with the same receptor as do endogenous and exogenous opioid agonists and to displace them from the receptor sites. However, it is now known that the effects of opioids are mediated by multiple opioid receptors, namely, mu-, kappa-, and delta-receptors. The affinity of the opiate antagonists naloxone and naltrexone for the mu-receptors is 10- to 20-fold greater than for kappa- or delta-receptors (Martin, Jasinski, & Mansky, 1984). The fact that these drugs have preferential affinity for mu-receptors and that they can reduce or eliminate self-injury suggests that maintenance of self-injury may be mediated by mu-receptors.

Naloxone and naltrexone are viewed as pure antagonists because they have no analgesic activity of their own. They have little or no effect when administered to resting animals because endogenous opioid systems are relatively inactive under normal circumstances (Holaday, 1985). Naloxone is a rapid-acting drug given parenterally to reverse (or prevent) the effects of opioid drugs, especially in the case of overdosage. It is capable of reversing many of the important effects of opioid drugs, including euphoria, analgesia, sedation, hypotension, respiratory depression, increase in cerebrospinal fluid pressure, miosis, and smooth-muscle spasm (Craig & Stitzel, 1990). Naltrexone is virtually identical to naloxone in its profile of activity but has a much longer half-life and is better absorbed when given by mouth.

## Therapeutic Effects on Self-injury

The genesis of the idea that self-injurious individuals may be addicted to their own endorphins and that opioid antagonists could be used to block the reinforcing effects of pain-induced release of endorphins was apparently first suggested by Richardson in 1979 (Richardson, personal communication, November, 1988). This hypothesis posits that self-injury itself causes the release of endogenous opioid ligands that attenuate pain. Thus, to maintain a state of self-reinforcement that is generated by the self-injury through the release of endogenous opioids, the person has to continue engaging in self-injury. A related formulation, the pain hypothesis, posits that "abnormalities in the endogenous opiate system results in an elevated pain threshold [which leads to] a reduced responsiveness to normal sensory stimulation" (Konicki & Schulz, 1989, p. 560). The treatment of choice suggested by these mutually nonexclusive hypotheses is the administration of an opioid antagonist.

The first trials of an opioid antagonist in the treatment of self-injury was undertaken in 1980 by Richardson and Zaleski, as well as by Sandman and his colleagues, although data from both trials were not published until 1983. The early trials of opioid antagonists used naloxone, but later trials used naltrexone. The literature on naloxone is reviewed first, followed by that on naltrexone.

*Naloxone*

Richardson and Zaleski (1983, 1986a, 1986b) reported an open, uncontrolled trial of naloxone (1 mg and 2 mg) with a 15-year-old boy who had a 12-year history of high-rate self-injury. The drug was dissolved in 30 ml of normal saline and given intravenously over a 6-hour period each day. When compared to predrug baseline, the frequency of self-injury increased during the administration of naloxone but decreased substantially in the evenings when the drug was discontinued. Furthermore, this effect endured for at least 2 days following the termination of the trial. Increased self-injury during drug administration was explained by the authors in terms of extinction of the reinforced response.

Sandman, Datta, Barron, Hoehler, Williams, and Swanson (1983) undertook a double-blind, crossover trial of naloxone (0.1 mg, 0.2 mg, 0.4 mg) with two adults who were profoundly mentally retarded. The suppressive effect of naloxone was very rapid, occurring within the first 10 minutes, but diminished by about 60 to 70 minutes after administration of the drug. However, unlike the previous study, there was no sign of an extinction burst of self-injury with either subject.

In a double-blind study, Davidson, Kleene, Carroll, and Rockowitz (1983) evaluated the effects of two doses of naloxone (0.15 mg and 0.075 mg) and a placebo with an 8-year-old boy who was severely mentally retarded. There was no clear effect of the drug on the boy's self-injury when compared to the predrug baseline or the placebo conditions. However, anecdotal observations suggested that while the rate of self-injury did not decrease, the actual intensity of the behavior did.

Sandyk (1985) reported a case study of the use of naloxone to control self-injury in an 11-year-old boy with mental retardation. Two studies were undertaken with this boy. In the first, after 1.2 mg of naloxone was administered intramuscularly as a bolus injection, self-injury ceased within 15 minutes of each of three administrations. In the second study, the same dosage was used but within a double-blind, placebo-controlled design. As in the open trial, self-injury ceased within 10 to 15 minutes of administration of the active drug but remained at high levels during placebo. In a further study, Gillman and Sandyk (1985) investigated the effects of naloxone (1.2 mg, i.m.) on the tics and self-injury of a 17-year-old man with Tourette's syndrome. Self-injury ceased within 10 minutes of administration of the active drug but remained at high levels during placebo.

The effects of three doses of naloxone (0.1 mg, 0.2 mg, 0.4 mg) and placebo were evaluated in a double-blind study on the self-injury of two women with profound mental retardation (Beckwith, Couk, & Schumacher, 1986). Naloxone did not affect the rate of self-injury, and no dose-dependent effects were observed. However, there appeared to be a placebo effect with one subject, who showed a decreasing trend in the rate of her self-injury. This study failed to replicate the results reported by Sandman et al. (1983), who used the same doses of naloxone.

Bernstein, Hughes, Mitchell, and Thompson (1987) attempted to replicate the findings reported by Richardson and Zaleski (1983), with an 18-year-old man who was severely mentally retarded and had engaged in self-injury for about 16 years. They used two doses of naloxone (0.5 mg and 1.0 mg) but gave the drug as a bolus injection every 30 minutes instead of a continuous drip, as used in the earlier study. There was a transient increase in self-injury following the first injection of 0.5 mg of naloxone, but this gradually decreased to below baseline level. The decreased level of self-injury was maintained for about 30 hours and then returned to baseline levels. There did not appear to be a dose-dependent correlation with self-injury. This patient was subsequently included in a trial of naltrexone (see next subsection).

In the most recent study, Barrett, Feinstein and Hole (1990) used a double-blind, placebo-controlled design to evaluate the effects of two doses of naloxone (0.2 mg and 0.4 mg) on the behavior of a 12-year-old girl who was moderately mentally retarded. The two doses, together with a placebo, were given within an alternating-treatments design (see Singh & Beale, 1986). When compared to the placebo condition, there was no significant decrease in self-injury under either active drug condition.

In summary, if these studies are taken in their best light, just over half reported a decrease in self-injury with the use of naloxone. However, the studies that reported positive outcomes were also the ones that typically lacked methodological rigor, with the better controlled studies suggesting little effect. Obviously, further research is necessary to resolve the question of treatment outcome with this drug.

### *Naltrexone*

Herman and her colleagues (Herman et al., 1985, 1986, 1987) reported an evaluation of the effects of naltrexone on the self-injury of three adolescents, two of whom were profoundly mentally retarded and the other had Tourette's syndrome. They were tested on placebo, and on 0.5, 1.0, 1.5, and 2.0 mk/kg of naltrexone. When compared to placebo, the initial three doses produced marked reductions in self-injury in all three subjects. The highest dose (2.0 mg/kg) was tested only on two subjects, and both showed no reduction in their rate of self-injury.

Bernstein et al. (1987) reported a double-blind, placebo-controlled trial of three doses of naltrexone (12.5, 25, and 50 mg/day) on the self-injury of an 18-year-old man with severe mental retardation. Self-injury decreased under the active drug conditions in a dose-dependent manner, with the largest decrease being evident under the highest dose (50 mg/

day). Further, the reduction in self-injury persisted after the active drug was stopped. This was probably due to the drug metabolites or prolonged endorphin-receptor blockade.

Szymanski, Kedesdy, Sulkes, Cutler, and Stevens-Orr (1987) used a double-blind, placebo controlled, withdrawal design to evaluate the effects of naltrexone (50 mg/day) on the self-injury of two young adults who were severely mentally retarded. In addition, one subject received a dose of 100 mg of naltrexone. No difference between the active drug, baseline, and placebo was reported in terms of the rate of self-injury in either subject. Further, no systematic changes were observed in several collateral behaviors as a function of the experimental conditions.

LeBoyer, Bouvard, and Dugas (1988) reported an open and acute dose trial of naltrexone (1.0, 1.5, and 2.0 mg/kg) with two young girls with autism. Self-injury decreased at the lower doses (1.0 and 1.5 mg/kg), as in the Herman et al. (1987) studies but not at the higher dose (2.0 mg/kg). In addition, positive changes in collateral behaviors, such as in hyperactivity and social behavior, also were observed.

Campbell, Adams, Small, Tesch, and Curren (1988) reported another open, acute-dose range tolerance study with a group of eight boys with autism. The subjects were withdrawn, and they engaged in aggression and stereotypy. Four of them also exhibited mild to moderate levels of self-injury. Although this study was not directly concerned with the effects of naltrexone (0.5, 1.0, and 2.0 mk/kg/day) on self-injury, the results showed that there was a slight reduction in self-injury under the drug conditions. No dose-dependent relationship between self-injury and naltrexone was reported. Data from an ongoing, double-blind, placebo-controlled study of the effects of naltrexone in children with autism have been reported by the same group of investigators (Campbell, Anderson, Small, Locascio, Lynch, & Choroco, 1990), but no direct measure of self-injury has been included in their assessment battery in this study.

Luiselli, Beltis, and Bass (1989) reported a double-blind, placebo-controlled trial of the effects of naltrexone on multiple forms of self-injury in a 16-year-old adolescent boy with mental retardation. When assessed within a reversal design, naltrexone (50 mg/day) failed to exert any therapeutic effects.

Barrett, Feinstein, and Hole (1990) conducted a double-blind, placebo-controlled evaluation of naltrexone (1.2 mg/kg/day), using a reversal design, with a 12-year-old girl with autism. Self-injury decreased substantially during the phases when naltrexone was in effect, and although it was higher during placebo conditions, the rate was still much lower than in the initial baseline. This suggests a carryover effect of the drug during the placebo period.

Walters, Barrett, Feinstein, Mercurio, and Hole (1990) conducted a double-blind, placebo-controlled study of naltrexone. They evaluated the effects of 1.0 mg/kg/day of naltrexone on self-injury and social relatedness, using a reversal design (Singh & Beale, 1986) with a 14-year-old boy with autism. Results showed that self-injury and panic outbursts decreased markedly, social relatedness increased, and social withdrawal decreased on naltrexone.

In the final study, Sandman, Barron, and Colman (1990) evaluated the effects of naltrexone (0, 25, 50, 100 mg/day) on the self-injury and collateral behaviors of four adults with severe or profound mental retardation. Results showed a dose-dependent relationship in three subjects, with self-injury decreasing with increasing dose. The other subject showed a decrease in self-injury only at the low and moderate doses but not at the high dose (100 mg/day). Naltrexone did not have a consistent effect either on collateral behaviors such as stereotypy and activity or on rating scales of behavior.

The naltrexone studies generally show a positive dose-dependent relationship, with self-injury being reduced at low and moderate doses (up to 1.5 mg/kg) but not at high doses (2.0 mg/kg). The current database is small and derived from a small set of single case studies. Large patient-sample studies are needed to confirm the potency of naltrexone in the treatment of self-injury.

## Side Effects

Opiate antagonists have few major subjective or physiological effects in the absence of opioid drugs.

### *Central Nervous System*

The direct actions of narcotic antagonists may result in drowsiness, dizziness, dry mouth, sweating, miosis, and respiratory depression. Loss of energy and mental depression have also been reported.

### *Gastrointestinal*

Nausea and abdominal pain have been reported secondary to naloxone and naltrexone administration.

## Antihypertensives (Propranolol)

No prevalence data on the use of antihypertensives in the management of problem behaviors in individuals with mental retardation is available. The antihypertensive drug of interest is propranolol, a beta-adrenergic blocker that is usually prescribed for hypertension, angina pectoris, and cardiac arrhythmias. It is not really a drug typically used for controlling problem behaviors in persons with mental retardation, although recently, it has been used in the treatment of psychiatric disorders, notably violent and explosive behaviors (e.g., Jenkins & Maruta, 1987; Ratey, Morrill, & Oxenkrug, 1983; Yudofsky, Williams, & Gorman, 1981). There is some suggestion in the recent literature that beta-blockers may be effective in controlling the aggressive and self-injurious behavior of individuals with mental retardation.

## Mode of Drug Action

The mechanism of action of propranolol and other beta-blockers in controlling aggressive and self-injurious behavior remains unclear. A major point of debate has been whether these drugs act peripherally (i.e., on the PNS) or centrally (i.e., on the CNS) in the reatment of aggression (e.g., see Ritrovato, Weber, & Dufresne, 1989; Sorgi, Ratey, & Polakoff, 1987; Whitman, Maier, & Eichelman, 1987). Propranolol is highly lipid-soluble and readily penetrates into the CNS to block receptor sites in beta-adrenergic, serotonergic and dopaminergic systems (Ritrovato et al., 1989). However, clinical success with nadolol, a less lipid-soluble drug (Woods & Robinson, 1981), led to the suggestion that peripheral mechanisms might also be involved in the ability of beta-blockers to affect aggression (Polakoff, Sorgi, & Ratey, 1986). The hypothesis postulates that the autonomic response to peripheral beta-blockade, resulting in a relative hypotension, bradycardia and other effects, reduces feedback of neural activity from peripheral to central nervous system. Apparently, however, nadolol does achieve appreciable levels in the cerebrospinal fluid, and central effects for the drug cannot be entirely ruled out (Whitman et al., 1987). Clearly, further study is needed to resolve whether beta-blockers affect aggressive behavior by central or peripheral mechanisms, or a combination of the two.

It has also been postulated that attenuation of aggressive behaviors following beta-blocker administration may be due to a pharmacokinetic interaction with neuroleptic medication (Whitman et al., 1987). Propranolol elevated thioridazine levels threefold to fivefold in aggressive individuals (Silver & Yudofsky, 1985) and increased serum concentration of chlorpromazine in schizophrenic patients (Peet, 1981). However, because propranolol is effective in reducing self-injurious behavior both alone and in the presence of neuroleptics, it is not clear whether the mechanism for propranolol's action is the same or different in the two situations.

## Therapeutic Effects on Self-injury

In one of the earliest studies to use individuals with mental retardation, Yudofsky et al. (1981) treated four patients (one with mental retardation) for irreversible CNS lesions, socially disabling aggressiveness, and outbursts of rage. The 22-year-old woman with mental retardation was treated with 510 mg/day of propranolol, and after 5 weeks on medication, her aggression, which included self-injury, ceased, and her social behavior improved substantially. She was able to return to her sheltered workshop employment for the first time in 6 months, after only 8 weeks on medication.

In multisite, open clinical trials, Ratey, Mikkelsen, Smith, Upadhyaya, Zuckerman, Martell, Sorgi, Polakoff, and Bemporad (1986) evaluated the effects of low-dose propranolol (120 mg/day) on the self-injurious and aggressive behavior of 19 individuals with severe or profound mental retardation. Given that the open trials were in four different settings, a number of different assessment instruments were used; most were clinical scales rather than standardized instruments. Overall, however, it was reported that 12 subjects showed a marked improvement in their self-injury and aggressive behavior, 4 showed moderate improvement, and 3 remained unchanged. The authors suggested that the improvement seen in these patients may have been due to the peripheral anxiolytic action of beta-blockers.

In another study, Ratey and his colleagues (Ratey, Mikkelsen, Sorgi, Zuckerman, Polakoff, Bemporad, Bick, & Kadish, 1987) treated eight individuals with autism, five of whom were mentally retarded, for self-injury and aggression. Of the eight subjects, the six who had self-injury showed marked improvement on propranolol (up to 160 mg/day) or nadolol (120 mg/day). In some cases, their self-injury ceased altogether, and in others it was reduced to very low levels. The latency of behavioral response on the drug was between 6 weeks and 3 months. However, comparatively low doses of the beta-blockers were used because the authors maintain that time on medication is a key factor rather than high dosage.

Ruedrich, Grush, and Wilson (1990) provided a brief case report of a 25-year-old man with severe mental retardation who exhibited a wide range of problem behaviors, including aggression and self-injury. He had been tried on a number of drugs and behavioral programs but with little effect. In an open trial, his treatment regimen was changed to propranolol (120 mg/day) and haloperidol (1.5 mg/day), and his behavior showed some improvement, including reduced levels of aggression and self-injury.

Finally, in a retrospective analysis of medical records, Luchins and Dojka (1989) reported on six individuals with mental retardation who had been treated with propranolol. All five subjects for whom data were provided showed a decrease in their rates of self-injury, but these changes were not as impressive as those reported by Ratey and his colleagues.

In summary, the general conclusion that can be reached is that retrospective studies and uncontrolled case reports attest to the efficacy of the beta-blockers in controlling self-injury and aggression in this population. However, the lack of well-controlled studies makes it hazardous to recommend the use of these drugs in daily clinical practice.

### Side Effects

The majority of the adverse effects related to the use of beta-adrenergic receptor-blocking agents are transient and mild.

#### *Cardiovascular*

Bradycardia and paresthesias of the fingers and hands (related to a decrease in peripheral circulation) are the most commonly seen adverse cardiovascular effects. Hypotension and congestive heart failure, especially in patients with prior myocardial dysfunction, are less common complications of propranolol usage.

#### *Central Nervous System*

Fatigue and weakness are commonly experienced side effects of propranolol, the incidence of which is increased with higher dosages. Other, less common, CNS effects that have been reported include insomnia, nightmares, dizziness, hallucinations, and mild symptoms of depression.

#### *Respiratory*

The increase in airway resistance resulting from the beta-adrenergic blockade can produce dyspnea, wheezing, and bronchospasm. This is a potentially life-threatening complication, especially for patients with asthma.

#### *Other*

Gastrointestinal distress including nausea, vomiting, and diarrhea, impotence in males, allergic reactions, augmentation and masking of hypoglycemia, and hematologic abnormalities also have rarely been reported.

## *GABA (Baclofen)*

No prevalence data on the use of baclofen is available.

### Mode of Drug Action

Baclofen acts within the spinal cord to suppress reflexes involved in the regulation of muscle movement. However, the precise mechanism of reflex attenuation is not known. Because it is a structural analogue of the inhibitory neurotransmitter GABA, there is speculation that baclofen may act by mimicking the actions of GABA, resulting in reduced motor activity, depressed brainstem reticular function, and hence sedation (Lehne, 1990).

### Therapeutic Effects on Self-injury

In the only published work using baclofen to treat self-injury in individuals with severe mental retardation, Primrose (1979) reported an open trial of baclofen (20–200 mg/day) with 22 individuals and a double-blind trial with 20 individuals. All but two of the subjects showed some improvement in the open trial, and these formed the subject pool for the double-blind trial. All individuals in the open trial improved while on baclofen (30–300 mg/day), and 9 of them were able to be taken off baclofen without increasing their rate of their self-injury. Further evaluation of baclofen appears warranted in the light of these findings.

### Side Effects

The most commonly observed adverse reactions associated with the use of baclofen are related to its CNS effects. Occasionally, these side effects will limit the use of the drug.

#### *Central Nervous System*

Transient sedation is the most frequently seen adverse effect in patients using baclofen. Other reported side effects include dizziness, weakness, confusion, headache, and insomnia. Hallucinations, ataxia, and mood alterations, including both euphoria and depression, are rare but have been observed with baclofen.

#### *Other*

Nausea, constipation, hypotension, and urinary frequency also are rare but have been reported as adverse effects related to baclofen use.

## *5-Hydroxytryptophan*

No prevalence data on the use of 5-hydroxytryptophan (5-HTP) in the management of problem behaviors in individuals with mental retardation is available. There is a strong interest in this drug for theoretical reasons because of its role in animal models of self-injury that show 5-HTP to be effective in blocking such behavior (Nyhan, 1976). Clinically, 5-HTP has been used in the treatment of several disorders related to low serotonin levels in both adults and children (Sokol & Campbell, 1988). Of interest here is its use with individuals with Lesch–Nyhan syndrome. This syndrome is caused by an inborn error of purine metabolism in which self-injury is the most notable feature. Studies have shown that the self-injury is related to hyposerotonemia and that treatment requires on increase of the patient's serotonin levels (see Chapter 3 of this volume).

### Mode of Drug Action

Because self-injury is related to hyposerotonemia, treatment requires raising the patient's level of serotonin (5-hydroxytryptamine) in the CNS. Direct administration of this drug is not feasible as it does not cross the blood–brain barrier. However, its metabolic precursor, 5-HTP is rapidly transported into the CNS where it is converted to serotonin by the action of the enzyme L-amino acid decarboxylase (van Praag, 1980).

### Therapeutic Effects on Self-injury

A few studies have used 5-HTP to treat self-injury in individuals with the Lesch–Nyhan syndrome. In an open trial, Mizuno and Yugari (1974, 1975) administered L-5-HTP to four patients for 36 weeks and reported that self-injury disappeared in all patients. Nyhan, Johnson, Kaufman, and Jones (1980) reported that a combination of 5-HTP, carbidopa, and imipramine was effective in reducing self-injury in seven of nine patients with the Lesch–Nyhan syndrome, although tolerance developed within 3 months of initiating the drug regimen. However, the efficacy of 5-HTP in reducing self-injury in the Lesch–Nyhan syndrome has not been replicated in other trials (Anders, Cann, Ciaranello, Barchas, & Berger, 1978; Anderson, Hermann, & Dancis, 1976; Ciaranello, Anders, Barchas, Bergers, & Cann, 1976; Frith, Johnstone, Joseph, Powell, & Watts, 1976). Given that the therapeutic effect of 5-HTP is outweighed by the rapid development of tolerance, its use in controlling self-injury is questionable. Furthermore, the fact that virtually no recent paper on it has been published in the past 10 years suggests that, at least for the present, 5-HTP, is not seen as a treatment of choice for this population.

### Side Effects

The effects and side effects of 5-HTP are related to the stimulation or inhibition of a variety of smooth muscles and nerves. The responses are often variable among individuals.

#### *Respiratory*

Bronchoconstriction may result in certain individuals, especially those with asthma. Other respiratory changes have also been noted.

#### *Cardiovascular*

Adverse effects are related to either vasoconstriction or vasodilation, resulting in variable blood pressure responses. The positive inotropic and chronotropic effects seen on the heart are of variable intensity.

#### *Gastrointestinal*

Both stimulation and inhibition of the motility of the stomach, small intestine, and large intestine can result in adverse effects.

#### *Endocrine*

Variable stimulatory and inhibitory effects on certain endocrine glands, including the pancreas, adrenal cortex, and adenohypophyseal may result in adverse effects related to the resulting abnormal glandular function.

#### *Central Nervous System*

Activation of vagal nerve endings in the coronary vascular bed may result in a reflex response triad consisting of bradycardia, hypotension, and hyperventilation. There is also evidence that sleep, aggression, and sexual behavior may be affected.

## *Antiepileptics (Anticonvulsants)*

Antiepileptics primarily are used for controlling seizures, but these drugs also have cognitive and behavioral effects (Stores, 1988). They are often used by clinicians for their psychotropic effects on behavior management, especially in those individuals who exhibit "episodic, violent outbursts of emotional, disruptive, or aggressive behavior" (Werry, 1982, p. 313).

Recent surveys have estimated that antiepileptic medication is prescribed for 36% to 42% of institutionalized individuals, and between 21% and 48% in community settings (Singh & Winton, 1989). What proportion of these prescriptions are for the control of epilepsy or for behavior management remains undetermined.

### Mode of Drug Action

The mechanism of action of carbamazepine is complex and incompletely understood. Recent studies suggest that events at the benzodiazepine–GABA receptor–chloride ionophore complex may provide a mechanism of action common to most of the anticonvulsants, including carbamazepine. The anticonvulsant action depends mainly on the ability of the drugs to restrict the spread of epileptic activity at the synaptic level (Eadie, 1987). Specifically, carbamazepine produces a dose-dependent fall in membrane conductance (Schauf, Davis, & Marder, 1974) and a decrease in brain GABA turnover, both of which would contribute to a reduction in neuronal activity.

## Therapeutic Effects on Self-injury

Typically, carbamazepine is the drug that is used for its psychotropic effects with individuals who exhibit behavior problems. Its efficacy in the treatment of behavioral and psychiatric disorders of patients without mental retardation has been reviewed by Berkheimer, Curtis, and Jann (1985), among others. A few studies with individuals with mental retardation also have shown that some of them show a marked behavioral improvement on carbamazepine (e.g., Langee, 1989; Reid, Naylor, & Kay, 1981). However, in the only study that included self-injury as a specific variable, carbamazepine (600 mg/day) had no apparent effect on the self-injury of a 15-year-old boy with profound mental retardation (Singh & Winton, 1984).

## Side Effects

Adverse effects are reported in up to one third of patients treated with carbamazepine, the majority of which are dose related.

### *Hematologic*

The most severe, although extremely rare, adverse effects associated with carbamazepine include the development of irreversible aplastic anemia and agranulocytosis. A transient and mild leukopenia is seen in approximately 10% of patients upon the initiation of treatment, and in 2% of patients, a persistent leukopenia is reported. A transient thrombocytopenia also has been noted in some cases.

### *Central Nervous System*

The most commonly reported side effects associated with carbamazepine usage are sedation, weakness, dizziness, disturbances of coordination, transient diplopia, and mild nystagmus. Visual hallucinations, confusion, abnormal involuntary movements and depression are rare but have been reported.

### *Gastrointestinal*

Symptoms including nausea, vomiting, abdominal pain, diarrhea, constipation, and anorexia can be related to carbamazepine usage.

### *Dermatologic*

Various types of skin eruptions have been reported, including pruritic and erythematous rashes, toxic epidermal neurolysis, photosensitivity reactions, alterations in skin pigmentation, and Stevens–Johnson syndrome.

*Other*

Cardiovascular symptoms including congestive heart failure, hypotension, hypertension, and lymphadenopathy have occasionally been reported. Abnormalities in liver function tests, hepatitis, genitourinary tract dysfunction, and inappropriate antidiuretic hormone secretion are rare but may occur.

## Current Status and Future Directions

Much has already been written about issues regarding the pharmacological management of individuals with mental retardation. For example, Mouchka (1985) and Schroeder (1985) raised a number of issues at the NIMH-sponsored workshop on pharmacotherapy and mental retardation. These issues include pharmacotherapy for those who are mentally retarded *and* mentally ill, the need for assessment instruments, withdrawal and tardive dyskinesias, measurement of drug blood levels in relation to behavioral outcome, ecobehavioral validity in drug research, and litigation regarding the use of drugs (Beyer, 1988; Golden, 1988; Lewis & Mailman, 1988; Singh & Aman, 1990). These are issues that need to be addressed regarding the entire field of pharmacotherapy for persons with mental retardation. In the remainder of this section, we present a few issues that affect the psychopharmacology of self-injury in this population.

### *Methodology*

This issue has been a problem with the field generally and continues to be a major factor in drug research. A majority of the studies reviewed did not meet the criteria for sound pharmacological research. The criteria outlined by Sprague and Werry (1971) and extended by a number of others (see Aman & Singh, 1991) still hold and should serve as the basis for all future research in this area. Too many studies are mere case reports without adequate experimental designs or controls. If the analysis is based on single subjects, then single-subject research designs should be used (Singh & Beale, 1986).

Virtually three fourths of the studies reviewed had one or more methodological flaw. Few studies were placebo-controlled and/or double-blind, and even fewer had subjects randomly assigned to different experimental groups. Indeed, often the subject sample was too small to allow the inclusion of some of the methodological niceties that a large sample size would have to offer.

Another problem is that a large number of studies did not control for additional treatments that were used together with the trial of the target drug. We have suggested elsewhere (Aman & Singh, 1980) that this is a major problem because of interactions or overlaps between treatments. For example, some drugs may interfere with the metabolism of other medications, thereby increasing the serum levels of these drugs without actually changing the drug dosage. For example, the serum level of thioridazine can be elevated if concurrent propranolol is administered (Silver, Yudofsky, Kogan, & Katz, 1986).

### Collateral Measures

Most of the studies did not include any measure of collateral behaviors or measures of learning. Given that drugs have a more general effect than on the target behavior alone, it behooves researchers to include social and maladaptive behaviors, as well as measures of learning. Further, these measures should be ecologically valid in terms of the individual and his or her environment (see Singh & Aman, 1990, on ecobehavioral analysis of pharmacotherapy).

### Dosage Effects

It is by now well established that drugs may have differential effects on a given behavior or given classes of behavior at different doses. Few studies reviewed in this chapter included more than one dose of the target drug. The best example of dose-dependent research work has probably been done with the opioid antagonists, naloxone and naltrexone, although dose-dependent relationships were explored only with self-injury rather than with a number of other behaviors as well.

### Heterogeneity of Subject Sample

The behavioral literature suggests that the motivation for a person's self-injurious behavior can be assessed through a functional analysis (O'Neill et al., 1990). Such an analysis provides at least four motivations for a given behavior, with any one or a combination being applicable to the behavior of a person within a given time period and setting. However, motivational factors are not taken into account when clinical decisions regarding drug therapy are made. This means that individuals exhibiting the same topography of behavior but having different motivations are all treated alike. The great heterogeneity of the sample of patients who engage in self-injury provides inherent difficulty in interpreting and comparing results across studies.

### Underreporting of Negative Results

We know that it is difficult to publish papers that report negative findings. However, this situation leads to an underreporting of negative results, thus making the marginal effects of some drugs look very positive. Well-controlled research that shows negative results should be published, as well as those with positive results.

### Targeting Self-injury as the Keystone Behavior

Virtually all of the older studies have included self-injury as a minor variable, if at all, and usually as a part of a class of behaviors (e.g., self-injury as a part of aggression), rather than a behavior of interest in its own right.

### Alternatives to Drugs

Few studies have incorporated or compared a drug regimen with another procedure, such as behavior modification. There are a small number of comparative or combined drug studies (e.g., Durand, 1982; Luiselli, 1986; Luiselli & Evans, 1987; Luiselli et al., 1986), and these should serve as models for future research on drug treatment for self-injury. Ackles (1986) and Schroeder, Lewis, and Lipton (1983) provide excellent discussions of the rationale and methodology pertinent to combined or comparative interventions using either group or single-subject designs.

### Rational Pharmacotherapy

The majority of the studies reviewed had no theoretical underpinnings. Rational pharmacotherapy for self-injury has to have a better basis than just trial and error. The recent flurry of activity on the theoretical or biochemical bases for some interventions is very promising. These include work on serotonin agonists for Lesch–Nyhan syndrome, endogenous opioids, and $D_1$ dopamine receptor supersensitivity (e.g., Deutsch, 1986; Goldstein, 1989; Goldstein, Anderson, Reuben, & Dancis, 1985; Konicki & Schulz, 1989).

## *Conclusions*

The experimental evidence attesting to the efficacy of pharmacological treatments for self-injury in individuals with mental retardation is not very strong. However, there is some optimism in the field as well. The recent studies are methodologically more robust and based more on rational pharmacotherapy than just trial and error, and there is some appreciation of the need for comparative and combined treatments.

## *References*

Abbott, P., Blake, A., & Vincze, L.(1965). Treatment of mentally retarded with thioridazine. *Diseases of the Nervous System*, *26*, 583–585.

Ackles, P. A. (1986). Evaluating pharmacological–behavioral treatment interactions. In M. Hersen (Ed.), *Pharmacological and behavioral treatment interactions* (pp. 54–86). New York: Wiley.

Adamson, W. C., Nellis, B. P., Runge, G., Cleland, C., & Killian, E. (1958). Use of tranquilizers for mentally deficient patients. *American Journal of Diseases of Children*, *96*, 159–164.

Aman, M. G. (1984). Psychoactive drugs in mental retardation. In J. L. Matson & F. Andrasik (Eds.), *Treatment issues and innovations in mental retardation* (pp. 455–513). New York: Plenum.

Aman, M. G., Field, C. J., & Bridgman, G. D. (1985). City-wide survey of drug patterns among noninstitutionalized retarded persons. *Applied Research in Mental Retardation*, *5*, 159–171.

Aman, M. G., & Singh, N. N. (1980). The usefulness of thioridazine for treating childhood disorders: Fact or folklore? *American Journal of Mental Deficiency*, *84*, 331–338.

Aman, M. G., & Singh, N. N. (1982). Methylphenidate in severely retarded residents and the clinical significance of stereotypic behavior. *Applied Research in Mental Retardation*, *3*, 345–358.

Aman, M. G., & Singh, N. N. (1988). *Psychopharmacology of the developmental disabilities*. New York: Springer-Verlag.

Aman, M. G., & Singh, N. N. (1991). Pharmacological intervention: Update. In J. L. Matson & J. A. Mulick (Eds.), *Handbook of mental retardation* (pp. 347–373). New York: Pergamon.

Aman, M. G., Teehan C. J., White, A. J., Turbott, S. H., & Vaithianathan, C. (1989). Haloperidol treatment with chronically medicated residents: Dose effects on clinical behavior and reinforcement contingencies. *American Journal of Mental Deficiency*, *93*, 452–460.

Aman, M. G., & White, A. J. (1988). Thioridazine dose effects with reference to stereotypic behavior in mentally retarded residents. *Journal of Autism and Developmental Disabilities*, *18*, 355–366.

Amin, P., & Yeragani, V. K. (1987). Control of aggressive and self-mutilative behavior in a mentally retarded patient with lithium. *Canadian Journal of Psychiatry*, *32*, 162–163.

Anders, T. F., Cann, H. M., Ciaranello, R. D., Barchas, J. D., & Berger, P. A. (1978). Further observations on the use of 5-hydroxytryptophan in a child with Lesch–Nyhan syndrome. *Neuropediatrie*, *9*, 157–166.

Anderson, L. T., Campbell, M., Grega, D. M., Perry, R., Small, A. M., & Green, W. H. (1984). Haloperidol in the treatment of infantile autism: Effects on learning and behavioral symptoms. *American Journal of Psychiatry*, *141*, 1195–1202.

Anderson, L. T., Hermann, L., & Dancis, J. (1976). The effect of L-5-hydroxytryptophan on self-mutilation in Lesch–Nyhan disease: A negative report. *Neuropediatrie*, *7*, 439–442.

Barrett, R. P., Feinstein, C., & Hole, W. T. (1990). Effects of naloxone and naltrexone on self-injury: A double-blind, placebo-controlled analysis. *American Journal of Mental Retardation*, *93*, 644–651.

Bates, W. J., Smeltzer, D. J., & Arnoczky, S. M. (1986). Appropriate and inappropriate use of psychotherapeutic medications for institutionalized mentally retarded persons. *American Journal of Mental Deficiency*, *90*, 363–370.

Beckwith, B. E., Couk, D. I., & Schumacher, K. (1986). Failure of naloxone to reduce self-injurious behavior in two developmentally disabled females. *Applied Research in Mental Retardation*, *7*, 183–188.

Berkheimer, J. L., Curtis, J. L., & Jann, M. W. (1985). Use of carbamazepine in psychiatric disorders. *Clinical Pharmacy*, *4*, 425–434.

Bernstein, G. A., Hughes, J. H., Mitchell, J. E., & Thompson, T. (1987). Effects of narcotic antagonists on self-injurious behavior: A single case study. *Journal of the American Academy of Child and Adolescent Psychiatry*, *26*, 886–889.

Beyer, H. A. (1988). Litigation and the use of drugs in developmental disabilities. In M. G. Aman & N. N. Singh (Eds.), *Psychopharmacology of the developmental disabilities* (pp. 29–57). New York: Springer-Verlag.

Briggs, R. (1989). Monitoring and evaluating psychotropic drug use for persons with mental retardation: A followup report. *American Jounal of Mental Retardation*, *93*, 633–639.

Burk, H. W., & Menolascino, F. J. (1968). Haloperidol in emotionally disturbed mentally retarded individuals. *American Journal of Psychiatry*, *124*, 1589–1591.

Burns, M. E. (1980). Droperidol in the management of hyperactivity, self-mutilation and aggression in mentally handicapped patients. *Journal of International Medical Research*, *8*, 31–33.

Caldwell, A. E. (1978) History of psychopharmacology. In W. G. Clark & J. Del Giudice (Eds.), *Principles of psychopharmacology* (2nd ed.). New York: Academic Press.

Campbell, M., Adams, P., Small, A. M., Tesch, L. M., & Curren, E. L. (1988). Naltrexone in infantile autism. *Psychopharmacology Bulletin*, *24*, 135–139.

Campbell, M., Anderson, L. T., Small, A. M., Locascio, J. J., Lynch, N. S., & Choroco, M. C. (1990). Naltrexone in autistic children: A double-blind and placebo-controlled study. *Psychopharmacology Bulletin*, *26*, 130–135.

Chandler, M., Gualtieri, C. T., & Fahs, J. J. (1988). Other psychotropic drugs: Stimulants, antidepressants, the anxiolytics, and lithium carbonate. In M. G. Aman & N. N. Singh (Eds.), *Psychopharmacology of the developmental disabilities* (pp. 119–145). New York: Springer-Verlag.

Ciaranello, R. D., Anders, T. F., Barchas, J. D., Berger, P. A., & Cann, H. M. (1976). The use of 5-hydroxytryptophan in a child with Lesch–Nyhan syndrome. *Child Psychiatry and Human Development*, *7*, 127–133.

Cooper, A. F., & Fowlie, H. C. (1973). Control of gross self-mutilation with lithium carbonate. *British Journal of Psychiatry*, *122*, 370–371.

Craig, C. R., & Stitzel, R. E. (1990). *Modern pharmacology* (3rd ed., pp. 537–538). Boston: Little Brown.

Creese, I., Burt, D. R., & Snyder, S. H. (1976). Dopamine receptor binding predicts clinical and pharmacologic potencies of antischizophrenic drugs. *Science*, *192*, 481–483.

Davidson, P. W., Kleene, B. M., Carroll, M., & Rockowitz, R. J. (1983). Effects of naloxone on self-injurious behavior: A case study. *Applied Research in Mental Retardation*, *4*, 1–4.

Davis, K. V., Sprague, R. L., & Werry, J. S. (1969). Stereotyped behavior and activity level in severe retardates: The effect of drugs. *American Journal of Mental Deficiency*, *73*, 721–727.

Dutsch, S. I. (1986). Rationale for the administration of opiate antagonists in treating infantile autism. *American Journal of Mental Deficiency*, *90*, 631–635.

Durand, V. M. (1982). A behavioral/pharmacological intervention for the treatment of severe self-injurious behavior. *Journal of Autism and Developmental Disorders*, *12*, 243–251.

Eadie, M. J. (1987). Mode of action of anticonvulsant drugs. In G. D. Burrows, T. R. Norman, & B. Davies (Eds.), *Antimanics, anticonvulsants and other drugs in psychiatry* (pp. 11–129). Amsterdam: Elsevier.

Farber, J. M. (1987). Psychopharmacology of self-injurious behavior in the mentally retarded. *Journal of the American Academy of Child and Adolescent Psychiatry*, *26*, 296–302.

Findholt, N. E., & Emmett, C. G. (1990). Impact of interdisciplinary team review on psychotropic drug use with persons who have mental retardation. *Mental Retardation*, *28*, 41–46.

Fox, L., & Westling, D. L. (1986). The prevalence of students who are profoundly mentally handicapped receiving medication in a school district. *Education and Training of the Mentally Retarded*, *21*, 205–210.

Frith, C.D., Johnstone, E. C., Joseph, M. H., Powell, R. J., & Watts, R. W. E. (1976). Double-blind clinical trial of 5-hydroxytryptophan in a case of Lesch–Nyhan syndrome. *Journal of Neurology, Neurosurgery, and Psychiatry*, *39*, 656–662.

Gadow, K. D. (1985). Prevalence and efficacy of stimulant drug use with mentally retarded children and youth. *Psychopharmacology Bulletin*, *21*, 291–303.

Gadow, K. D., & Poling, A. G. (1988). *Pharmacotherapy and mental retardation*. Boston: College-Hill.

Galambos, M. (1965). Long term clinical trial with diazepam on adult mentally retarded persons. *Diseases of the Nervous System*, *26*, 305–309.

Gillman, M. A., & Sandyk, R. (1985). Opiatergic and dopaminergic function and Lesch–Nyhan syndrome. *American Journal of Psychiatry*, *142*, 1226.

Golden, G. S. (1988). Tardive dyskinesia and developmental disabilities. In M. G. Aman & N. N. Singh (Eds.), *Psychopharmacology of the developmental disabilities* (pp. 179–215). New York: Springer-Verlag.

Goldstein, M. (1989). Dopaminergic mechanisms in self-inflicting biting behavior. *Psychopharmacology Bulletin*, *25*, 349–352.

Goldstein, M., Anderson, L. T., Reuben, R., & Dancis, J. (1985). Self-mutilation in Lesch–Nyhan disease is caused by dopaminergic denervation. *Lancet*, *1*, 338–339.

Grabowski, S. W. (1973). Safety and effectiveness of haloperidol for mentally retarded behaviorally disordered and hyperkinetic patients. *Current Therapeutic Research*, *15*, 856–861.

Grossett, D. L., Williams, D. E. (1988, May). *Psychopharmacological intervention for the treatment of self-injurious behavior in a person with profound mental retardation and a psychiatric disorder*. Paper presented at the annual convention of the Association for Behavior Analysis, Philadelphia.

Haegeman, J., & Duyck, F. (1978). A retrospective evaluation of pipamperon (Dipiperon) in the treatment of behavioral deviations in severely mentally handicapped. *Acta Psychiatrica Belgica*, *78*, 392–398.

Heistad, G. T., Zimmerman, T. L., & Doebler, M. I. (1982). Long-term usefulness of thioridazine for institutionalized mentally retarded patients. *American Journal of Mental Deficiency*, *87*, 243–251.

Herman, B. H., Hammock, M. K., Arthur-Smith, A., Egan, J., Chatoor, I., Werner, A., & Boeckx, R. L. (1986). Role of opioid peptides in self-injurious behavior. *Society for Neuroscience Abstracts*, *12*, 412.

Herman, B. H., Hammock, M. K., Arthur-Smith, A., Egan, J., Chatoor, I., Werner, A., & Zelnick, N. (1987). Naltrexone decreases self-injurious behavior. *Annals of Neurology*, *22*, 550–552.

Herman, B. H., Hammock, M. K., Egan, J., Feinstein, C., Chatoor, I., Boeckx, R., Zelnick, N., Jack, R., & Rosenquist, J. (1985). Naltrexone induces dose-dependent decreases in self-injurious behavior. *Society for Neuroscience Abstracts*, *11*, 468.

Hill, B. K., Balow, E. A., & Bruininks, R. H. (1985). A national survey of prescribed drugs in institutions and community residential facilities for mentally retarded people. *Psychopharmacology Bulletin*, *21*, 279–284.

Holaday, J. W. (1985). *Endogenous opioids and their receptors*. Kalamazoo: Upjohn.

Huessy, H. R., & Ruoff, P. A. (1984). Towards a rational drug usage in a state institution for retarded individuals. *Psychiatric Journal of the University of Ottawa*, *9*, 56–58.

Insel, T. R., Ninan, P. T., Aloi, J., Jimerson, D.C., Skolnick, P., & Paul, S. M. (1984). A benzodiazepine receptor-medicated model of anxiety. *Archives of General Psychiatry*, *41*, 741–750.

Intagliata, J., & Rinck, C. (1985). Psychoactive drug use in public and community residential facilities for mentally retarded persons. *Psychopharmacology Bulletin*, *21*, 268–278.

Iwata, B. A., Vollmer, T. R., & Zarcone, J. R. (1990). The experimental (functional) analysis of behavior disorders: Methodology, applications, and limitations. In A. C. Repp & N. N. Singh (Eds.), *Perspectives on the use of nonaversive and aversive interventions for persons with developmental disabilities* (pp. 301–330). Sycamore, IL: Sycamore Publishing.

Jakab, I. (1984). Short-term effect of thioridazine tablet versus suspension on emotionally disturbed/retarded children. *Journal of Clinical Psychopharmacology*, *4*, 210–215.

Janicak, P. G., & Vadis, J. M. (1987). Clinical usage of lithium in mania. In G. D. Burrows, T. R. Norman, & B. Davies (Eds.), *Antimanics, anticonvulsants and other drugs in psychiatry* (2nd ed., Vol. 7, pp. 46–74). New York: Basic Books.

Jenkins, S. C., & Maruta, T. (1987), Therapeutic use of propranolol for intermittent explosive disorder. *Mayo Clinic Proceedings*, *62*, 204–214.

Konicki, P. E., & Schulz, S. C. (1989). Rationale for clinical trials of opiate antagonists in treating patients with personality and self-injurious behavior. *Psychopharmacology Bulletin*, *25*, 556–563.

Lacny, J. (1973). Mesoridazine in the care of disturbed mentally retarded patients. *Canadian Psychiatric Association Journal*, *18*, 389–391.

Langee, H. R. (1989). A retrospective study of mentally retarded patients with behavioral disorders who were treated with carbamazepine. *American Journal of Mental Deficiency*, *93*, 640–643.

LeBoyer, M., Bouvard, M. P., & Dugas, M. (1988). Effects of naltrexone on infantile autism. *Lancet*, *1*, 715.

Lehne, R. A. (1990). *Pharmacology for nursing care*. Philadelphia: W. B. Saunders.

Le Vann, L. J. (1969). Haloperidol in the treatment of behavioral disorders in children and adolescents. *Canadian Psychiatric Association Journal*, *14*, 217–220.

Lewis, M. H., & Mailman, R. B. (1988). Drug blood levels: Measurement and relation to behavioral outcome in mentally retarded persons. In M. G. Aman & N. N. Singh (Eds.), *Psychopharmacology of the developmental disabilities* (pp. 58–81). New York: Springer-Verlag.

Lipman, R. S. (1970). The use of psychopharmacological agents in residential facilities for the retarded. In F. J. Menolascino (Ed.), *Psychiatric approaches to mental retardation* (pp 387–398). New York: Basic Books.

Llorente, A. F. (1969). The management of behavior disorders with thioridazine in the mentally retarded. *Journal of the Maine Medical Association*, *60*, 229–231.

Luchins, D. J., & Dojka, D. (1989). Lithium and propranolol in aggression and self-injurious behavior in the mentally retarded. *Psychopharmacology Bulletin*, *25*, 372–375.

Luiselli, J. K. (1986). Behavior analysis of pharmacological and contingency management interventions for self-injury. *Journal of Behavior Therapy and Experimental Psychiatry*, *17*, 275–284.

Luiselli, J. K., Beltis, J. A., & Bass, J. (1989). Clinical analysis of naltrexone in the treatment of self-injurious behavior. *Journal of the Multihandicapped Person*, *2*, 43–50.

Luiselli, J. K., & Evans, T. P. (1987). Assessing pharmacological and contingency management interventions with mentally retarded adolescents in a residential treatment program. *Behavioral Residential Treatment*, *2*, 139–152.

Luiselli, J. K., Evans, T. P., & Boyce, D. A. (1986). Pharmacological assessment and comprehensive behavioral intervention in a case of pediatric self-injury. *Journal of Clinical Child Psychology*, *15*, 323–326.

Malseed, R. T., & Harrigan, G. S. (1989). *Textbook of pharmacology and nursing care*. Philadelphia: J. B. Lippincott.

Marholin, D., Touchette, P. E., & Stewart, R. M. (1979). Withdrawal of chronic chlorpromazine medication: An experimental analysis. *Journal of Applied Behavior Analysis*, *12*, 159–271.

Martin, J. E., & Argran, M. (1985). Psychotropic and anticonvulsant drug use by mentally retarded adults across community residential and vocational placements. *Applied Research in Mental Retardation*, *6*, 33–49.

Martin, W. R., Jasinski, D. R., & Mansky, P. A. (1984). Naltrexone, an antagonist for the treatment of heroin dependence: Effects in man. *Archives of General Psychiatry*, *28*, 784–791.

Micev, V., & Lynch, D. M. (1974). Effect of lithium on disturbed severely mentally retarded patients. *British Journal of Psychiatry*, *125*, 110.

Mikkelsen, E. J. (1986). Low dose haloperidol for stereotypic self-injurious behavior in the mentally retarded. *New England Journal of Medicine*, *315*, 398–399.

Millichamp, C. J., & Singh, N. N. (1987). The effects of intermittent drug therapy on stereotypy and collateral behaviors of mentally retarded persons. *Research in Developmental Disabilities*, *8*, 213–227.

Mizuno, T., & Yugari, Y. (1974). Self-mutilation in Lesch–Nyhan syndrome. *Lancet*, *1*, 761.

Mizuno, T., & Yugari, Y. (1975). Prophylactic effects of L-5-hydroxytryptophan on sclf-mutilation in the Lesch–Nyhan syndrome. *Neuropadiatrie*, *6*, 13–23.

Mouchka, S. (1985). Issues in psychopharmacology with the mentally retarded. *Psychopharmacology Bulletin*, *21*, 262–267.

National Institute of Mental Health. (1989). *Draft report of the consensus development panel on treatment of destructive behaviors in persons with developmental disabilities*. Washington, DC: Author.

Naylor, G. J., Dick, D. A. T., Dick, E. G., & Moody, J. P. (1974). Lithium therapy and erythrocyte membrane cation carrier. *Psychopharmacology*, *3*, 81–86.

Nyhan, W. L. (1976). Behavior inh the Lesch–Nyhan syndrome. *Journal of Autism and Childhood Schizophrenia*, *6*, 235–252.

Nyhan, W. L., Johnson, H. G., Kaufman, I. A., & Jones, K. L. (1980). Serotonergic approaches to the modification of behavior in the Lesch–Nyhan syndrome. *Applied Research in Mental Retardation*, *1*, 25–40.

O'Neil, R. E., Horner, R. H., Albin, R. W., Storey, K., & Sprague, J. R. (1990). *Functional analysis of problem behavior: A practical assessment guide*. Sycamore, IL: Sycamore Publishing.

Ortiz, A., Dabbagh, M., & Gershon, S. (1984). Lithium: Clinical use, toxicology and mode of action. In J. C. Bernstein (Ed.), *Clinical psychopharmacology* (pp. 111–144). Boston: John Wright PSG.

Peet, M. (1981). Is propranolol antischizophrenic? *Neuropharmacology*, *20*, 1303–1307.

Poindexter, A. R. (1989). Psychotropic drug patterns in a large ICF/MR facility: A ten-year experience. *American Journal of Mental Retardation*, *93*, 624–626.

Polakoff, S. A., Sorgi, P. J., & Ratey, J. J. (1986). The treatment of impulsive and aggressive behavior with nadolol. *Journal of Clinical Psychopharmacology*, *6*, 125–126.

Primrose, D. A. (1979). Treatment of self-injurious behavior with la GABA (gamma—aminobutyric acid) analogue. *Journal of Mental Deficiency Research*, *23*, 163–173.

Ratey, J. J., Mikkelsen, E. J., Smith, B., Upadhyaya, A., Zuckerman, S., Martell, D., Sorgi, P., Polakoff, S., & Bemporad, J. (1986). Beta-blockers in the severely and profoundly mentally retarded. *Journal of Clinical Psychopharmacology*, *6*, 103–107.

Ratey, J. J., Mikkelsen, E., sorgi, P., Zuckerman, S., Polakoff, S., Bemporad, J., Bick, P., & Kadish, W. (1987). Autism: The treatment of aggressive behaviors. *Journal of Clinical Psychopharmacology*, *7*, 35–41.

Ratey, J. J., Morrill, R., & Oxenkrug, G. (1983). Use of propranolol for provoked and unprovoked episodes of rage. *American Journal of Psychiatry*, *140*, 1356–1357.

Reid, A. H., Naylor, G. J., & Kay, D. S. G. (1981). A double-blind, placebo controlled crossover trial of carbamazepine in overactive severely mentally handicapped patients. *Psychological Medicine*, *11*, 109–113.

Repp, A. C., Felce, D., & Barton, L. E. (1988). Basing the treatment of stereotypic and self-injurious behaviors on hypotheses of their causes. *Journal of Applied Behavior Analysis*, *21*, 281–289.

Repp, A. C., & Singh, N. N. (1990). *Perspectives on the use of nonaversive and aversive interventions for persons with developmental disabilities*. Sycamore, IL: Sycamore Publishing.

Richardson, J. S., & Zaleski, W. A. (1983). Naloxone and self-mutilation. *Biological Psychiartry*, *18*, 99–101.

Richardson, J. S., & Zaleski, W. A. (1986a). Endogenous opiates and self-mutilation. *American Journal of Psychiatry*, *143*, 939.

Richardson, J. S., & Zaleski, W. A. (1986b). On the role of endogenous opioids in the maintenance of self-mutilation. *International Journal of Neuroscience*, *31*, 129.

Ritrovato, C. A., Weber, S. S., & Dufresne, R. L. (1989). Nadolol in the treatment of aggressive behavior associated with schizophrenia. *Clinical Pharmacy*, *8*, 132–135.

Ruedrich, S. L., Grush, L., & Wilson, J. (1990). Beta adrenergic blocking medications for aggressive or self-injurious mentally retarded persons. *American Journal of Mental Retardation*, *95*, 110–119.

Sandman, C. A., Barron, J., & Colman, H. (1990). An orally administered opiate blocker, naltreoxone, attenuates self-injurious behavior. *American Journal of Mental Retardation*, *95*, 93–102.

Sandman, C. A., Datta, P. C., Barron, J., Hoehler, F. K., Williams, C., & Swanson, J. M. (1983). Naloxone attenuates self-abusive behavior in developmentally disabled clients. *Applied Research in Mental Retardation*, *4*, 5–11.

Sandyk, R. (1985). Naloxone abolishes self-injury in a mentally retarded child. *Annals of Neurology*, *17*, 520.

Schauf, D. L., Davis, F. A., & Marder, J. (1974). Effects of carbamazepine on the ionic conductances of Myxicola giant axons. *Journal of Pharmacology and Experimental Therapeutics*, *189*, 538–542.

Schroeder, S. R. (1985). Issues and future research directions of pharmacotherapy in mental retardation. *Psychopharmacology Bulletin*, *21*, 323–326.

Schroeder, S. R. (1988). Neuroleptic medications for persons with developmental disabilities. In M. G. Aman and N. N. Singh (Eds.), *Psychopharmacology of the developmental disabilities* (pp. 82–100). New York: Springer-Verlag.

Schroeder, S. R., & Gualtieri, C. T. (1985). Behavioral interactions induced by chronic neuroleptic therapy in persons with mental retardation. *Psychopharmacology Bulletin*, *21*, 310–315.

Schroeder, S. R., Lewis, M. H., & Lipton, M. A. (1983). Interactions of pharmacotherapy and behavior therapy among children with learning and behavioral disorders. In K. D. Gadow (Ed.), *Advances in learning and behavioral disabilities* (Vol. 2, pp. 179–225). Greenwich, CT: JAI Press.

Schroeder, S. R., Rojahn, J., Hawk, B., Kanoy, R. C., Thios, S. J., Mulick, J. A., & Stephens, M. (1982). environmental antecedents which affect management and maintenance of programs for self-injurious behavior. In J. H. Hollis & C. E. Meyers (eds.), *Life threatening behaviors: Analysis and intervention* (pp. 105–159). Washington, DC: American Association on Mental Deficiency.

Schroeder, S. R., Rojahn, J., Mulick, J. A., & Schroeder, C. S. (1990). Self-injurious behavior. In J. L. Matson (Ed.), *Handbook of behavior modification with the mentally retarded* (2nd ed., pp. 141–180). New York: Plenum Press.

Silver, J. M., & Yudofsky, S. C. (1985). Propranolol for aggression: Literature review and clinical guidelines. *International Drug Therapy News*, *20*, 9–12.

Silver, J. M., Yudofsky, S. C., Kogan, M., & Katz, B. L. (1986). Elevation of thioridazine plasma levels by propranolol. *American Journal of Psychiatry*, *143*, 1290–1292.

Singh, N. N. (1981). Current trends in the treatment of self-injurious behavior. In L. A. Barness (Ed.), *Advances in pediatrics* (Vol. 28, pp. 377–440). Chicago: Year Book Medical Publishers.

Singh, N. N., & Aman, M. G. (1981). Effects of thioridazine dosage on the behavior of severely mentally retarded persons. *American Journal of Mental Deficiency*, *85*, 580–587.

Singh, N. N., & Aman, M. G. (1990). Ecobehavioral assessment of pharmacotherapy. In S. Schroeder (Ed.), *Ecobehavioral analysis in developmental disabilities* (pp. 182–200). New York: Springer-Verlag.

Singh, N. N., & Beale, I. L. (1986). Behavioral assessment of pharmacotherapy. *Behavior Change*, *3*, 34–40.

Singh, N. N., & Millichamp, C. J. (1985). Pharmacological treatment of self-injurious behavior in mentally retarded persons. *Journal of Autism and Developmental Disorders*, *15*, 257–267.

Singh, N. N., Parmelee, D. X., Sood, A., & Katz, R. (in press). Collaboration of disciplines. In J. L. Matson (Ed.), *Handbook of hyperactivity in children*. New York: Pergamon Press.

Singh, N. N., & Repp, A. C. (1988). Current trends in the behavioral and psychopharmacological management of problem behaviors of mentally retarded persons. *Irish Journal of Psychology*, *9*, 362–384.

Singh, N. N., Sood, A., Sonenklar, N., & Ellis, C. R. (1991). Assessment and diagnosis of mental illness in persons with mental retardation: Methods and measures. *Behavior Modification*, *15*, 418–442.

Singh, N. N., & Winton, A. S. W. (1984). Behavioral monitoring of pharmacological interventions for self-injury. *Applied Research in Mental Retardation*, *5*, 161–170.

Singh, N. N., & Winton, A. S. W. (1989). Behavioral pharmacology. In J. K. Luiselli (Ed.), *Behavioral medicine and developmental disabilities* (pp. 152–179). New York: Springer-Verlag.

Skolnick, P., & Paul, S. M. (1983). New concepts in the neurobiology of anxiety. *Journal of Clinical Psychiatry*, *44*, 12–20.

Snyder, S. H. (1981). Dopamine receptors, neuroleptics and schizophrenia. *American Journal of Psychiatry*, *138*, 460–464.

Sokol, M. S., & Campbell, M. (1988). Novel psychoactive agents in the treatment of developmental disorders. In M. G. Aman & N. N. Singh (Eds.), *Psychopharmacology of the developmental disabilities* (pp. 146–167). New York: Springer-Verlag.

Sorgi, P., Ratey, J., & Polakoff, S. (1987). Beta-adrenergic blockers for aggressive behavior in schizophrenia. *American Journal of Psychiatry*, *144*, 539. Letter.

Sovner, R., & Hurley, A. (1981). The management of chronic behavior disorders in mentally retarded adults with lithium carbonate. *Journal of the Nervous and Mental Disease*, *169*, 191–195.

Sprague, R. L., & Werry, J. S. (1971). Methodology of psychopharmacological studies with the retarded. In N. R. Ellis (Ed.), *International review of research in mental retardation* (pp. 147–210). New York: Academic Press.

Stone, R. K., Alvarez, W. F., Ellman, G., Hom, A. C., & White, J. F. (1989). Prevalence and prediction of psychotropic drug use in California developmental centers. *American Journal of Mental Retardation*, *93*, 627–632.

Stores, G. (1988). Antiepileptic drugs. In M. G. Aman & N. N. Singh (Eds.), *Psychopharmacology of the developmental disabilities* (pp. 101–118). New York: Springer-Verlag.

Szymanski, L., Kedesdy, J., Sulkes, S., Cutler, A., & Stevens-Orr, P. (1987). Naltrexone in the treatment of self-injurious behavior: A clinical study. *Research in Developmental Disabilities*, *8*, 179–190.

Tesar, G. E. (1982). The role of stimulants in general medicine. *Drug Therapy*, *12*, 186–193.

Tu, J., & Smith, J. T. (1983). The Eastern Ontario survey: A study of drug-treated psychiatric problems in the mentally handicapped. *Canadian Journal of Psychiatry*, *28*, 270–276.

Tyrer, S. P., Walsh, A., Edwards, D. E., Berney, T. P., & Stephens, D. A. (1984). Factors associated with a good response to lithium in aggressive mentally handicapped subjects. *Progress in Neuro-Psychopharmacology and Biological Psychiatry*, *8*, 751–755.

Vaisanen, K., Kainulainen, P., Paavilainen, M. T., & Viukari, M. (1975). Sulpiride versus chlorpromazine and placebo in the treatment of restless mentally subnormal patients: A double-blind crossover study. *Current Therapeutic Research*, *17*, 202–205.

Vaisanen, K., Rimon, R., Raisanen, P., & Viukari, M. (1979). A controlled double-bling study of haloperidol versus thioridazine in the treatment of restless mentally subnormal patients: Serum levels and clinical effects. *Acta Psychiatrica Belgica*, *79*, 673–685.

Vaisanen, K., Viukari, M., Rimon, R., & Raisanen, P. (1981). Haloperidol, thioridazine and placebo in mentally subnormal patients: Serum levels and clinical effects. *Acta Psychiatrica Scandinavica*, *63*, 262–271.

van Praag, H. M. (1980). Central monoamine metabolism in depression. *Comprehensive Psychiatry*, *21*, 30–54.

Varga, E., & Simpson, G. M. (1971). Loxapine succinate in the treatment of uncontrollable destructive behavior. *Current Therapeutic Research*, *13*, 737–742.

Walters, A. S., Barrett, R. P., Feinstein, C., Mercurio, A., & Hole, W. (1990). The treatment of self-injury and social withdrawal in autism with naltrexone. *Journal of Autism and Developmental Disabilities*, *20*, 169–176.

Werry, J. S. (1982). Pharmacotherapy. In B. B. Lahey & A. E. Kazdin (Eds.), *Advances in clinical child psychology* (Vol. 5, pp. 283–321). New York: Plenum Press.

Whitman, J. R., Maier, C. J., & Eichelman, B. (1987). Beta-adrenergic blockers for aggressive behavior in schizophrenia. *American Journal of Psychiatry*, *144*, 538. Letter.

Wolfensberger, W., & Menolascino, F. (1968). Basic considerations in evaluating the ability of drugs to stimulate cognitive development in retardates. *American Journal of Mental Deficiency*, *73*, 414–423.

Woods, P. B., & Robinson, M. L. (1981). An investigation of the comparative liposolubilities of beta-adrenoceptor blocking agents. *Journal of Pharmacy and Pharmacology*, *33*, 172–173.
Yudofsky, S., Williams, D., & Gorman, J. (1981). Propranolol in the treatment of rage and violent behavior in patients with chronic brain syndromes. *American Journal of Psychiatry*, *138*, 218–220.
Zaleski, W. A. (1970). Clinical evaluation of mesoridazine in mentally retarded patients. *Canadian Psychiatric Association Journal*, *15*, 319–322.

# 13
# Peer Review and Human Rights Committees

Walter P. Christian, Stephen C. Luce, and Eric V. Larsson

The protection of clients' rights to safety and effective treatment is a basic goal of any human service agency. These rights are ensured through effective organizational, staff-training, and management practices. Professional peer reviews and human rights committee reviews are two activities that are undertaken to (1) underscore the protection of clients' rights during the clinical decision-making process, and (2), assure the consumers, the trustees of the agency, and the public that the basic rights are protected.

The treatment of severe dysfunctional behavior such as self-injury involves potential risk to the client and potential liability for the service program and practitioner. If self-injury is allowed to occur or if treatment is inadequate or ineffective in reducing injury to the client, the client's rights to treatment and safety may be violated. If the procedures employed in the treatment of self-injury are judged to be too restrictive or aversive, the client's right to the most appropriate, least restrictive treatment may be violated. In addition, there is always the risk of clients seriously injuring themselves regardless of the treatment procedures employed. For these reasons, programs and practitioners involved in work with self-injurious clients are advised to arrange for ongoing monitoring and evaluation to ensure that their treatment practices are consistent with the accepted societal and professional standards of care.

Of course, the need for review of such treatment is not totally left to the discretion of the program manager or the practitioner. For example, the Education for All Handicapped Children Act of 1975 (Public Law 94–142) provides for parent involvement and review of a student's educational program prior to its implementation. In *Wyatt v. Stickney* (1972), the court ordered that a Human Rights Committee be created "to review all research and habilitation programs to ensure that the dignity and human rights of residents are protected" (see also Christian, 1983a; Katz-Garris & Garris, 1983). The Joint Commission on the Accreditation of Health Care Organizations (JCAHO) conducts site reviews of human service programs prior to their certification. Finally, review by peers and human rights committees has come to be recognized as an essential component of human service programming, particularly when severe behavior problems are being treated and restrictive or aversive treatment procedures are being employed (Christian, 1983c, 1983d; Czyzewski, Sheldon, & Hannah, 1986; Hannah, Christian, & Clark, 1981; Mahn, Maples, Murphy, & Tubb, 1975; Martin, 1981; May et al., 1975; Morris & Brown, 1983; Sheldon-Wildgen & Risley, 1982).

Specifically, two types of review are required: professional peer review and human rights committee review. As is discussed in this chapter, these are independent review mechanisms that cannot be consolidated without compromising the goals and procedures of each.

The chapter provides a detailed outline of standard policy and procedure in a hands-on format, in the hope that what we are describing can be readily incorporated into practice. Essential references and rationales are also provided but at times may simply be implicit in the content of the procedural outlines. Following a presentation of standard practices for peer review and human rights review, a discussion of common obstacles to effective implementation of these practices is provided.

## Peer Review

Peer review is designed to determine the extent to which a service program or a specific treatment procedure is consistent with the prevailing *professional standard of care* for the client being served and the behavior being treated. The most frequent forms of peer review are case consultation and program review, although peer review can also be employed to assess the competence and ethical conduct of a particular practitioner. *Case consultation* involves a review of a particular client's plan of service, with consideration as to how it might be revised so that services and treatment procedures are more effective. *Program review* is more comprehensive than a case consultation, involving off-site review of documentation (e.g., policy and procedure manuals, procedures for training and supervising staff), typically followed by an on-site review.

In the case of a program involved in the treatment of self-injurious clients, case consultation and program review should be conducted by independent licensed professionals with demonstrated expertise in an approach to the treatment of self-injury which has a documented history of effectiveness with similar clients exhibiting similar behavioral topographies. Because a single reviewer is not always sufficient, a *peer review committee* can be established to ensure that a review is sufficiently representative and comprehensive. Most important, each reviewer must know the professional standard of care for self-injury and be able to determine whether that standard is being met by the program or procedure being reviewed.

## *Planning for Peer Review*

Planning for peer review begins with preliminary considerations concerning identification and recruitment of the membership of the peer review committee, determination of policy and procedure for a particular review, and preparation of staff for the review (as in Appendix 13A).

Planning for peer review also involves identifying the standards or criteria for the review and developing the forms and procedural guidelines to be used by reviewers. Standards or criteria are identified through a review of pertinent legislation and regulatory guidelines, relevant ethical standards, current research literature regarding services for the client population and the treatment of self-injury, and individual service plans.

Reviewers also must know what to look for and what questions to ask in their efforts to determine whether criteria are being met. The *Organizational Analysis and Development Survey* (Christian, 1984) was developed to provide peer reviewers and consultants with a listing of these questions and indicators. The *OAD Survey* is a 94–item checklist for structuring the reviewer's observation and evaluation of three aspects of program operation: Management, service programming, and legal safety. Guidelines more specific to programs and procedures for the treatment of self-injurious behavior have been developed by Judith Favell and are presented in Appendix 13B. Another useful device is the "Peer Reviewer's Evaluation Form," shown in Appendix 13C. It can be used to facilitate the reviewer's task and to ensure that he or she obtains the kind of information most likely to result in a representative evaluative report.

These surveys help to ensure that review activity is sufficiently systematic and comprehensive and to facilitate the preparation of written reports of findings and recommendations. It also is useful to have key staff complete selected items on the survey as part of off-site planning for the review. Reviewers can then use their on-site ratings to check the reliability of information obtained from staff. Low reliability of these ratings would raise questions about whether the program's communication systems are adequate and whether staff and management are sufficiently trained and supervised in the appropriate treatment methodology.

## *Off-Site Review*

Unless it is limited to a review of a sample document or service plan, off-site review is typically preliminary to on-site activity. In fact, the scope and focus of on-site review activity is frequently determined following a review of supporting documentation. Therefore, as much pertinent documentation as possible should be reviewed prior to the site visit, taking care to ensure that the program has obtained the necessary consent to share the information. In addition to the survey data described in the previous section, documentation needed for a thorough off-site review is included in Appendix 13D.

Not every review will require such extensive review of documentation, but reviewers should at least have access to such information. Additional information can be requested, and communication between reviewers concerning their preliminary findings and recommendations can be conducted by telephone.

## *On-Site Review*

On-site review is most efficient when reviewers are assigned office space, as well as a member or members of the program staff to assist them in getting around the facility, interviewing staff, observing clients, and examining documents. In our experience, the more competent the staff assisting the reviewers, the more accurate the reviewers' findings. A typed agenda should also be developed and provided to reviewers and program staff in advance of on-site activity. Christian and Hannah (1983) have described procedural steps for on-site program review and, to a lesser extent, case consultation (see Appendix 13E). Any necessary orientation and training on these procedures should be provided for reviewers prior to the site visit.

## *Reporting Findings and Recommendations*

An accurate, well-organized, comprehensive report serves as the permanent product data of review activity. The quality of the report is an indication of the general competence of the reviewer (i.e., the reviewer's understanding of the pertinent professional standard of care) and the relevance of the reviewer's findings and the appropriateness of his or her recommendations. A poor report can actually serve to compromise or even invalidate an otherwise competent review.

For these reasons, it is a good idea for program staff and reviewers to consider the format of the written report *prior* to the review. For example, reports of case consultation should include the information listed in Appendix 13F.

Reports of program review should include a comprehensive overview of the setting and its facilities, staff, and services, as well as specific findings and recommendations concerning the aspect of the program that was the primary focus of review activity. There are several formats for writing such a report, but in general, several key sections should always be included (Christian & Hannah, 1983). A sample is presented in Appendix 13G.

### *In-House Review*

In our experience, effective in-house review strategies are critical to obtaining satisfactory results from any type of external program or human rights review. Strategies such as regular observation and recording of client behavior, observation and recording of staff behavior, case record review, client tracking systems, and professional advisory boards are particularly valuable in settings providing services to clients at risk. These strategies are also consistent with JCAHO guidelines that require in-house monitoring of various aspects of program operation and service delivery by staff committees (e.g., monitoring of seclusion and restraint by the "Executive Committee of the Professional Staff").

For example, Christian and Romanczyk (1986) have described how task-analyzed orientation and training, performance contracting, effective supervision, and peer review (e.g., treatment team meetings) can be used to develop and maintain reliable observation and recording of client behavior. Dyer, Schwartz, and Luce (1984) have shown how *pla-check* ratings (Doke & Risley, 1972) and contingent feedback can be used to improve the quantity and quality of staff interaction with clients. Christian, Norris, Anderson, and Blew (1984) used case-record review procedures and contingent feedback to monitor and improve the record-keeping performance of direct service staff in a residential treatment setting. Gruber, McGrale, Blew, Luce, and Christian (1982) found guidelines (agenda for meetings), prompts, and performance feedback to be effective in increasing staff participation, data presentations, and data-based revision of service plans at residential treatment team meetings. Christian, Clark, and Luke (1981), and Christian and Hannah (1983) have described how client tracking systems can help to ensure that (a) each client receives services and treatment procedures consistent with his or her needs; (b) periodic reviews of client progress are conducted; (c) services for the client are adequately planned, documented, and evaluated; and (d) service programming is consistent across staff and settings. Finally, Christian (1983b) has described how a professional advisory board of expert consultants can be established to provide program staff with ongoing, informal evaluative feedback with a minimum investment of time, effort, and money.

## Human Rights Committees

Whereas peer review is concerned with the extent to which a program or procedure is consistent with the professional standard of care, human rights review is concerned with the *societal standard of care*, as defined in laws and regulations. As the major vehicle of human rights review, the human rights committee (HRC) is designed to provide safeguards sufficient to protect clients from inhumane and improper treatment and to ensure that treatment is as efficient, appropriate, and minimally restrictive as possible. In the case of the self-injurious client, the HRC must determine whether proposed treatment procedures are acceptable in light of the totality of circumstances (i.e., given the severity of the self-injury and whether the behavior can be reduced or eliminated using a treatment procedure less restrictive than that which has been proposed). In short, the HRC is concerned with the legal safety of service programming—namely, how clients can *receive effective treatment* without infringing on their constitutional right to be *free from unnecessarily restrictive treatment.*

Before proceeding with a discussion of HRC membership and function, however, it is important to note that an effective HRC should be considered part of an overall system for developing a legally safe service program. Such a system includes the following strategies: (a) identifying criteria for the protection of client rights within a human service setting; (b) assessing the status of the program relative to legal safety criteria; (c) educating staff, clients, and client guardians about rights issues and the program's commitment to protect client rights; (d) obtaining informed consent for any assessment and treatment the client receives; (e) maintaining confidentiality about all aspects of the client's involvement with the service program; (g) using internal and external peer review to track client progress and evaluate program effectiveness; (h) providing task-analyzed orientation, training, supervision, and evaluation of program staff in client rights issues and legal safety requirements; and (i) working with the HRC to provide orientation, training, and performance contracting for the program's human rights officer (HRO) and to ensure that the HRO and program staff work cooperatively to monitor client rights and legal safety. A list of questions for use by program staff in assessing the status of its legal safety policy and procedure is provided in Appendix 13H.

## *Establishing the Committee*

### Membership

In many cases, the membership and function of a program's HRC are dictated by state regulation and/or the requirements of certifying/licensing agencies. Most important, the HRC should be representative of societal standards and capable of making *objective* decisions. Therefore, while at least 25% of HRC membership can be program staff, 75% should be made up of volunteers who are representative of the local community. For programs serving self-injurious clients, HRC membership should include one or more lawyers, physicians, clergy, client guardians or advocates, psychologists, and educators. Care should be taken to ensure that the HRC is not dominated by a special interest, whether it be that of staff and supportive professionals or of parents and advocates. If objectivity is compromised, the HRC will be ineffective and unresponsive to the needs of either the client or the program.

#### Policy and Procedure

It is common for the HRC to meet a minimum of once a month, with the agenda developed and distributed at least 2 weeks prior to the meeting. At each meeting, a specified number of randomly selected client records should be reviewed. Each member should serve as a representative for certain clients and should present information obtained from each client's case record and/or from his or her own observations of, and interview with, the client receiving services, providing of course the client has given consent for the release of this information. In addition, a member of the program staff should present the rationale and justification for the client's treatment. The HRC should also consider proposals for all moderately restrictive treatment procedures, determining whether the overall treatment goals and procedures are appropriate and whether the goals are being reached.

In our experience, an effective HRC is one that has specific policies and procedures and that provides orientation and training to ensure that its members' performance is consistent with procedural guidelines. Sample policies and procedures for the HRC are presented in Appendix 13I. Sample guidelines for use by the HRC in specifying levels of restrictiveness for treatment procedures are provided in Appendix 13J.

### *Interacting with the Committee*

In our experience, the major problem encountered by human service staff in their work with an HRC is not in how the HRC operates but how staff members interact with the HRC. The HRC functions much like a computer, with the quality of its decision-making being largely dependent on the quality of the information it is provided. In other words, there should never be an occasion where the HRC rejects a proposed treatment procedure (i.e., approval is formally requested only when approval has been implicitly obtained by adherence to accepted procedures). For these reasons, several procedures should be followed when seeking a positive review or approval from an HRC (Appendix 13K).

## Obstacles to Implementation

A number of obstacles to effective implementation may be evident when peer review and HRC review procedures are implemented in the human service setting. In our experience, obstacles are most common in the areas of committee membership, definition of terms, and agency implementation.

## Committee Membership

As discussed previously, the different policies and procedures for peer review and for HRC review require different membership for each review committee. The purpose of the HRC is to provide social validation for the proposed treatment procedures, from the point of view of the lay public. The purpose of the peer review committee is to provide expert validation. However, in our experience, HRCs are often found to be composed of experts rather than members of the lay public. This is problematic because the participation of the experts is subject to parochial professional bias and special clinical interests. We have seen how HRC discussions can deteriorate into the provision of recommendations for programming and theoretical disputes rather than focus upon judgments of the social validity and appropriateness of treatment procedures. In these situations, lay persons on the HRC may be intimidated by their own lack of experience in the professional realm and may provide little participation. Because the members are volunteers, and there is often much to be accomplished, such digressions may result in ineffective, inefficient HRC meetings and may ultimately result in inadequate committee function and resignation of frustrated committee members.

Of course, the lay membership of the HRC may also be a source of difficulty (i.e., the inexperience of these individuals, while necessary to ensure their objectivity, may contribute to inefficient HRC function). Without adequate orientation and training, lay members are unlikely to appreciate the intended purpose of their participation and may not easily focus on the necessary activities. Therefore, in order to accomplish the goals of the HRC, sufficient orientation, training, and coordination must be provided. An effective HRC must have a well-trained chair, who can develop a structured agenda and manage the meetings tightly enough to complete the agenda within a reasonable time period.

Regarding the membership of the peer review committee, peer reviewers should be thoughtfully recruited, the agency should contract with the reviewers for specific activities, and the agency should monitor reviewers' performance to ensure that they meet the terms of their contract. Typically, peer reviewers are paid consultants whose excess time can become very expensive if the goals of the review are not clearly specified and adhered to. It is also important, however, that the agency be thoroughly prepared for the review to ensure that the reviewer has access to the written materials, facilities, personnel, and clients necessary to ensure that the reviewer can fulfill the requirements of his or her contract.

Thoughtful recruitment of members for the HRC is also important but may be considerably more difficult. The HRC members cannot be paid or otherwise induced to participate without compromising their objectivity. On the other hand, open invitations to the public rarely result in inquiries from appropriate members. Parents and relatives, while serving one important role on the committee, may have personal motives that conflict with the long-term interests of the clients. Therefore, some manner of locating persons who do not have some vested interest in the treatment procedures is necessary. The most common route is to work through the clinician's network of associates in the community to find volunteers who already have a record of reliable participation in similar activities.

Another avenue is to recruit HRC members from the agency's board of trustees. When these persons have little or no involvement in the day-to-day programming and treatment planning at the service agency, they can prove to be a valuable addition to the HRC. Not only do they provide the input of the lay public, but they also have a personal stake in the professional and legal validity of the agency's clinical practices. This practice has precedence in the literature (Sheldon-Wildgen & Risley, 1982) and in the regulations of states such as Massachusetts (Office for Children, 1989). However, the use of individuals who are in any way affiliated with the agency as HRC members is likely to receive careful scrutiny from regulatory agencies and advocates and must be utilized cautiously.

## *Definitional Issues*

A written policy and procedure manual is basic to effective review of human rights and professional practice. It is essential to translate due process from a solid base of policy into practice. However, an obstacle to ensuring the rights of clients comes in the ambiguity of the terms chosen to describe the reviewed procedures. A variety of euphemisms, for example, are commonly employed by agencies in order to describe procedures that might meet with less approval if more specific terminology were used. For example, many contingent-effort (Luce, Christian, Lipsker, & Hall, 1981) procedures, especially those involving considerable physical guidance, may warrant human rights review. However, the same procedure is frequently implemented without human rights review and is described as "prompting on-task behavior" or a similar euphemism. Similarly, the procedure of movement-suppression time-out (Rolider & Van Houten, 1985) may warrant human rights review, while comparable procedures are being applied without review in the form of "prompting a client to remain in a corner" time-out procedure. Solutions to these problems are discussed subsequently.

In considering the extent to which a procedure should be reviewed by an HRC, a number of dimensions may be identified. These dimensions include the intensity of the procedure, the duration of the procedure, the level of client effort required by the procedure, the topography of the effortful response, the level of client resistance, the relation of procedures and target behaviors, the combination of component treatment procedures, and the definition of the target behavior.

In defining the *intensity* of treatment procedures, the challenge is to ensure that the procedures are defined along the critical dimensions of restrictiveness. The *duration*, or length of application, of each procedure is the most objectively definable dimension and therefore each procedure should have clear duration guidelines specified. The *acceptable level of effort* of a procedure and the amount of *client resistance* should also be specified but may remain subject to misinterpretation. In these cases, procedural guidelines should be written as conservatively as possible. For example, the definition of physical resistance by the client might include any action by a client being physically guided that (1) might result in an injury such as bruising, or (2) may be misinterpreted by any observer.

Another dimension concerns when the treatment procedure is administered. The clarity of the specific target response required to initiate the contingency and the exact procedure can dramatically affect the restrictiveness of the procedure under peer review. An unclear contingency or one that lacks specificity leads to inconsistent application, application to untargeted behaviors, or consequences that are ineffectively delayed. A suppressive procedure that is not delivered contingently is unlikely to be effective in reducing the rate of the behavior. Therefore, the lack of a contingency would be likely to cause an otherwise acceptable procedure to be completely unacceptable as an unnecessary intrusion into the life of the client.

In some cases, there may not be a contingency in which a specific target response is required to cue the procedure. For example, a device such as a padded brace or a helmet that is applied noncontingently as part of a plan for preventing the risk of injury to a client may be viewed as much less restrictive than the contingent application of the same device as an aversive consequence for a target behavior. In fact, it is essential to minimize the risk of self-injury while the effects of a contingent procedure are developing. Medication that is prescribed as an ongoing prophylactic may be viewed as much less restrictive than the same medication when administered contingently as a chemical restraint.

Some extinction and negative-reinforcement strategies present clinicians with another condition involving exposing clients to a potentially unpleasant stimulus noncontingently. These procedures sometimes involve noncontingently exposing a client to a subjectively aversive stimulus in order either to extinguish fearful or escape behavior or to develop escape or avoidance behaviors. In these cases, HRC review may be essential to reconcile the value of exposing a client to a subjectively noxious, fearful stimulus, as opposed to the value of continuing to maintain a probability of debilitating emotional responses. To the extent that the stimulus of concern is normally found in naturalistic settings, controversy is diminished.

Another definitional problem arises when the treatment procedure is composed of multiple components. The procedure may be identified and categorized on the basis of one salient aspect (e.g., restitution), but closer scrutiny of the various unlabeled components of the procedure (e.g., graduated guidance) may result in a radically different reading of restrictiveness. A problem of this kind also exists when one procedure (e.g., physical restraint) is contingent upon the client's lack of compliance with a primary procedure (e.g., positive practice). In this case, traditional monitoring methods and forms that are designed for one-component procedures may not be sophisticated enough to accurately report complete data on multiple component procedures. The secondary procedure will often be much more restrictive but may be much less carefully documented. Also, the level of its implementation may be hidden in summary data on the primary procedure.

This situation is most likely to exist when the client is first trained to participate in the restrictive procedure. For example, in the early stages of a treatment plan, the client may be physically prompted through a procedure. The treatment plan to be reviewed by others must describe and propose measurement strategies for all stages of the procedure. Indeed, in most cases, the procedures implemented in the training phase will be much more restrictive in duration and intensity than those implemented once the client has been repeatedly exposed to treatment. In other cases, restrictiveness may increase if multiple treatment applications are needed. For example, some forms of medication and effort have greater risk if administered over a long period of time.

Further, with multiple component procedures, one or more components may be unnecessary, despite the fact that the total package may be effective. In some cases, the unnecessary component may involve the increased risk of the package, while in other cases, it might obscure the risks that the package contains. For example, an overcorrection procedure might contain forms of manual guidance that come to resemble physical restraint. The manual guidance procedure may not be obvious to a reviewer unless the prompting component were completely described. Obviously such a package could lead one to conclude that a procedure is more or less effective than it really is. This could result in the client being given unnecessary exposure to ineffective procedures or a procedure with greater risks than are necessary.

The definition of the target behavior is also a major issue. The actual topography of the behavior may not warrant the restrictiveness of the intervention. For example, a self-injury definition may include some mild behaviors that are not severe or dangerous enough to warrant restrictive procedures. However, the label assigned to the definition may sound so dangerous as to allow a procedure to be continued when it is actually contingent upon innocuous behaviors. Often, this problem arises because a treatment procedure, to be effective, must be designed with a wide enough target definition to encompass the full class of severe and mild self-injurious behaviors. In our experience, the self-injurious behavior will often respond to treatment and result in an elimination of the severe forms of the behavior, but a residual rate of the mild forms will continue. In this case, the relatively mild forms of the behavior, still referred to by the severe label, can perpetuate an unnecessarily restrictive procedure. In such a case, a thorough review is needed to fade to a less restrictive procedure.

A final dimension concerns how the treatment procedure fits with the context of the behavior. The actual level of restrictiveness of a procedure may depend on the context of its application rather than on a simple description of the procedure itself. A treatment procedure that consists of an activity that is unrelated to or that interferes with the ongoing activity that was scheduled for the client would be likely to be judged more restrictive than one that is related to the ongoing activity. For example, moderately restrictive procedures for the treatment of self-injury might involve prompting a client through a sorting task during a scheduled time to watch television. Alternatively, a less-restrictive procedure might involve prompting a client to sit on his or her hands. Another form of contingent effort may involve prompting a client to clean the floor after misusing instructional materials. Being given new academic materials during an instructional period would be less disruptive and therefore less restrictive.

## *Implementation*

The most well-organized human rights and peer review activities will be ineffective if the activities are not functionally integrated into the day-to-day responsibilities of the direct-care staff. For example, the agency may generate very appropriate paperwork to document the protections that were afforded to various clients in various situations, but other instances of lack of due process are not precluded by this. A situation of this kind can be very difficult to detect at the level of agency review.

Procedures that may help to ensure the protection of client rights include assigning the direct-care staff the responsibilities of one-to-one case managers for each client; task-analyzing the responsibilities of these case managers to act as personal human rights officers for each client; and assigning the case managers' direct supervisor with the responsibilities of staff training and monitoring human rights compliance and treatment adherence (Christian & Reitz, 1986). In particular, training and organizational prompts may be provided to staff so that they will routinely initiate due process at the appropriate junctures and will follow up on the results of the reviews. For example, one common lack of adherence to due process occurs when clients receive emergency restraint for self-injurious behaviors. While these interventions may closely adhere to the standards for emergency practice, they may come to be applied as a routine to control a specified behavior without being subjected to formal review as a part of the client's treatment plan. Such abuses are very difficult to uncover in an external review. Comprehensive staff training and direct on-site supervision by personnel who have demonstrated skills in the procedures being used are much more likely to prevent such problems.

A related issue concerns the validity of the agency's procedures. While a program may have written treatment procedures and methods for reliable and objective data collection, which are state-of-the-art, these activities may not be consistently or accurately implemented by staff. As mentioned previously, statements of policy and procedure may contain many points of definitional ambiguity. The only certain protection of the rights of the clients in these cases rests on the quality of the decisions made by the direct-care staff, both during the implementation of the procedure and in prompting a review. Once again, comprehensive staff training and direct supervision is much more likely to ensure the protection of human rights than is an external review activity. This does not mean that the review is redundant; rather, the review becomes functional when the staff members consistently address the review and its outcomes in a timely manner.

This also raises the issue of staff satisfaction with the review procedures. In many agencies, review activities are commonly viewed as needless red tape and a contributing source of staff attrition. This view may result in a serious lack of adherence to standards. However, if the review activities are functionally integrated into the program, the benefits may be more readily appreciated by the staff and communicated to the consumers.

## Summary

Programs and practitioners involved in the education and treatment of self-injurious clients must take steps to ensure that their policies and procedures are consistent with professional and societal standards of care. The professional standard of care is defined by the research literature and professional codes of ethics. The societal standard of care is defined by laws and regulations, which are reflective of the values and concerns of the general public.

This chapter has described how compliance with each of these standards can be evaluated and promoted, using peer review and human rights committees. Policies and procedures specific to each type of review are presented, as well as information concerning how program staff can be supportive of and cooperative with each type of review activity. As described throughout the chapter, peer review and human rights committees will be most effective when used in conjunction with a well-coordinated system of in-house legal safeguards and program evaluation strategies.

## References

Christian, W. P. (1983a). Legal issues relevant to child development and behavior. In M. D. Levine, W. B. Carey, A. C. Crocker, & R. T. Gross (Eds.), *Developmental-behavioral pediatrics* (pp. 1175–1190). Philadelphia: W. B. Saunders.

Christian, W. P. (1983b). Managing the performance of the human service consultant. *The Behavior Therapist*, *6*, 47–49.

Christian, W. P. (1983c). Professional peer review: Recommended strategies for reviewer and reviewee. *The Behavior Therapist*, *6*, 86–89.

Christian, W. P. (1983d). Protecting client rights in mental health programs. *Administration in Mental Health*, *11*(2), 115–123.

Christian, W. P. (1986). *Assessing the structure and process of mental health and retardation services: The Organizational Analysis and Development Survey*. In Fuoco, F. J. & Christian W. P. (Eds.), *Behavior therapy in residential treatment environments* (pp. 168–188). New York: Van Nostrand Reinhold.

Christian, W. P., Clark, H. B., & Luke, D. E. (1981). Sefeguarding clients' rights in the provision of clinical counseling services to children. In G. T. Hannah, W. P. Christian & H. B. Clark (Eds.), *Preservation of clients' rights: A handbook for practitioners providing therapeutic, educational, and rehabilitative services* (pp. 19–41). New York: Free Press.

Christian, W. P., & Hannah, G. T. (1983). *Effective management in human services*. Englewood Cliffs, NJ: Prentice-Hall.

Christian, W. P., Norris, M. B., Anderson, S. R., & Blew, P. A. (1984). Improving the record-keeping performance of direct service personnel. *Journal of Mental Health Administration*, *11*(2), 4–7.

Christian, W. P., & Reitz, A. (1986). Administration. In F. J. Fuoco & W. P. Christian (Eds.), *Behavior analysis and therapy in residential programs*. New York: Van Nostrand Reinhold.

Christian, W. P., & Romanczyk, R. G. (1986). Evaluation. In F. J. Fuoco & W. P. Christian (Eds.), *Behavior analysis and therapy in residential programs* (pp. 145–193). New York: Van Nostrand Reinhold.

Czyzewski, M. J., Sheldon, J., & Hannah, G. T. (1986). Legal safety in residential treatment environments. In F. J. Fuoco & W. P. Christian (Eds.), *Behavior analysis and therapy in residential programs* (pp. 194–228). New York: Van Nostrand Reinhold.

Doke, L. E., & Risley, T. R. (1972). The organization of day-care environments: Required vs. optional activities. *Journal of Applied Behavior Analysis*, *5*, 405–420.

Dyer, K., Schwartz, I., & Luce, S. C. (1984). Improving the quality of planned activities through staff feedback. *Journal of Applied Behavior Analysis*, *17*, 249–259.

Griffith, R. G., & Henning, D. B. (1981). What is a human rights committee? *Mental Retardation. 19*(2), 61–63.

Gruber, B. K., McGrale, J. E., Blew, P. A., Luce, S. C., & Christian, W. P. (1982, May). *Increasing the efficiency of client review meetings*. Paper presented at the annual convention of the Association for Behavior Analysis, Milwaukee.

Hannah, G. T., Christian, W. P., & Clark, H. B. (Eds.). (1981). *Preservation of client rights: A handbook for practitioners providing therapeutic, educational, and rehabilitative services*. New York: Macmillan/Free Press.

Katz-Garris, L., & Garris, R. P. (1983). Litigation and legislative regulations impacting on the treatment of the developmentally disabled. In J. L. Matson & F. Andrasik (Eds.), *Treatment issues and innovation in mental retardation* (pp. 97–128). New York: Plenum.

Luce, S. C., Christian, W. P., Lipsker, L., & Hall, R. V. (1981). Response cost: A case for specificity. *The Behavior Analyst. 4*, 75–80.

Mahn, S., Maples, S., Murphy, S., & Tubb, G. (1975). A mechanism for enforcing the right to treatment: The Human Rights Committee. *Law & Psychology Review*; Spring, 131–149.

Martin, R. (1981). Legal issues in preserving clients rights. In G. T. Hannah, W. P. Christian, & H. B. Clark (Eds.), *Preservation of client rights: A handbook for practitioners providing therapeutic, educational and rehabilitative services* (pp. 3–13). New York: Free Press.

May, J. G., Jr., Risley, T. R., Twardosz, S., Friedman, P., Bijou, S. W., & Wexler, D. (1975). *Guidelines for the use of behavioral procedures in state programs for retarded persons* (Monograph). Arlington: National Association for Retarded Citizens Advisory Research Committee.

Morris, R. J., & Brown, D. K. (1983). Legal and ethical issues in behavior modification with mentally retarded persons. In J. L. Matson & F. Andrasik (Eds.), *Treatment issues and innovation in mental retardation* (pp. 61–95). New York: Plenum.

Office for Children, Commonwealth of Massachusetts. (1989). *Regulations for Licensure or Approval of Group Care Facilities for Children*. Report No. 603 CMR 3.00 et seq.

Rolider, A., & Van Houten, R. (1985). Movement suppression time-out for undesirable behavior in psychotic and severely developmentally delayed children. *Journal of Applied Behavior Analysis, 18*, 275–288.

Sheldon-Wildgen, J., & Risley, T. R. (1982). Balancing clients' rights: The establishment of human rights and peer review committees. In A. Bellack, M. Hersen & A. Kazdin (Eds.), *International handbook of behavior modification* (pp. 263–289). New York: Plenum.

Wyatt v. Stickney, 325 F. Supp. 781, 784, aff'd on rehearing 344 F. Supp. 341 (M. D. Ala. 1971), aff'd on rehearing 344 F. Supp. 373, aff'd in separate decision, 344 F. Supp. 781, 784, aff'd on rehearing 344 F. Supp. 341 (M. D. Ala. 1971), aff'd on rehearing 344 F. Supp. 373, aff'd in separate decision, 344 F. Supp 387. 390, 392, 394–407 (M. D. Ala. 1972), aff'd sub nom, Wyatt v. Aderholt, 530 F. 2d 1305 (5th Dir. 1975).

# Appendix 13A Preparation for Peer Review: Agency Self-evaluation

1. Is the review proactive or reactive? What crisis or problem has prompted the reactive review? What is the proactive review intended to provide (e.g., professional validation for some program or procedure, supplemental program evaluation efforts, and/or facilitation of organizational planning and development)?
2. Are program staff likely to be cooperative and supportive of the review? Which staff should participate in the review? Do staff know how to conduct themselves during a review?
3. Is the review likely to be controversial? Is there likely to be some involvement by the courts or federal/state regulatory agencies?
4. Have there been previous reviews similar to the one proposed? What was the outcome?
5. What activity is the review likely to involve (e.g., case consultation, procedure review, program review, off-site review of documentation, on-site review)?
6. What product is the review expected to yield (e.g., desired format of written report), and how is that product to be used and/or disseminated?

# Appendix 13B
# Guidelines for Designing and Evaluating Treatment Programs for Self-injurious Behavior (SIB)[1]

I. Planning

_____ 1. Is the designer of the program competent in the area of behavioral treatment of SIB?

_____ 2. Has appropriate consultation been sought/received?

_____ 3. Is the program devised in the context of an interdisciplinary process and regarded as clinically important for this client?

II. Treatment Program

Does the intervention program specifically include

_____ 1. Prioritization and limitation of goals, with self-injury ranked as one of the first targets for intervention?

_____ 2. Objective description of, and data on the targeted self-injurious behaviors(s) (including topography, rate, and intensity)?

_____ 3. Provision for protection of the individual during treatment (e.g., by manual blocking of the SIB, or some form of physical protection)?

_____ 4. Documentation that a thorough medical exam was conducted and appropriate medical treatment applied (e.g., with otitis media or impaction)?

_____ 5. Rationale for use of psychotropics, if used, and provision for frequent behavioral evaluation of the drugs' effects?

_____ 6. Description, based on direct observation and caregiver reports, of

Conditions under which SIB occurs?
Conditions under which SIB does not occur?
Typical consequences of SIB?

[1] Favell, J. E. Unpublished manuscript, used by permission.

Complete listing of appropriate behavior and the usual consequences for such behavior?

_____ 7. Based on Item 6, provision for altering or eliminating conditions that are associated with the SIB (e.g., noise, fatigue, demands)?

_____ 8. Based on Item 6, provision for use of conditions associated with little or no SIB as a distraction and/or as reinforcer?

_____ 9. Procedures for strengthening appropriate, noninjurious behavior, including

Provision for a humane, enriched environment in which alternative activities and opportunities for social interaction are available at all times?

Formal or informal evidence that the reinforcers to be used are powerful?

Provision for reinforcement for periods of noninjury (differential reinforcement of other behavior)?

List of at least 15 behaviors to be reinforced, which are at least approximations of appropriate behavior and which hold promise as being incompatible with SIB (e.g., communication, compliance, independent play (differential reinforcement of incompatible behavior)?

Specification of contingencies, schedules of reinforcement and other specific information on when, how, and for what behavior reinforcers will be delivered?

_____ 10. Attempts to identify and minimize reinforcement for SIB:

Positive reinforcement, especially attention?

Negative reinforcement (i.e., the opportunity to escape or avoid unpleasant situations)?

Sensory stimulation?

_____ 11. Explicit attention to redistributing relative reinforcement toward appropriate, noninjurious behavior and away from SIB?

_____ 12. If relevant, justification for use of punishment (e.g., insufficient effects with differential reinforcement procedures by themselves, lack of feasibility of differential reinforcement procedures due to severity, frequency, or topography of SIB)?

_____ 13. Documentation of appropriateness and effectiveness of specific punishment procedure proposed:

From the research literature?

Rationale for its appropriateness with this individual?

_____ 14. Research support for *any* proposed intervention that departs from the preceding (Items 1 through 13)?
_____ 15. Explicit program plans for generalizing improvement to all situations?
_____ 16. Explicit program plans for maintaining improvement over time?
_____ 17. Provision for frequent (e.g., daily) review and, if necessary, revision of these procedures by the program's designer?

III. Review
_____ 1. Was the treatment plan reviewed and approved by the program's administration?
_____ 2. Was the treatment plan approved by an HRC composed of consumer representatives, lawyers, and clients?
_____ 3. Was the treatment plan approved by a peer review committee composed of qualified behavioral psychologists who are independent of the program under review?
_____ 4. Was informed consent obtained from the appropriate legal guardian (or, if appropriate, the client himself or herself)?

IV. Implementation Plan
_____ 1. Are sufficient and appropriate staff identified to conduct treatment?
_____ 2. Is a specific schedule of staff coverage devised and updated daily?
_____ 3. Does staff training include
Training by a qualified behavioral psychologist?
Training to criteria in the actual conduct of the program?
_____ 4. Has the physical environment been arranged so that treatment can occur (e.g., are the appropriate recreational materials and reinforcers *always* available; is space created where the client can be treated and monitored)?
_____ 5. Have social and programmatic features of the environment been arranged so that treatment can occur (e.g., are special meal schedules arranged, are other clients who disrupt treatment or agitate the self-injurer occupied elsewhere)?
_____ 6. Can treatment occur in this overall situation (e.g., with this staff, in this physical and social environment)?

V. Management and Evaluation of Treatment

____ 1. Are provisions made for daily, direct observation of treatment by

Management (especially the direct supervisor)?

Appropriate professional staff (especially the psychologist)?

____ 2. Are provisions made for regular, direct observation of treatment by

Human rights committee members or their representatives?

Peer review committee members or their representatives?

____ 3. Are arrangements made for review of the data on SIB and appropriate, noninjurious behavior at least weekly by professional, administrative, and direct-service staff?

____ 4. Are consequences brought to bear on compliance with treatment procedures:

If staff are complying, are they receiving, for example, positive feedback, credit for promotions, or merit raises?

If staff are not complying, are they receiving corrective feedback, or transfers, or termination?

# Appendix 13C
# Peer Reviewer's Evaluation Form[2]

Program reviewed: ______________________________
Program area: ______________________________
Program personnel interviewed (name and title): ______________________________
______________________________
______________________________
______________________________

1. What are the program's strengths in this areas? ______________________________
______________________________
______________________________
______________________________

2. What are the program's weaknesses in this area? ______________________________
______________________________
______________________________
______________________________

3. What improvements/program changes in this area might be recommended? ______________________________
______________________________
______________________________
______________________________

4. Additional comments (use back of form if necessary) ______________________________
______________________________
______________________________
______________________________

Reviewer's name ______________________________ Date ______________

[2] Data from Christian, W. P., & Hannah, G. T. (1983).

# Appendix 13D
# Documentation for Off-Site Review

1. Policy and procedure information (including a policy and procedure manual, if available, current organizational charts, performance standards for key positions, and information regarding personnel practices): This should include a detailed description of how program staff are oriented, trained, supervised, and evaluated; special attention should be given to orientation, training, and so on, in the use of restrictive treatment procedures
2. Demographic data concerning clients (age, presenting problems, length of stay) and staff (academic qualifications, certifications, previous experience)
3. Description of strategies utilized to ensure that the program is legally safe (e.g., human rights committee policy and procedure, minutes from HRC meetings, procedures for obtaining informed consent and ensuring confidentiality, etc.)
4. A sample treatment plan considered to be representative of the clients presently served in the program; for case consultation, a copy of the treatment plan for a self-injurious client; examples of progress notes and behavior change data appropriate to such a treatment plan
5. Copies of reports (findings and recommendations) by external consultants and peer reviewers who have evaluated the program during the past 12 months
6. A detailed description of all program evaluation strategies presently employed by the program, including a copy of the program's most recent annual report, if available
7. Finally, copies of any documentation indicating the effectiveness of the program, satisfaction of its consumers and funding agencies, satisfaction of its staff, and so on (e.g., summaries of satisfaction ratings, data for clients presently served by the program indicating the extent to which their needs are being met, follow-up data for clients discharged from the program) (Christian, 1983d)

# Appendix 13E
# Outline of On-Site Program Review

A. Initial conference with key program staff
   1. Introduction of reviewers and program staff; assignment of staff to assist reviewers
   2. Discussion concerning purpose, goals, and objectives for review
   3. Discussion of agenda for review activity
   4. Clarification and additional information, as necessary (e.g., answering questions from program staff)

B. Review activity
   1. Examination of pertinent program descriptions, records, etc. (as previously described)
   2. Examination of human rights committee minutes
   3. Tour of facility
   4. Observation of staff performance and client behavior
   5. Interviews with key staff (using forms and guidelines previously described)
   6. Interviews with clients (if possible), representatives of local social services agencies, members of the local community, etc.

C. Wrap-up meeting of review committee
   1. Brief summary by each reviewer
   2. Preparation for debriefing program staff

D. Debriefing of program staff
   1. Purpose of review
   2. Findings
      a. Exemplary areas
      b. Areas in need of improvement
   3. Recommendations

E. Preparation and dissemination of written reports

F. Follow-up by peer reviewers
   1. Obtaining satisfaction ratings from key staff of program reviewed

2. Obtaining feedback from reviewers concerning how to improve future reviews
3. Monitoring program concerning follow-through on reviewers' recommendations
   a. Written reports
   b. Telephone contacts
   c. Additional on-site review (if necessary)

# Appendix 13F
# Components of Case Review Report

1. An assessment of the client's present plan of treatment (i.e., what it includes and why it is or is not effective)
2. An appraisal of the legal and ethical safeguards presently in effect and how they might be improved (e.g., human rights committee review, in-house peer review)
3. A revised plan of treatment (if necessary)
4. References to the professional literature supporting a recommended revision of the treatment plan
5. Description of a method for evaluating and providing a follow-up review of the revised treatment plan
6. A discussion of future programming strategies, where appropriate (e.g., arranging for eventual transition of the client to a less-restrictive treatment setting, working with a therapist in the local area capable of providing expert consultation on an ongoing basis, seeking the assistance of state agencies, and/or obtaining additional on-site peer review services)

# Appendix 13G
# Components of Program Review Report

A. Summary
   1. Purpose of the review
   2. Findings
   3. Recommendations

B. Table of contents

C. Peer review committee
   1. Names and affiliations
   2. Areas of expertise

D. Acknowledgments

E. Body of report
   1. Purpose of review
   2. Focus (areas of program reviewed)
   3. Procedures (observation, evaluation, etc.) employed in the review
   4. General description of the program
      a. Physical plant
      b. Program mission (goals and objectives)
      c. Client population
      d. Staffing (qualifications, staff-to-client ratio)
      e. Services; philosophy of treatment
      f. Pertinent licensing/regulatory agencies
   5. Exemplary aspects of the program
   6. Recommendations for improvement
   7. Plans for follow-up
   8. Concluding comments

F. References (for publications cited in report)

G. Appendixes (supporting documents)

# Appendix 13H
# Legal Safety Assessment[3]

1. Does the program provide information for each new client that lists and explains his or her rights as a consumer of the program's services? Is this information written in a language that the client can understand?
2. Has the program developed a policy statement concerning legal safety in human service programming and the role of program staff in ensuring that those guidelines are followed?
3. Do program staff members receive orientation and training in legal safety issues and procedures and the skills necessary to provide legally safe programming to the program's clients?
4. Does placement of the client in the program subject him or her to unequal or unfair circumstances?
5. Is written consent obtained from the client (or proper representative) concerning the goals, objectives, potential risks/benefits, and procedural strategies of the services he or she is to receive?
6. Have procedures been established for protecting the client's privacy and the confidentiality of his or her involvement with the program?
7. Is written consent obtained from the client (or proper representative) to seek and/or give referral information from/to other agencies?
8. When possible, is feedback obtained from the client regarding his or her own perception of needs and treatment goals?
9. Is there an opportunity for the client (or proper representative) to air any dispute about procedures?
10. Does the client receive services as part of an individualized plan based on his or her special needs?
11. Does the program employ a mechanism for ensuring that the client receives the services called for in his or her service plan (e.g., record review systems, client tracking systems, peer review procedures)?

---

[3] Data from Christian, W. P. (1984).

12. Have specific, measurable intermediate and long-range goals and objectives been specified regarding the client's needs and strengths?
13. Does a method of evaluation exist for each goal and objective on the client's service plan?
14. Has there been a full assessment of any medical, neurological, physiological, or psychological causes for the client's presenting problem that might suggest an alternative approach?
15. Does the client (or proper representative) have access to his or her plan of services (treatment plan)?
16. Have procedures been established for periodic review of the client's plan of service (treatment plan)?
17. Have program staff received in-service training regarding new developments in legal policy, treatment methodology, and strategies for evaluating client progress?
18. Do staff members utilize treatment procedures with a documented history of effectiveness when used with similar clients in similar settings?
19. Does the program have a functional human rights committee?
20. Does the human rights committee (HRC) function to provide an external, unbiased review of the services each client receives?
21. Do HRC members make periodic quality-of-life tours of the program's facilities?
22. Are written reports of the HRC function available for inspection?
23. Have policies and procedures been established that regulate the use of seclusion, restraint (physical, mechanical, and chemical), physical isolation, and other coercive or restrictive treatment procedures?
24. Have due process procedures been established to ensure that each client is served, using the least restrictive alternative possible?
25. Are adequate written records maintained?
26. Are allegations of abuse investigated?
27. Are program staff members sensitive to client rights issues, attempting to improve services while minimizing possibilities for client abuse?
28. Are potentially controversial aspects of the program (e.g., use of restrictive treatment procedures) routinely reviewed by external consultants with appropriate/sufficient expertise?
29. Is there a member of the program's staff who is responsible for monitoring the program's compliance with legal safety guidelines?

# Appendix 13I
# Sample Policies and Procedures for the Human Rights Committee[4]

I. Statement of purpose
   A. Provide sufficient and adequate safeguards for the clients of a human service program to ensure humane treatment
   B. Ensure that appropriate treatment is accomplished as quickly as possible in the least restrictive manner

II. Specification of goals
   A. Review (number) restrictive treatment procedures and/or program policies per meeting, following the functional guidelines for the review process
   B. Observe all areas of the program facility [*number*] times per month, following functional guidelines for review processes
   C. Set up specific guidelines for receiving client, staff, and/or guardian concerns pertaining to clients' rights
   D. Educate clients, guardians, staff, and members of the local community as to the purpose and function of the HRC
   E. Additional goals to be determined by each HRC

III. Members
   A. Composition
      1. Twenty-five percent of the membership from within the organization
      2. Seventy-five percent of the membership from outside of the organization (when possible, a higher percentage of external membership should be recruited)
      3. Client membership
         a. Dependent upon functioning level and capability of client
         b. Additional to internal and external membership

[4] Adapted from Czyzewski, M. J., Hannah, G. T., Risley, T. R., & Sheldon-Wildgen, J. (1981) A sample policy for the human rights committee. Unpublished manuscript; used by permission.

B. Training
  1. Tour of facility, including overview of facility's program and goals
  2. Suggested readings: Griffith and Henning (1981); Hannah, Christian, and Clark (1981); Sheldon-Wildgen and Risley (1982)
  3. Overview of relevant rights issues, regulatory guidelines, program policies and procedures (lecture), and role and function of program's human rights officer

C. Appointing members
  1. Program manager appoints internal members
  2. Manager appoints external members from a pool of volunteers recommended by external sources (see "Recruitment")
  3. Program manager appoints clients and/or their guardians or advocates to membership on the committee

D. Recruitment
  1. Internal members recruited by program manager
  2. External members
     a. Special interest groups (local chapters of professional associations, advocacy groups, and so on) are contacted to suggest names of interested members
     b. Advertisements are run in local newspaper to recruit volunteers from the community at large
     c. Community advisory board and professional advisory board members are contacted for suggestions
  3. Client members recruited by staff and/or by a client advocate, through verbal notification, posting signs, and memoranda

E. Committee size
  1. Approximately 8 to 15 members (not including client members)
  2. Subcommittees not necessary unless required for special projects

F. Membership time limits
  1. Suggested minimum time period for active membership: 2 years
  2. Maximum time period for active membership: 5 years

G. Visibility
  1. Clients, their parents, spouses, and/or guardians, and staff are informed about the human rights committee and its functions
  2. A written fact sheet, briefly describing the purpose and function of the human rights committee, with the name and address of the committee chairperson should be dis-

tributed to each client/guardian upon admission to the program
3. Articles are run in local newspapers explaining the function of the committee and its current membership

H. Compensation: reimbursement for travel

I. Confidentiality
1. Statutes governing confidentiality vary from state to state. Each program should be aware of its state's particular statutes, as well as applicable licensing and accreditation standards. For example:
    a. Disclosure of any records to the human rights committee may require the prior consent of the client and/or guardian
    b. Committee members may be required to sign a pledge not to disclose the name of any client
    c. The program manager may be required to issue a statement granting members who have signed a pledge of confidentiality access to client records for the purpose of review
2. If noncommittee members are present at meetings, pseudonyms should be assigned for each client to be discussed

IV. Access to consultants
- A. Internal (consultants employed as members of the program staff)
- B. External
    1. Professional advisory board: Leading experts in a variety of specialty areas are available for telephone consultations with human rights committee members; they can inform members whether procedures are professionally justified
    2. Professional peer review

V. Mechanisms for internal operations
- A. Quorum
- B. Visitor (nonmember) policy
- C. Meeting frequency
    1. Called by program manager
    2. Called by committee chairperson
- D. Agenda-setting process
- E. Decision-making process

VI. Functional guidelines (review process)
- A. Review of policies and procedures
    1. Selection of [*number*] programs or procedures to review

2. Specific requirements by subtypes of programs (see Appendix 13J):
   a. Develop list of procedures requiring no approval from the human rights committee before, during, or after use
   b. Develop list of procedures that can be implemented prior to committee approval but require post hoc review
   c. Develop list of procedures that require committee approval prior to implementation
3. Review programs or procedures
   a. Program staff presents rationale for procedure
   b. Committee member plays "devil's advocate," suggesting either less restrictive alternative or more restrictive procedure; staff member justifies the choice of procedure
4. Complete human rights committee due process summary report (see Christian & Hannah, 1983)
   a. Circulate report to program manager
   b. File copy of completed report in notebook maintained by committee
   c. Enter case note in client's record
5. Grant permission for a specific staff member to pilot a specific procedure with an individual client for a limited time period prior to filing a formal review for the procedure to be used with the client by program staff
   a. Allows procedure to be tested without delay
   b. Allows parameters of procedures to be adjusted prior to full implementation by all staff
   c. Once tested, approves/vetoes continued use of procedure based on data of initial trial period
6. Review program policies

B. Ongoing monitoring of living environment and observation of treatment procedures, and client–staff interactions
   1. Each ward, unit, or therapy group is assigned to a team of one to three committee members (actual number of team members depends on size of facility and size of human rights committee)
   2. Team randomly visits its assigned ward, unit, or therapy group (each human rights committee determines what is an appropriate number of visits to make)
   3. Team members complete checklist sensitizing them to areas of rights and quality-of-life issues
      a. How does the unit look?

i. What, if anything, makes it attractive?
ii. What does it need?

b. How do the clients look (for example, are the clothes socially acceptable)?
c. If the client was your child or relative, would you be comfortable with the staff–client interaction you saw?
d. Interview the clients (depends on functioning level of client)
e. Did the staff members you observed respect the client's privacy (for example, knock on the door and wait for a response)?
f. In your opinion, is the staff behavior appropriate, given the age and functioning level of clients?
g. Were toys, magazines, etc. accessible to all clients? Was a staff member's presence necessary to remove items from high shelves, locked boxes, etc.?
h. What percentage of the clients observed were engaged in appropriate activity when you entered the ward or unit?

4. Copies of checklist results are circulated to program manager and to the unit staff

VII. Committee members complete a summary report of the service plan for each client reviewed (see Christian & Hannah, 1983)

VIII. Other responsibilities

A. Exit interview with client/guardian
B. Exit interview with staff
C. Grievances
   1. If complainant is not satisfied with the action taken by program management, a formal complaint is filed with the human rights committee
   2. Committee makes recommendation
D. Investigation of abuses
   Manager substantiates (committee does not coordinate or conduct investigation)

# Appendix 13J
# Sample Guidelines for HRC Review of Treatment Procedures[5]

A. Identification of nonrestrictive procedures (procedures exempt from HRC approval)
   1. *Positive reinforcement*: Immediately following a behavior, client receives praise, edibles, or other reinforcer to increase the frequency of the behavior
   2. *Nonreinforcement* (*except* in the case of health-threatening or dangerous behavior): Withholding reinforcement (ignoring, disregarding) contingent upon a behavior in order to decelerate that behavior.
   3. *Differential reinforcement*: Positive reinforcement of one class of behavior and not another, or positive reinforcement in one stimulus condition and not another; all schedules, including
      Differential reinforcement of other behaviors (DRO)
      Differential reinforcement of high rates of responding (DRH)
      Differential reinforcement of low rates of responding (DRL)
      Differential reinforcement of incompatible behaviors (DRI)
   4. *Manual guidance/prompt*: Compliant client guided by hand to perform a sequence of movements designed to teach or improve adaptive skills (e.g., in a toothbrushing program, compliant client aided in grasping the toothbrush and reaching all areas of his/her teeth).

B. Identification of Restrictive Procedures
   Assignment to levels is based on these criteria: (1) The degree of intrusiveness into the life of the client, (2) the potential for abuse, (3) the degree of risk to the client, (4) the professional acceptance of

[5] These guidelines may be dictated by state law or by the requirements of regulatory agencies. Care should be taken to ensure that the sample presented here is modified so that it is completely consistent with pertinent statutes and regulations and that it is approved by program management and the program's HRC.

the procedure; and (5) similar assignments made in professional reports. In all cases, the use of any aversive or deprivational procedures should be the least restrictive procedure necessary to produce effective client treatment gains.

*Level 1*: Procedures requiring no HRC approval before, during, or after use.

a. *Contingent loss of reinforcement*: A procedure to decrease the strength of a behavior by removing a reinforcer, contingent upon that behavior. For example, a predetermined number of token points or stickers is removed from those already earned, contingent upon occurrence of a specified behavior (such as hitting), or nonperformance of a specified behavior (such as refusal to particpate in an educational activity). Tokens may *not* be used to purchase basic goods and services, but may be used to purchase certain extra or nonrequired snacks, privileges, etc.
b. *Meal delay*: Temporary interruptions of a client's meal (e.g., removal of plate) contingent upon a specified behavior that occurs *in conjunction with the meal*; no more than 60 seconds per infraction. *At no time can this procedure result in the client's missing a meal*. Example: Client's plate of food is removed for 10 seconds contingent upon throwing a spoon.
c. *Withdrawal of nonessential goods or services*: Denial of activities or items the client may normally receive. Example: Contingent withholding of normally received but nonessential items, such as coffee, tea, or dessert. Note: Under Level 1, clients *may not be denied* activities or items that are considered "basic goods or services," or are called for in the client's individual service plan.
d. *Time-out from positive reinforcement*: Behavior-dependent *activity time-out* durations (e.g., 30 seconds sitting without tantrumming) where the average time-out duration needed to meet behavioral criteria is less than 5 minutes (averaged across the first 2 weeks of program implementation and monthly thereafter) and which includes an unobstructed view of the client.
e. *Contingent effort*: Required performance of a task or physical exercise for less than 60 seconds (per application), which is *not* physically enforced against active resistance.

*Level 2*: Procedures that can be implemented prior to HRC approval but require post-hoc review of data indicating the frequency and duration of procedural implementation.

a. *Time-out from positive reinforcement*: Behavior-dependent *activity time-out* where the average time-out duration needed to meet behavioral criteria does not exceed 20 minutes (averaged across the first 2 weeks of program implementation and monthly thereafter).

b. *Contingent effort* (contingent exercise, correction, overcorrection, positive practice): Required performance of (a) a particular behavior or (b) multiple repetitions of a behavior for a period likely to exceed 60 seconds per application and which may be physically enforced against active resistance. Example: Client required to make a specific number of beds after a tantrum during which he pulled sheets and blankets off a bed.

c. *Physical prompt/restraint*: The gentle prompting/restraint of the client for less than 60 seconds, which may be enforced against active client resistance.

d. *Physical prompt plus verbal reprimand*: This procedure involves physically prompting the client's head and body toward the trainer, who simultaneously provides a sharp, firm "No."

*Level 3*: Procedures that require HRC approval prior to implementation and HRC review of frequency and duration data during their implementation.

a. *Extinction* of health-threatening or dangerous behaviors. Example: Withdrawing attention contingent upon severe head-banging.

b. *Physical restraint* (immobilize a client's arms, legs, head, and/or body), which exceeds 60 seconds or is enforced against active resistance.

c. *Time-out from positive reinforcement*: Behavior-dependent *environmental time-out.* Example: contingent upon a specified aggressive behavior, the client is physically brought to a time-out room and required to stay there 5 mintues or until calm for 30 seconds. His or her egress is physically blocked (e.g., door to a time-out room held shut until client is calm). *Note:* Environmental time-out is not to be employed with clients who may engage in severe self-injury.

d. *Noxious or aversive stimuli*, contingently applied, that elicit a startle response, but are not injurious to the client. Examples of noxious stimuli include water mist from a spray bottle, unpleasant tastes or odors. Example: contingent upon biting, client is squirted in the mouth with a solution of lemon juice and water.

e. *Mechanical restraints*: Procedures using a mechanical device to limit freedom of movement in order to reduce severely aggressive or self-destructive behavior. Example: The contingent application of a restraint device on a client who engages in self-injurious behavior, or placing an aggressive client in a restraint chair until calm for 2 minutes.

f. *Medication* used to control dysfunctional behavior: The administration of a drug to reduce the level of a client's dysfunctional behavior (e.g., aggression) and to make the client more amenable to special education.

# Appendix 13K
# Preparation for Human Rights Review

1. Develop a thorough understanding of client rights and pertinent legal requirements and current research regarding the target behavior and proposed treatment procedures.
2. Obtain as much information as possible about the committee's current membership, policy, and procedure. If possible, attend an HRC meeting and observe how the meeting is conducted.
3. Obtain HRC approval of guidelines for reviewing treatment procedures (such as those presented in Appendix 13J) and of the form that is to be used in submitting any proposed treatment for HRC review. Provide orientation and training for HRC members sufficient for them to have a working knowledge of treatment philosophy, methodology, and terminology.
4. Obtain a preliminary review (no formal approval requested) by the HRC of any treatment that is likely to be controversial.
5. Submit proposal to HRC members in advance of their scheduled meeting, using the approved form. Attach documentation from the research literature, which is supportive of the proposed procedure.
6. Prepare a formal presentation for the HRC meeting, which might include the showing of audiovisual recordings of the target behavior. In the case of controversial treatment procedures, an expert consultant may be asked to participate in the presentation (with prior approval of the HRC). The results of case consultation and program review conducted by outside experts can also be presented.
7. Negotiate for HRC approval (e.g., If the procedure cannot be approved as presented, under what conditions would it be approved?).
8. Provide the HRC with utilization reports for restrictive treatment procedures (frequency, duration, context) that are timely, concise, and accurate, using a format approved by the HRC.
9. Monitor HRC function; read minutes of each meeting, and attend meetings when possible.

10. Prepare for facility or quality-of-life tours by the HRC, using the same procedures that have been recommended for preparing for peer review (Appendix 13I, part VI-B).
11. Model professionalism and a personal commitment to promoting legal safety and preserving client rights in all interactions with the HRC.

# Index

MIX
Papier aus verantwortungsvollen Quellen
Paper from responsible sources
FSC® C105338

If you have any concerns about our products,
you can contact us on
**ProductSafety@springernature.com**

In case Publisher is established outside the EU,
the EU authorized representative is:
**Springer Nature Customer Service Center GmbH**
**Europaplatz 3, 69115 Heidelberg, Germany**

Printed by Libri Plureos GmbH
in Hamburg, Germany